Selfhood, identity and personality styles

Selfhood, identity and personality styles

Giampiero Arciero and Guido Bondolfi

WILEY-BLACKWELL

A John Wiley & Sons, Ltd, Publication

Wiley-Blackwell is an imprint of John Wiley & Sons, formed by the merger of Wiley's global Scientific, Technical and Medical business with Blackwell Publishing.

Registered office: John Wiley & Sons, Ltd, The Atrium, Southern Gate, Chichester, West Sussex, PO19 8SQ, UK

Editorial Offices: 9600 Garsington Road, Oxford, OX4 2DQ, UK
The Atrium, Southern Gate, Chichester, West Sussex, PO19 8SQ, UK
111 River Street, Hoboken, NJ 07030-5774, USA

For details of our global editorial offices, for customer services and for information about how to apply for permission to reuse the copyright material in this book please see our website at www.wiley.com/wiley-blackwell.

Library of Congress Cataloguing-in-Publication Data

Arciero, Giampiero.
Selfhood, identity and personality styles / Giampiero Arciero and Guido Bondolfi.
p. ; cm.
Includes bibliographical references.
ISBN 978-0-470-51719-2 (cloth), 978-0-470-67022-4 (paper)
1. Personality disorders. 2. Personality. I. Bondolfi, Guido. II. Title.
[DNLM: 1. Identification (Psychology) 2. Personality. 3. Self Psychology. WM 460.5.I4 A674s 2009]
RC554.A73 2009
616.85'81–dc22

2009018187

A catalogue record for this book is available from the British Library.

This book is published in the following electronic formats: ePDF 9780470749364 Wiley Online Library 9780470749357

Set in 10/12pt Times by Thomson Digital, Noida, India
Printed in Singapore by Markono Print Media Pte Ltd

First Impression 2011

To Viridiana and Nathalie

Contents

Foreword: Philosophy from the Clinic

One might think that "finding oneself in the world", the title of one of the sections contained in this book, would not be problematic. On the one hand, setting aside momentarily some of the fascinating pathologies that Arciero and Bondolfi discuss in this work, on an existential or pragmatic level, it is no problem, and indeed we might say it's unavoidable. We are in-the-world in a very strong sense – fully embodied and embedded – and this is how we find ourselves on a pre-reflective, ecological level, as well as on the level of our everyday reflective engagements. On the other hand, theoretically and scientifically, this facticity is often something that gets lost. Without rejecting the rightfully enthusiastic welcome with which we embrace the advances of brain sciences, for example, explanations of human behavior are nonetheless often made exclusively in terms of neural mechanisms in the individual brain. Discussions of how one person comes to understand and interact with another person are often reduced to discussions of what brain mechanisms can account for an individual's capacity. Likewise in psychology and philosophy of mind, arguments revolve around questions about subpersonal innate mechanisms or individual mechanisms that enable learning. Frequently accompanied by the dismissal of phenomenology as unable to explain anything that matters, science presents us with a reified picture of ourselves: we just are a collection of neurons (see, e.g., Crick 1995); a self is nothing but a functional model generated by brain processes (see, e.g., Metzinger 2003); our sense of agency or free deliberation is an illusion (see, e.g., Wegner 2002). In much of this, then, the person and the personal level are simply eliminated.

Arciero and Bondolfi's broad-ranging analyses reminds us that whether we are meeting in cafes, or congregating in institutional labs, we are first of all, *persons*, with first-person experiences that are shaped in second-person, intersubjective encounters – not with other brains, but with other persons. If science eliminates the personal level, the level where we find ourselves in the world, where selfhood, identity, and personality have important effects, in favor of subpersonal processes, then it would be impossible to say what such processes explain. For example, if mirror neurons are to play a role in explaining intersubjectivity, then it seems incumbent that we understand the complexities of intersubjective experience at the level of personal interaction – an interaction that takes place in a world that is diversely shaped by social, cultural, and institutional practices. Neurons are responsible to no one; this cannot mean that there is no such thing as moral responsibility. The meaning of personal responsibility is entirely a personal one – which is to say, an interpersonal one. Indeed, that's the general rule about meaning: meaning is something that occurs on the level of the person.

Arciero and Bondolfi lead us through detailed scientifically and phenomenologically informed expositions that relate subpersonal and personal level accounts, and that trace out the lines that tie personal to interpersonal and more broadly social phenomena, starting with the most basic experiential domain of pre-reflective awareness, moving through basic action-oriented interactions to communicative and narrative practices that build a meaningful lifeworld. One of the main principles they defend is that our perception and interactive engagement with others and with the world is never without implications for the self, and vice versa. We can call it the principle of mutual implication. This applies not only for the most basic, embodied, ecological dimension, where movement registers information about both world and self, but for higher-order levels that involve aspects of complex emotion and personality. Thus, for example, in their own fMRI studies, Arciero and Bondolfi show that differences in styles of emotional processing correlate to different areas of neural activation. That is, different areas of the brain are activated for highly self-related stimuli depending on whether one tends to be externally oriented (emotionally Outward prone) or introceptively oriented (emotionally Inward prone).

Arciero and Bondolfi are psychiatrists first, even if they prove themselves to be philosophers and neuroscientists as well. One could interpret their goal in *Selfhood, Identity and Personality Styles* in the following way. If philosophically we can rethink the fundamental conceptions of what it means to be a person and what emotion means, and do so fully informed by current neuroscience, then this should have important implications for our understanding of various pathologies – including eating disorders, obsessive-compulsive disorder, hypochondria, phobias and depression. In that case, philosophy and cognitive neuroscience are in service to psychiatry. But equally one can read this book productively in the other direction. In that respect, I suggest we think of this book with the subtitle: "Philosophy from the Clinic." The various disorders and the vignettes presented by the authors challenge philosophical presuppositions about the nature of self and personhood, and help us to see possibilities for a non-reductive neuroscience.

The authors define a number of personality styles, and consider a number of disorders in light of the principle of the mutual implication of self with others and the world. The forces that enter into this relation are not always well balanced; in some cases others and/or the worldly arrangements that characterize institutions and modern technologies come to dominate so that certain degrees of autonomy and self-authorship (which are in any case never absolute) are threatened or actually extinguished. The effects on an individual's life of such ill-balanced arrangements are reflected both in clinical cases and in literary expressions, and this dual reflection bespeaks not simply individual tragedies, and literary tragedies, but problems that pervade social structures and practices. Arciero and Bondolfi point to the increase in the velocity of cultural and technological changes and the effect this has on emotional responses, which can go in either opposition or conformity to such processes.

The role of narrative (both of the literary and clinical type) is important for Arciero and Bondolfi, and rightly so. We become thoroughly familiar with stories very early, and we learn to use narrative frameworks to make sense out of our own actions and the actions of others, as well as our joint actions. Our early narratives are focused on action and they translate actions into language. The narrative framing of actions also tends to invade our everyday engagements and conversations with each other, providing templates to help us make sense of behavior. We listen to stories, or we act them out; we can see them acted out in play and in cultural productions, in plays, on television, or in our family house, or in the street. Everyday personal narratives, as well as cultural narratives, are formed and understood intersubjectively—and they help to form us in our self-understanding. This view is consistent with hermeneutical approaches, and, for example, with the views of Charles Taylor (1989), who suggests that reductionistic science cannot tell us the full story since humans are self-interpreting beings whose self-understandings constitute their being. Narratives (which are much more particularistic than theory or folk psychology, and in any case are necessary for the application of theory) help us to frame specific situations and their meaning in a way that gives us an understanding of what others in those situations are about. They contribute to and shape the knowledge background necessary for understanding ourselves and others; they teach us what to expect or not expect; what is appropriate or not appropriate; they provide knowledge of what actions are acceptable and in what circumstances, and when, and by whom, and what sort of events are important and noteworthy, and what kind of explanations constitute the giving of good reasons.

Narrative operates *both* as a force that reproduces traditions and interpretive patterns and pre-reflectively reinforces the established power structures, *and* as a critical reflective tool for undermining such forces, whether in political and cultural contexts or specifically in psychoanalytic contexts. Narratives serve to mediate intersubjective relations. They can map out the immediate and deeper contexts of action and understanding, provide detailed descriptions of events, objects and persons, help to coordinate complex tasks, define the identities and roles of individuals and groups, and express agreement among individuals. Narratives can also generate a reflective attitude about new or different possibilities. Narrative literature (like art generally) often plays this role. Narratives provide an important source for staking out new social arrangements, and for pushing the boundaries of what is acceptable and what is not.

We can encounter someone in the highly contextualized situations of everyday life and recognize and acknowledge them for who they are only if we have a narrative that we can use to make sense of them, or they or someone else gives us the narrative which constitutes their own story. How, otherwise, would we be able to diagnose the kind of distortions that clinical work is supposed to address? None of this can involve a theory-of-mind simulation-style reduction of the other's narrative to the model of one's own self-narrative. Putting myself in the other person's shoes will be difficult if the other person wears a different size, a different style, or doesn't wear shoes at all. The diversity of narratives reflects a diversity of lifeworlds.

Of course, just as the lifeworld can be colonized by systems (e.g., just as technologies and economic factors can shape our lives), so systems can invade narratives and put them to the service of established relations. But systems can do the same with theory. Theory has no advantage over narrative in this regard. Moreover, if the force of such colonization depends on most of it remaining hidden (the less we know of it, the more power it has), then the capacity for narrative to set out and explicate such hidden powers will be critical.

Importantly, narrative is better able to do this in the very language of the lifeworld—in terms that focus on people, and motives, and events, and actions, and interactions—and in a way that avoids the abstractions and the often reductionist leanings of theory. In that case, narrative practice will run less of a risk of dehumanizing and alienating the participants. In the clinic we need to stay close to everyday experience—we need to capture the everyday interaction as it really happens among people. What we need to avoid is the abstraction and generalization that often happens via theory, which includes the use that theory makes of reifying and reductionistic science.

Arciero and Bondolfi make it clear that our understanding of others is not a matter of mental states flying through thin air between minds; human feelings, intentions, thoughts and beliefs are deeply embedded in backgrounds and contexts, in embodied social interactions and communicative practices in the everyday lifeworld, and all of these phenomena are characterized by a great many differences that need to be recognized and acknowledged. Just because these backgrounds and contexts are rich and complex, narrative is a relevant and unavoidable tool for understanding others. Competency with different kinds of narratives—literary narratives, clinical narratives, and everyday narratives—enables us to understand others in a variety of ways, as they live in a diversity of situations. That needs to be part of clinical work: the recognition of difference and the irreducible nature of such differences.

Shaun Gallagher

References

Crick, F. 1995. *The Astonishing Hypothesis: The Scientific Search for the Soul.* New York: Scribner.

Metzinger, T. 2003. *Being No One. The Self-Model Theory of Subjectivity.* Cambridge, MA: MIT Press.

Taylor, C. 1989. *Sources of the Self: The Making of Modern Identity.* Harvard University Press.

Wegner, D. M. 2002. *The Illusion of Conscious Will.* Cambridge, MA: MIT Press.

About the Authors

Giampiero Arciero, M.D., Ph.D. is Director of the Institute of Constructivist Psychology and Psychotherapy of Rome (IPRA) and consultant at the Department of Psychiatry of the Geneva University Hospitals (Switzerland). He collaborates with the Psychiatric Neuroscience Group, University of Bari (Italy). He has worked as a visiting researcher at the University of Fribourg (Switzerland), as Associate Director of the Personal Development Laboratory at the University of California, Santa Barbara (USA) and as Professor of Psychotherapy at the University of Siena (Italy).

In addition to several peer reviewed publications, he is the author of the following books:

Studi e dialoghi sull'identità personale (2002)
Estudios y Dialogos sobre la identidad personal (2° ed., 2005)
Sulle Tracce di Sè (2006)
Tras las huellas de sí mismo (2009).

Guido Bondolfi is a psychiatrist, psychotherapist and a mindfulness instructor (MBCT and MBSR). He is *Chargé de Cours* at the Medical School of the University of Geneva (Switzerland) where he teaches Psychiatry and Psychotherapy. As head of a *Secteur* and of a specialized programme for depressive disorders at the Department of Psychiatry of the Geneva University Hospitals, Guido Bondolfi's research interests include cognitive psychotherapy, mood disorders and pathological gambling.

He is the author of more than 50 peer reviewed publications and of a book: *Traitement intégré de la dépression : de la résistance à la prévention de la rechute* (2004).

Introduction

The title of a book, like a proper name, defines its identity. There are three interweaving themes informing this text. The first is selfhood, which, in line with the continental hermeneutic–phenomenological tradition, we have termed ipseity – thus emphasizing the need to account for the way in which each person, in dealing with others and the different circumstances of everyday life, is present to himself and pre-reflexively conscious of himself. This perspective of selfhood emerges from the ontological need to grasp individuals from their ways of being rather than by conceptualizing them according to the same categories that are applied to objects.

It is this very need that underlines the second theme of the book, identity, which in relation to action and feeling raises the question of 'who' to a new level: that of temporality. Stating who a person is implies that all individual passions and actions be understood within the framework of a historical dimension characterized by the permanence of the person, designated by its proper name, as being the same over time. In line with the work of Ricoeur, we have come to envisage narrative as the act by means of which personal identity takes shape while events interweave to form a plot. It is through the various forms of narrative that the person acquires his historical identity, which we term 'narrative identity'.

If narrative is what enables the individual to recognize his own experiences as personal experiences, and hence to identify himself, narrative variances can be seen to reflect different ways of experiencing one's own life. It is on the basis of these reflections on the relation between the pre-reflexive dimension and its narrative configuration that we have approached the third theme of the book: the psychological typifying of personality according to different emotional tendencies which crystallize in the course of a person's life and are reflected in the construction of his personal story. This is where we turn to the neurosciences and develop a psychopathology that can take account of continuity with normal personality. From this perspective, our appeal to literary (as well as clinical) examples should be regarded as an engagement with an experimental field within which we can observe the variations and boundaries of the narrative and of its characters: a sort of laboratory allowing us to analyse the heterogeneous 'experiments' performed on identity, thus drawing literature and psychology closer together.

It was our wish for the cover of the book to be embellished by the reproduction of a painting: Francis Bacon's 'Study of George Dyer'. This original choice was due to the ontological perspective that informs our work – and which Bacon grasps in his painting: a perspective that sees the living body as a way of being in the world, and its happening as a wholly original phenomenon. We too, like Bacon, see the perceiving flesh and the perceived body as one. Unfortunately, although we did our best to elucidate the reasons why we wished to make use of this reproduction, the Bacon Estate did not grant us permission.

The text comprises two parts. Part One, in four chapters, explores the first two themes of the book. In the five following chapters, Part Two discusses the various styles of personality and the pathologies these may engender.

Chapter 1 focuses on the difference between the typically modern conceptualization of the Self and a view of ipseity that by placing one's way of feeling in the world at the centre of its analysis reverses both the perspective on the meaning of experience and that on reflection and personal identity. Chapter 2 engages with the relation between ipseity and language, starting from the problem of individual understanding of the other, which has been addressed in developmental psychology and the neurosciences. The importance and limits of the Mirror Neuron System (MNS) as a means to explain the relation between experience and language represents the driving motive behind our argument. Chapter 3 introduces the question of how to account, by means of language, for the permanence of Self over time. Personal identity dynamically takes shape through the narrative act: through language, it reflects different emotional inclinations which, when configured into a story, allow the person to perceive himself as stably situated over time. These dispositions may be defined on a continuum that extends from the Inward to the Outward polarity, depending on whether the frame of reference adopted by the individual in his search for personal stability is predominantly based on the body or on an externally anchored system of coordinates.

Chapter 4, which ends the first section, turns to the psychology of emotions to explore the distinction traced in the previous chapter between Inward and Outward, showing how the different possible combinations along the continuum demarcated by these polarities correspond to different ways of feeling emotion. This emotional basis will be the foundation on which to present the different styles of personality that characterize the five chapters making up the second section of the book. Each style may thus manifest those characteristics that mark one of the two polarities in a more or less prevalent way, thereby finding a place within the continuum.

In the context of the Outward polarity, Chapter 5 explores issues surrounding the type of personality prone to eating disorders, while Chapter 6 examines the style prone to obsessive-compulsive disorders.

Unlike the previous styles of personality, the style prone to hysteria and hypochondria – the object of Chapter 7 – may be considered a sort of combination of the two polarities, as both are here used in the search for personal stability.

In the context of the Inward polarity, the styles of personality prone to phobias and depression are analyzed in Chapters 8 and 9, respectively.

Arguments fixed in the written form cannot but show the influence of the conversations, debates and exchanges of ideas that have accompanied us during the writing of this text: in particular, our meetings and walks with Vittorio Gallese, in whose company we spent many late nights discussing the meaning of experience and its neural substrate – an experience often enriched by our discussions on phenomenology and the philosophy of science with Corrado Sinigaglia. To these we should add our weekly reflections on research methodology, genetics, psychiatry and neurosciences with Alessandro Bertolino; our daily dialogues on developmental psychology, the neurosciences and psychotherapy with Viridiana Mazzola; our pondering on the themes of ancient philosophy with Michele Alessandrelli and on hermeneutics with Elizbieta O'Bara.

On the day on which this introduction was written, one of our pupils, Martina Grilli, lost her life in a car accident. She too took part in the conversations that contributed to shape this book. We express our most profound and sincere gratitude to Martina and all our students for their curiosity and eagerness to learn, and for the confidence they placed in us by choosing us as their teachers.

We warmly wish to thank the many people who have supported us, or have otherwise contributed to the writing of this book. Both of us would particularly like to thank:

Professors Mario Maj and Norman Sartorious, for their strong support towards the fulfilment of this project;
Professor Marcello Nardini, for having supported the empirical researches that enrich this volume through his discrete presence;
Professors Francois Ferrero and Gilles Bertschy, who have been constant sources of encouragement and support and, above all, have allowed us to meet regularly during the preparation of the manuscript;
our friend Maurizio Bigioni, for his warm and generous support of Ipra research;
our Ipra colleagues in Rome, Bari, Reggio Emilia and Tenerife, our colleagues at the Slop of Tortona and those at the post-rationalist centres of Santiago and Buenos Aires;
the members of the Depression and Bipolar Programs of the Department of Psychiatry of the University Hospitals of Geneva, and particularly Jean-Michel Aubry, Lucio Bizzini, Francoise Jermann and Béatrice Weber, whose pragmatism, wisdom and wit have been an inspiration in times of self-doubt;
our families, for their unwavering support, and especially Marie, Julie and 'Leopardo' for their kindness and patience.

Finally, special thanks goes out to Sergio Knipe and Steve McKend for their hermeneutical sensitivity in helping us to put the work into the final English form and to Fiona Woods for her professional competence and unconditional support.

Part One

1 Subjectivity and Ipseity

Dasein *works in the how of its being-now.*[1]

Robert is thirty years old. Over the last ten years he has done odd jobs, including holiday village entertainer, ski instructor and skipper. He has travelled a great deal, he has had many love affairs and he has passionately sought to realize one of the dreams of his youth. Robert wanted to be a pilot. In order to achieve this goal he studied hard, he acquired pilot licenses, he went to live in different countries, he spent a lot of money. Nevertheless, today, despite having completed his training, and despite having received promises, commitments and assurances from various companies, he still does not have a job. This, in his opinion, is what has led him to seek help. Indeed, he feels his life is meaningless, that he has no stimuli and that he is incapable of taking any initiative whatsoever, even the simplest. He remains closeted at home all day long.

In actual fact, on reconstructing the origin of Robert's current problem, the onset of this malaise appears to be related to the coming to an end of Robert's relationship with a woman: Sarah, the girl he was living with, disappeared suddenly from Robert's life. Robert had met Sarah two years earlier in a discotheque. Before that he was feeling just as he is feeling now – tired and bored by his existence, bitterly disappointed by the fact that he could not find any work, suffering through a life which was scattered with periods of emptiness, in which his only problem was how he could get through the day.

Sarah is twenty-three years old and works in a bar. When Robert first sees her he is stunned by her physical beauty: her green eyes, her slender figure, her blonde hair – a set of features which seizes his imagination. He has only just seen her and he is already in love with her.

From that night on his only thought is how he can manage to meet her again. He tries to meet people who know her, he approaches her friends, he talks with the owner of the discotheque to try to obtain information about her, he returns to the discotheque in order to meet her – until he manages to organize a dinner to which he invites her in the company of mutual friends. As in the film which Robert has constructed in his imagination, from that evening on their encounters become more frequent and intense. However, something happens which shatters Robert's expectations. As the two become more deeply acquainted, Robert experiences an increasing sense of anxiety and malaise; he

Selfhood, identity and personality styles Giampiero Arciero and Guido Bondolfi

finds he is unable to talk about his life, and he feels she is not close to him. Perhaps it's their difference in age, perhaps because they have reached different stages of maturity, or probably because they have different types of sensibilities. This distance, which is a sign that intimacy between the two is impossible, dashes his hopes. The body which drew him like a magnet does not possess the qualities he desires in a woman. Despite this fact, he suggests they live together.

After all, despite the distance between them, she is beautiful, attentive to his needs, quick at reading his thoughts and anticipating his desires. And what is more, he no longer has the strength to live alone, to fall, shut up in his room, into that painful condition of total loss of meaning which he experiences every day.

Since he met Sarah, those days destroyed by emptiness have disappeared. Sarah manages to keep him away from the precipices of solitude by constantly seeking him out. This is the most important effect which the girl has produced on his life, and this is the reason why he has asked her to live with him.

When Sarah enters Robert's world, he has already been a 'remote control man' for several years, a man who spends his days moving from the settee to the television, to the PlayStation, to the computer. Thus, for Sarah, choosing to live with Robert means joining this seesaw, moving from one screen to another, tuning in to his expectations, but at the same time camouflaging herself in Robert's daily life. The only interval between changing screens is a raid on the shopping centres to lose themselves among the crowds, to buy some unimportant object or other . . . and so on, day in day out.

After a few months she gives up her job in the discotheque, even though it is only part-time. Every second of the day her life is absorbed into Robert's and becomes indistinguishable from his; while he navigates through his technological spaces she concentrates her attention on him, eliminating any possibility of emptiness that might occur.

Gradually, even those escapes to the shopping centres become rarer and rarer, as does sexual intercourse; she becomes ashen, he observes her dying away.

This is one year after their relationship began.

Suddenly she start being a little less attentive, 'less devoted', in his words. In other words, Sarah begins to be no longer exclusively attuned to Robert's life. One of her old friends makes an appearance, then she timidly goes out for the first time, almost as if guilty of committing some heinous crime, then she goes out for a pizza, then to the cinema, then to the discotheque, then . . . her absences become more frequent . . . she is less considerate, and when she goes out, in an incredible crescendo, he seeks her out, he is worried, he fears he will lose her, he is terrified in case she leaves him. Emptiness reappears on the horizon.

Robert attempts to stem the haemorrhage of meaning caused by Sarah's abandoning him in every way possible. He attempts bribery: he buys her increasingly costly gifts; then come the threats, the arguments, the violent fights. He feels Sarah is on the point of leaving him. Her periods of absence become longer and longer until, one day, she disappears without leaving any word.

He falls into the abyss. 'I seemed to exist no longer, I couldn't feel myself anymore'. His sense of identity dissolves into thin air. For the first time in his life, he realizes just how important Sarah is to him: 'She was my mirror so while she was there, I was there too, then she went away and suddenly I didn't exist any longer.' He disappears, drawn into nothingness.

1.1 From Kant to cybernetics

What is the origin of this painful displacement, of this disappearing into nothingness, of this being absorbed by the void? What structures underlie the ordinary and the extraordinary experiencing of Self? What is the origin of the so-called sense of Self?

Most people could probably provide an intuitive answer to this question. At bottom, the sense of Self corresponds to that experience of ownership and impenetrability of one's thoughts, of one's internal dialogues, of one's affective states, that many – but not all – of us have from infancy. This 'mental solitude' is held as constituting the basis of our sense of personal uniqueness, of identification and of demarcation from others. It is perhaps that very same solitude that Descartes had in mind when he redefined the concepts of subject and subjectivity.

Ultimately, being oneself means that the faculty of knowing lies within the subject, in his head, and the subject has such a status by dint of being enclosed within himself, separate and distinct from the world and from others.

Doesn't common sense tell us the same thing? Isn't it true that we say 'What's got into you?' to express surprise at, and disapproval of, unexpected and bizarre behaviour? And again, doesn't common sense tell us that strange behaviour is signalled by tapping one's forehead with one's forefinger?

'Why the Mind is in the Head' is the title of one of the lectures delivered at the 1951 Hixon Symposium, a landmark in the history of cybernetics (McCulloch, 1965); half a century later modern neuroscience has definitely not rejected the idea of locating the mind in the head (Amodio and Frith, 2006).

But Robert's case presents us with a strange dilemma. Robert loses his sense of Self, he disappears as a person, when Sarah leaves him. He thus possesses a discontinuous sense of Self, which comes into being only through the presence of the other and which disappears when the other disappears. Being alone 'in one's own head', dialogue with oneself without the other, corresponds to the loss of meaning, to the dissolution of the sense of Self. Naturally, when dealing with experiences of this nature, a chorus of voices is raised by those who question the very existence of the Self understood as a self-contained individual, which modernity had recognized as a subject.

One of the most authoritative voices in this chorus is Ken Gergen's (1999: 122), who asks the question: 'can we compellingly reinscribe what it is to be a person in a way that moves us away from the individualist premise and toward the relational?' In this way a new topic comes on stage in contemporary psychology: Self as Relationship. One of the foundation stones of the modern mode of conceptualizing the Self, being enclosed within the confines of one's own mental sphere, is shattered. In one fell swoop the gulf of sense between the subject and reality is overcome. The Self as solitary lord and master of *cogitationes* becomes the public co-constructor of meaning; its constitutive dimension is social, like the discourses through which it emerges: socially distributed selves animated by socially-constructed emotions. This is the stance taken by social constructivists.

The Relational Self has had a significant impact on contemporary psychology and psychotherapy. This new hot topic, which made its appearance a few decades ago on a psychological stage that was lifeless and lacking in ideas,[2] has managed to group together various trends, which go from constructionism to constructivism, from family therapy to narrativism, from cognitivism right up to Buddhist psychology.

Robert's experience, however, touches upon another, even more pressing, central conceptual issue that occupies philosophers, neuroscientists, sociologists and scholars of literature: the problem of the sense of unity of the human experience. That is, the relationship between the multiplicity of the individual's actions and passions and the unity of the Self, or as James believed, the relationship between the Self as known (Me) and the Self as knower (I).

When Robert passes from the chat line to the PlayStation, from films to shopping centres, from the discotheque to compulsive shopping, when, in the intervals between different contexts, he is lost in a meaningless emptiness, when he perceives himself only when he is tuned in to an external source of reference, the way Robert perceives himself does not appear to be ascribable to a sense of unity which knows itself (is conscious of itself) as the basis of its own actions. It is difficult to understand an experience of Self of this nature in the light of that type of subjectivity which modern thought conceives of as what remains identical despite wide variations in conduct.

The inability to account for a mode of experiencing life such as Robert's is connected to the very characteristics which define the Self as it is conceived of by modernity: the Self's privacy even to itself, the unity of the multiplicity of experiences and the continuity of the sense of Self.

These aspects, which are constitutive of the modern Self, also correspond to the account common sense offers of first-person experience. For, when one thinks of oneself, who would not say that he is certain that his thoughts are private (privacy), that he feels he is always himself in the different situations he encounters in daily life (unity) and that he feels that his experiences are linked together by an uninterrupted sense of being himself (continuity)?

Robert, on the contrary, does not experience his own Self as being stable over time. He might say he does not have a sense of unity, a stable image of the Self, but that in fact he has many, all of which are different. He would say he is not sure whether he is thinking or acting in a certain way to please the other person or whether he really does believe what he is saying and doing; he would be uncertain both of the authorship of his states and of their privacy. He would admit that he can feel and can think things which are the complete opposite with regard to the current situation, without these different experiences of Self being coherently connected to each other.

Our questions start here, from clinical practice with people. Although these questions obviously spill over into contiguous scientific domains in the search for comparisons, contaminations, dialogic exchanges, they are nevertheless posed from the standpoint of the psychiatrist and the therapist: that is, the point of departure is the investigation of people's stories and the ultimate objective is to provide therapy.

The search for a solution to the problems set by the case of Robert constitutes the itinerary for this first chapter.

The first step will be to analyse the origins of the three characteristics of the modern Self and to show why these origins continue to constitute the basis of the way we conceive of the Self today. To produce an overall picture of this first step, we will draw a brief outline of the Kantian concept of Self, showing that this framework is present in systems theory, in the neurosciences, in most branches of contemporary psychology and psychiatry. In particular, I will analyse the perspective taken by nonlinear systems, which underpins Cloningher's approach to the study of personality, and then pass on to the view of closed systems adopted by the constructivists, concentrating principally on the psychology of the Self. The element which these different perspectives have in common, from Kant to nonlinear systems, up to closed systems, is the same mode of conceptualizing the Self: the Self is understood as a thing: in Kant as a ordering mechanism in the cyberneticians as a computational object.

We shall see that it is only the domain of hermeneutic phenomenology that proposes a new method of investigating the Self, or rather, of being oneself. And it is this perspective that will enable us to discover that the classic mode of conceptualizing the Self has always implicitly conceived it as a thing, an object, with object-like characteristics and with the capacity to serve as an object in relation to other objects. This change in viewpoint will enable us to grasp the fact that the continuity between Kant and cybernetics is buttressed by the understanding – and the study – of the Self, through the deployment of those categories which are applied to objects that are produced, to things. In modern thought, the Self has the ontological status of a thing that is produced.

But the Self cannot be explained as if it were an object with properties such as, for instance, the weight of a bag. Instead, it appears through possible ways of being. One feels like this or like that in one situation or in another. Adopting this vision, which places the experience of being oneself centre stage, with all it entails, thus means asking a novel question: what happens if, instead, we consider the Self not as a thing, but as a 'who'.

The second part of the chapter attempts to answer this question. A serious enquiry into this issue implies that the starting point is the awareness that the sole phenomenon in real flesh and blood to which we have access when we study the Self is the experience each of us has of always living in the present. What distinguishes one's experience of being oneself is how one feels now, every single time. If this fact, this phenomenon, constitutes our starting point, how can we make sense of those fundamental features that characterize both the modern Self and the common-sense Self: continuity, unity and privacy? The development of these topics involves a scrutiny of Heidegger's phenomenology, above all the phenomenology of his early years, from 1919 to 1929. Our goal is to discover whether the nature of ipseity that we can derive from Heidegger's philosophy will enable us to grasp the dilemma set by Robert.

1.2 The sense of self and the variety of experience

The relationship between the diversity, the multiplicity, of one's experience – of one's actions and feelings – and the concurrent sense that every experience is perceived as belonging to oneself implies two polarities. On the one hand, something (the Self as subject) that remains one and invariable in the course of time: the sense, that is, that the different events in one's life belong to the subject experiencing them: the Self as a knower (I) of James. On the other hand, the Self as object, which corresponds to the diversity of one's experiences, and which, on the contrary, changes continuously in relation to its interactions with the external world and with others; in other words, in relation to the 'affections': the Self as known (Me) of James.

Kant (1977, 1980) welds these two polarities into a unity. He conceives of the former, the Self as subject, as invariable and as the unifying ground of the latter, the Self as object, which is changeful. The relationship between these two polarities of the Self may be compared, from a logico-grammatical standpoint, to the relationship between subject and predicate. The subject, that is, may be viewed as the base which unifies all its predicates. For example, we may state that Robert is intelligent, a sportsman, a scholar and so forth. We may state, using different words, that the one and invariable Self consists in the combining of the manifold changing experiences into a unity. Kant terms this unity the 'I-think'.

What this means is that even during the simplest possible experience, for instance my perception of the page I am writing on the computer screen, I not only grasp the content I am perceiving as I write (the Self as object), but 'I think', I apprehend myself along with what is perceived (the Self as subject). Subjectivity, understood as self-consciousness, lies in this property: namely, in the combining which unifies all the single experiences. That is, the subject is conscious of his own experience in the thousands of actions he carries out in the course of his daily existence. The subject is thus conscious of himself inasmuch as he perceives himself as constituting the foundation, the unifying ground by which his manifold acts are combined – following the determinations of the categories.

With regard to the relationship between the I of consciousness (the Self as subject) and the experiencing I (the Self as object), Kant has this to say:

> *'The I think expresses the act of determining my existence. The existence is thereby already given but the manner in which I am to determine it, the way I am to posit in myself the manifold pertaining to it, is not yet thereby given' (Kant, 1967).*

That is, the meaning of my experience is related to how I connect the multiplicity of my experiences. The I think is this very order.[3]

This being an I, which is identical for every living subject, is thus what remains when the I (the Self as subject) is divested of all its determinations (the Self as object). If we take away from Robert his intelligence, his being a sportsman and a scholar, what remains is Robert as a thinking thing, a *res cogitans*. That is to say, when we remove all the predicates from the subject, when we purify the unity of its multiplicity, what remains is the pure I. But while the multiplicity of one's experiences may be determined by the I think, the latter can in no way be determined: it remains unknowable. Such an asymmetry at the heart of identity is the aporia which this view of the Self leads to, a view which goes from cybernetics, without ever constituting a topic in that domain, to psychiatry, to cognitive psychology and to constructivism.

1.3 Nonlinear systems and the construction of the self

Nonlinear systems

It is both extremely interesting and, as we shall see, extremely surprising to discover that some of the aspects of Kant's conception of subjectivity are to be found as cornerstones of the cognitive sciences right from one of the two articles that lay the foundations of first-order cybernetics.[4] I am referring to 'A Logical Calculus of the Ideas Immanent in Nervous Activity' by Warren McCulloch and Walter Pitts (in McCulloch, 1965). Let us get straight to the heart of the matter by quoting the authors themselves:

> *The all-or-none law of nervous activity is sufficient to insure that the activity of any neuron may be represented as a proposition. Physiological relations existing among nervous activities correspond, of course, to relations among the propositions (p. 21).*

Hence, starting (a) from the state of activity or inactivity of every single neuron which correspond respectively to the logical values true or false (0 or 1), (b) from their connections – so that if two neurons tend to be active together, connecting up is facilitated, whereas the opposite state inhibits any connection (the rule governing the change is a [Boolean] function of two arguments [such as 'and' 'or'] – Varela et al., 1991), we obtain c) the brain is comparable to a machine operating by deduction.

The spirit is embodied in the mechanism. Starting from basic operational rules, a machine would be capable of ordering concrete experience, that is, it would be capable of 'thinking'.

See also Figure 1, from McCulloch (1965).

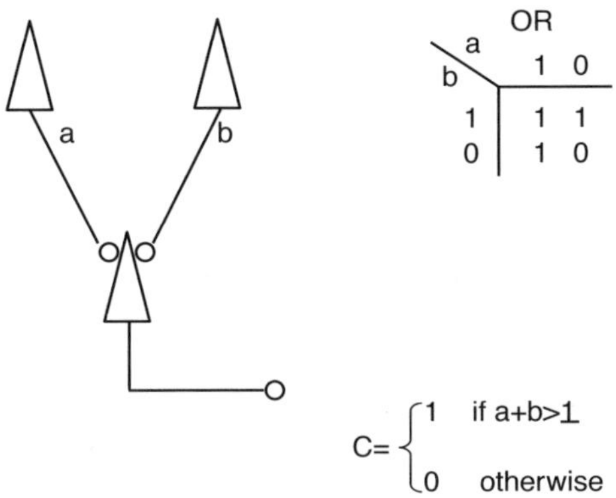

Figure 1 McCulloch, Warren S. Introduction by Seymour A. Papert., Embodiments of the Mind, figure, © 1965 Massachusetts institute of Thechnology, by permission of the MIT Press.

McCulloch's philosophical stance is a bold one. He offers a vision of the brain as an embodied logico-mathematical machine, thereby furnishing the neuroanatomical and neurophysiological bases to an a priori synthetic judgement (Dupuy, 1985), that is, to that knowledge which, in Kant's view, we possess a priori and in conformity to which every determination, every definition of experience, must come about. As is well known, in philosophy the so-called Copernican revolution is founded on the a priori synthetic judgement.[5]

Starting from the second half of the 1970s,[6] along the pathway inaugurated by McCulloch there developed a new perspective with regard to the issue of cognition: the standpoint of self-organized systems. From the behaviour of the single neuron, attention moved on to the analysis of the coherence of the system as a whole, that is, to the investigation of those global structures which emerge as a result of the cooperation taking place among all the units that constitute the system. It is the connectedness of the system that matters! This accounts for the origin of the name (neo)connectionism which characterized this branch of research, especially in its early stages.

In this view, the organism is conceived of as a self-organized system which, starting from an initial state, moves along a certain transformative trajectory as a result of the cooperation in a given context among the elements of which it is composed (Thelen, 2002; Thelen and Smith, 1994). In the course of its development, and in relation to each specific situation, every system will 'settle into' states of dynamic stability, termed 'attractors', which resist perturbations and to which the system tends to return when perturbed. That is, each organism 'prefers' a certain landscape of attractors, a coherent space state around which it fluctuates and which characterizes the system.

This new approach to the study of the system introduces both a synchronic and a diachronic dimension. If, from the perspective of real time, the behaviour of the system appears to be the result of the global dynamics of the system within the context in which it acts, from the standpoint of duration, the emergence of new structures is consolidated by the tendency of the components of the system to activate themselves in a coherent fashion. The connectedness of the system is thus indivisible from the history of its transformations. The position that was occupied in Kant by the 'I think', understood as the link which unifies the wide variety of behaviours exhibited by the system (according to the categories), is taken by the ordering mechanism.

Construction of the self

We must leave aside the extraordinary history of cybernetics, which comes right up to the present and which has brought about tremendous changes in all our lives,[7] in order to focus our attention on the application of the theory of nonlinear systems to the conceptualization of the Self in psychiatry.

One example of dynamic systems – or complex systems, or nonlinear systems – which has met with great success in psychiatry is the approach of Cloninger and his colleagues to the study of personality (Cloninger, 1993, 1999). Cloninger's theory of personality posits that the Self is actually a mechanism. Let us see how.

Cloninger and his colleagues believe personality is a complex system that evolves over time and which is a combination of two constitutive elements: temperament and character. These two constitutive dimensions give rise to the respective differentiations into four temperament traits and three character traits, all of which can be specified objectively and can combine dynamically. This approach furnishes a 'table of elements' enabling the construction of a typology of personality and its psychopathology.

The four temperament traits ('Harm Avoidance', 'Novelty Seeking', 'Reward Dependence' and 'Persistence'), are correlated with four neural systems that influence stimulus-response patterns and are associated with four different psychobiological profiles. Each trait is made up of specific components, called 'facets', which refer to an individual's emotional predispositions, that is, to the inheritable differences underlying one's automatic response to danger, novelty and types of reward. Each trait may be inherited independently of the other traits, but not in such a way as to be mutually exclusive. Hence, all combinations are possible.

The three character traits ('Self-directness', 'Cooperativeness' and 'Self-transcendence'), which concern the higher individual cognitive functions, are inherited to a lesser degree and are moderately influenced by social learning, culture and random personal life events.[8]

How does the system work? The mechanism is constituted by two classes, temperament and character, whose dimensions – the traits – acting in synergy, structure and strengthen their connections. When they operate independently, however, they decrease and weaken the connections. Given these premises, personality development may be seen as a dynamic system which, starting from the initial temperament configuration, proceeds through the maturational stages as a consequence of a peculiar form of cooperation among the elements of which it is constituted.[9] The state of the system may be envisaged moment by moment as a tendency to gravitate around conditions of dynamic stability – the attractors. The latter correspond to particular structures of relationships between the temperament traits and the character traits in a given maturational context.

What this means is that each organism 'prefers' a certain mosaic of attractors, a coherent space state around which it fluctuates and which characterizes it. This applies not only to normality but also to pathological conditions. For instance, the chronicity and difficulty of treating a personality disorder may be accounted for by the fact that, once personality has stabilized a certain dynamic configuration, it tends to maintain that stability, even if it does not correspond to the best possible form of adaptation for that individual.

In the view of Cloninger and his colleagues, who see personality development as a walk in an adaptive landscape made up of areas of high (hills) and low (valleys) adaptive value, attractor states correspond to the hills, while the valleys correspond to states of great instability, so much so that even the slightest perturbation may drive the system away from this point of low fitness. When the system is perturbed, it will respond spontaneously to internal or external constraints by seeking adaptive changes of personality, motivated by the optimization of fitness.

When a state of high stability is achieved, that state remains virtually invariable unless the system is subjected to external or maturational pressures. For the stability of the system to change, fitness must decrease by a slippage toward a valley. Only at that point will the organism spontaneously seek a new configuration capable of meeting both external and internal constraints. On the other hand, as we mentioned earlier, stability itself may become a trap, as is the case when a given disturbance becomes chronic: 'Such local maxima correspond to arrests in character development and may lead to practical termination of search' (Cloninger and Svrakic, 1999).

How can we understand the relationship between the unity and the multiplicity of the Self as seen by Cloninger?

Perhaps the clearest answer lies in their definition of personality.

Cloninger and Svrakic (1999) employ the terms of Gordon Allport (1937) to define personality as the 'dynamic organization within the individual of those psychophysical systems that determine his or her unique adjustment to the environment'. And in the paragraph which follows, they specify that by dynamic organization they mean 'an organized system ("*unitas multiplex*") that is constantly evolving and changing', while the expression they borrow from Allport, 'within the individual', means that 'personality is what lies behind a specific individual's acts'.

This definition is reflected in Marc D. Lewis' application of the principles of self-organization to the development of dynamic cognitive-emotional systems. Lewis (Lewis, 2005: 173) writes: 'cognitive systems construed as dynamic systems do not process information transduced from the outside world; they reconfigure themselves in response to an ongoing stream of sensory events'.

Hence, the unifying principle, which gathers and determines the multiplicity of experiences, may be located in organizational dynamics, in real activity, which is structured at the level of connections. The system's connectedness is the *unitas*, which is continuously reorganized in relation to the multiplex of experience. This is why

Cloninger can claim that at the base of every act there lies the entire unit. Every act is determined by the unity of the system, which, by conserving the traces of the structures that have emerged in the course of its history, integrates the dimension of duration with the ongoing event through the continuous recomposition of connectivity. The system adjusts itself moment by moment in relation to the external and internal constraints. That is to say, every current act, every current experience, is defined by the principle of order which – like the Kantian I think – determines the present state of the system, the difference being that in Kant, this unifying connection is not a subject but a mechanism. On this count, we might state what Ricoeur stated about structuralism: 'a transcendentalism without a subject' (1969); a Kantism without the I think.

1.4 The organization of living systems and constructivism of the self

But why should it be surprising that aspects of the Kantian conception of subjectivity constitute the basis of these views? What has Kant got to do with dynamic self-organizing systems?

Heidegger once said that cybernetics is the metaphysics of the atomic age. What does this mean? Can Heidegger's words indicate a direction, or are they simply the condemnation of technical knowledge by a philosopher whose border town was Freiburg?

Perhaps the most significant clue to fully understanding what Dupuy called the Heideggerian anathema in his noteworthy study of the first stage of cybernetics has been provided by Lettvin, one of McCulloch's collaborators. Speaking of McCulloch's intellectual development, he writes: 'He devoted himself to discovering how the brain works in the same way that an inventor knows exactly every single cog in the machine he has created. The key to such knowledge lies, not in observation, but in the construction of models which are then compared to the data available . . . And McCulloch preferred to run the risk of failure in his attempts to create a brain, rather than succeed in furnishing an improved description of existing brains' (Dupuy, 1985: 78).

The cybernetician as Plato's Demiurge! Like the craftsman who, the *Timaeus* argues, imposes a pre-existing form on as-yet formless material.

Is there a thread linking ancient philosophy, Kant and contemporary science?

In a work which is so closely linked to the research developed in *Sein und Zeit* that it appears to be the continuation of the latter,[10] Heidegger provides an extraordinarily clear reply. The trait which connects ancient philosophy with modernity is the fact that the being of consciousness is considered in exactly the same way as the being of an object: an *ens creatum*. That is, like a thing whose specific way of life, its autonomous existence, belongs to it on the basis of having been produced; like the vase which, once it has been moulded by the Demiurge from a pre-existing form, stands for itself.

Thus, there is no difference between the ways of existing of a vase, of a mouse and of a man. Clearly, existence refers back to an act of creation, hence to an *ens increatum*. And this is the fundamental theme which constitutes the meeting ground of ancient ontology with Christian theology in the Middle Ages and which then enters the modern age via Descartes. Descartes is the thinker who directs philosophical enquiry toward the subject, interpreting subjectivity through the employment of the ontological categories of ancient and medieval philosophy. In other words, existence is conceived of as the specific way of being of a thing which belongs to that thing exclusively by dint of the fact that it has been produced.

This perspective also offers us a better grasp of the Kantian view of subjectivity. The one and invariable Self is that created thing (like the vase), a *res cogitans* to be precise, which lies at the base, which connects, which is the subject of all possible determinations. With Kant, for the first time the thinking thing becomes quite simply that 'I' which, being in possession of the multiplicity of its determinations, is the knowledge of its own identity. In thinking or in perceiving, in acting or in suffering, in judging or in loving – that is, in the multiplicity of its determinations – the thinking thing, the 'I think', grasps itself; it is conscious of its own Self, it is self-conscious, hence it stands for itself. In actual fact, however, starting out from the theme of the subject did not constitute a fundamental step forward inasmuch as the ontological difference between the way of being of the subject, which understands itself through living, and the mode of presence at hand of the object was never clarified (Heidegger, 1988: 123).

Does this indistinctiveness still permeate contemporary science? Does that very same ontology which never permitted the subject's way of being to be investigated still lie at the heart of scientific thought?

The organization of living systems

A second approach that may be identified within the domain of the study of self-organization constitutes the foundation of radical constructivism. The basic postulate of this perspective is 'The nervous system is organizationally closed' (Riegler, 2003).

What does 'organization' mean and what does 'closure' mean? Organization is the heuristic description of the behaviour of the system: it enables the identification of the invariant features ('eigenbehaviour'), according to which the processes constituting an autonomous natural system (i.e. metabolic processes, developmental processes, processes of the nervous system), are so closely interconnected as to form a whole.

Operational closure refers, instead, to that mechanism which, as a result of its functioning, allows the generation of a variety of internal transformations. The nervous system thus appears as a closed network of interacting neurons where any change in the state of relative activity of a collection of neurons leads to a change in the state of relative activity of another, or the same, collection of neurons (Riegler, 2003).

A system thus organized has its own internal coherence whose features are distinct and relatively independent of the environment. The internal coherence of the system defines an autonomous system inasmuch as it constitutes a whole, while the complexity of the system is manifested in the configuration of the landscape of its possible behaviours.

Evidently, since in this view the system is considered impermeable to environmental input (which explains why it is a closed system), the relationship with the external world is maintained by structural changes in the system coupled with perturbations in the medium in which it lives. This means that, in order to come to terms with a change in the environment, a system changes continuously its internal structure but conserves its organization.

This is why Varela says 'Internal transformations are the main thread which allow us to comprehend the dynamics of the system; the coupling (of the two independent series of events – those taking place in the system and those occurring in the environment) only intervenes if certain unforeseen events or circumstances help us to better understand a given transformational pathway' (Varela, 1983: 149). The ultimate regulation of adaptation is assigned to structural changes that are subordinated to the invariance of the living organism.

Extending the biological interpretation to include relationships with the environment brings psychology on to centre stage; and, more generally, cognition. A cognitive act is then defined as the actual action undertaken by a living organism in its environment and it can only be explained by having recourse to the organizational dynamics of the system. Being a Self implies the maintenance of the organization of the system through continual structural changes coupled with the perturbations originating in the environment in which it lives. In this way everything that takes place is brought forth by the living organism in its praxis of living.

This interpretation of cognition gives rise to the epistemological aphorism which has characterized the Santiago school and second-order cybernetics: 'Everything said is said by an observer to another observer that could be him or herself' (Maturana, 1988).

In actual fact, this aphorism can only be fully understood if one bears in mind the other manoeuvre which accompanies the emphasis on the biological ontology of the observer, a manoeuvre whose flavour and terminology are explicitly phenomenological: placing objectivity within brackets. It consists in suspending every postulate regarding the experience of things and of the world (inasmuch as they refer to the internal dynamics of the system), leaving one's consciousness pure (the organization of operations), which is very similar to what remains when one suspends real experience. This so to speak residual consciousness is thus the absolute foundation of all positing of being, of objects, of swans, of plants and of people. In it, the world is defined by means of the invariances pertaining to the organism's internal operations. It is the place of the biology of knowledge.

Constructivism of the self

The most striking aspect of this mode of conceiving self-organizing systems is undoubtedly that of organizational closure. This mechanism establishes an absolute distinction between the sphere of lived experience, of the dynamics of change, which is necessarily coupled with the conservation of organization – which Guidano (1991) identifies with that of personal meaning – and the external world.

The domain of personal meaning is a coherent unity closed to any information that might come from the external world. Hence, the question that must be asked is: How is the sphere of personal meaning constituted?

The starting point to investigate this aspect is the immediate experience of daily life: for example, my immediate experience of the table I am writing on. This experience is embodied in a stream of experience which constitutes the flowing of individual experience. From the standpoint of the internal dynamics of the system, this corresponds to the succession of internal configurations of coherence within the system itself: that is, it consists of structural changes.

In a well-known adage, Maturana says that at the level of immediate experience there can be no difference between perception, illusion and hallucination (Maturana, 1988). It is only when we examine immediate experience by means of reflection, therefore through another act of the same nature as the act preceding it (from the viewpoint of closed systems, this corresponds to the coordination of the coordination of actions), that we can distinguish between the various modes of gaining immediate experience of something; it is the relationship between the praxis of living and its explanation.

This interdependent polarity is the backbone of the model of the Self produced by Guidano, who has been one of the most subtle representatives of constructivism (Guidano, 1987, 1991). In his work, Guidano posits that this polarity corresponds to a circular process of mutual regulation between the immediate experiencing of oneself (the acting and experiencing I) and the more abstract and explicit sense of Self that emerges as a result of self-referring the ongoing experience (the observing and evaluating Me). Guidano thus combines the perspectives of Maturana and James.

It is interesting to note that the object of reflection (immediate experience) and the act of reflecting (explaining) belong to the same flow, to the same domain (coherence of the operations of the system).

The embodied consciousness, which continuously constructs and reconstructs itself as the organization of the acts and of the reflection on those acts, is totally separated from the real world and from any contamination on the part of that world. This is the deep significance behind operational closure: in terms of the mechanisms organizing the process, it founds the closed unit of experience. The entire world is banished from this unit and it can only constitute a transcendental domain.

At the level of CNS, what the observer may see is changes in relations of activities between neurons as they interact, determining changes in the properties of the components of the neuronal network, which in their turn bring about changing relations of activities. Translating this into an example: from the standpoint of sensorimotor activity, an environmental perturbation X (for instance, the hand approaching a source of heat) stimulates structural changes in the sensory surface. Since the sensors are part of the neural network, structural changes in the sensory surface trigger structural changes of the effectors, changing relations of activities between the components of the system. (To the observer, such changes in the internal dynamics of the network appear to take the form of postural changes, such as the removal of the hand.) In their turn, changes in effectors trigger changes in relations of activities between the elements of the system, thereby determining structural changes in the sensory surface and, consequently, in the range of perturbations that are significant for the system.

When anything that is outside the system comes into contact with the system, the only reaction it can cause is that of a perturbation to the dynamics of the system. Consequently, within this dimension defined through recursive circularity, a real object can only arise as a perturbation of the dynamics of the system. As such, and unlike input, a perturbation cannot specify the way in which a given transformation of the system itself can come about – the transformation can only be determined by the global organization of the system.

Returning to the previous problem (to my immediate perception of the table I am writing on), the table I am writing on might present itself to me as perception, hallucination, illusion by means of memory, or of an imaginary scenario, or in other ways, but no matter what form this experience takes, the experience in itself does not contain the table. The table and the entire material world belong to a domain that is totally different from that of consciousness – and of the objects of consciousness – which, instead, constitutes a unitary context in itself.

The close connection with Husserl's phenomenology is crystal clear. In one extract from *Ideas I* (Husserl, 1962), he makes an extremely lucid distinction between reality and the abyss which divides it from the domain of consciousness, over which the term 'disturbance' builds a bridge: 'We are aware of things not only in perception, but also consciously in recollections, in representations similar to recollections, and also in the free play of fancy; and this in "clear intuition" it may be, or without noticeable perceptibility after the manner of "dim" presentations, they float past us in different "characterizations" as real, possible, fancied, and so forth'; and shortly afterwards we find the extract: 'We shall not think of confusing the *objects of which we are aware* under these forms of consciousness with the conscious experiences themselves which are a consciousness *of* them' (Section 35, page 106, original emphasis). In terms of the mechanisms operating, it is the consciousness of this or that ... that the system grasps.

This approach is especially evident in a psychology of the Self, such as that championed by Guidano, which is not outdated in the domain of constructivism and which assigns to these concepts the role of founding presuppositions for clinical practice. On the basis of these concepts Guidano has identified four invariant types of organization of the Self understood as the internal coherence of the system. He has dubbed these types Organizations of Personal Meaning. He has also traced their origins in the development of an equal number of forms of attachment. These correspond to four basic configurations of operations ordering experience, to four unitary categories for the organization of acts and of reflections on acts, which are structured, in Guidano's view, by different developmental pathways.

He writes (Guidano, 1991: 33): 'an Organization of personal meaning is to be interpreted as a unitary ordering process in which continuity and internal coherence are sought in the specificity of the formal, structural properties of its knowledge processing (flexibility, generativeness, and abstracting level) ... This leads to the adoption of a systems process-oriented methodology that can identify the deep syntactic rules ("I") capable of generating a coherent range of surface, semantic representations ("Me") according to an ever-changing interaction with the world.'

The therapist employs this model to seek principles which the patient uses to order his experience. Such principles – which remain constant throughout the patient's life – enable the patient to consistently recognize and appraise his experience as unitary and continuous in time. This analysis, which is guided by the four organizational principles and by the ways they combine, takes shape through the therapist's trying to 'cleanse' the patient's experiences of all those elements which are extraneous to the structural invariants hypothesized by the therapist as constituting the patient's organizational structure, in order to confirm the therapist's hypothesis.

One of the techniques which Guidano developed, the so-called 'moviola' technique, consisted in interrupting the flow of consciousness, bringing the experience into focus, amplifying it and running over it again in order to grasp the meaning attributed by the patient to what he had seen and done, and going slowly back and forth in order to extrapolate the principles ordering experience.[11]

The most striking aspect of this approach, and one which becomes even more obvious in the course of clinical practice, is that by placing experience within brackets, hence by opening out on to the perspective of the internal dynamics of the system and of the coherence of the system, real experience is taken as corresponding to the configuration of the organism's internal processes. As in Kant, the one and invariable Self consists in the connection of manifold changing experiences in a unity.

This brings about the concurrent cancellation of two extremely important aspects. First of all, by placing it within brackets, the reality (*realis*) of consciousness, or factual consciousness, is set aside: precisely that state of being involved in things and in the material world which concerns man in facts, from a concrete viewpoint. Consciousness thus appears the presupposition, the a priori condition, on the basis of which objects – to use a Kantian metaphor – come to be regulated and reality can manifest itself and thus become significant.

On the other hand, the 'mineness' of acts, the occurring singularization of experience, is eliminated. This being mine of acts and experiences is elided or simplified in order to grasp the organization, the configuration of internal coherence. Such deletion suppresses the history of the person, and with it, the person's identity. Identity thus becomes a portrait. It constitutes the organization of personal meaning (Guidano, 1987, 1991).

What does the expression 'identity thus becomes a portrait' mean? Let us deal with this question by analysing the story that we are using as a testing ground for our investigation of the Self.

1.5 Robert's self from a systemic perspective

As we have stressed before, the model produced by Cloninger and his colleagues would have identified such unity in multiplicity by relating Robert's real experience to the combination of the features (temperament and character) which defined, at the given moment x, the dynamics of the system in its landscape of states. When Robert asked for our help, we could have analysed him by taking into account a combination of features; we could have evaluated the high or low dispositions for each temperament trait in combination with a high or low score of character dimensions in relationship to his lifestyle. In that case, we would have examined Robert's world with a neutral attitude, trying to identify those regularities in the phenomena of Robert's life experiences in the light of the model. That would have enabled us to cleanse the experiences analysed of the personal residual experiences, those foreign to the structural organization of the personality, and, consequently, to formulate a diagnosis. This is the perspective on which the natural sciences are founded.

Things are more complicated from the point of view of closed systems.

From this perspective, unity arises through the flowing of experience: unity itself is the self-organization of the multiplicity of experiences. Unity is the process itself. This corresponds to the continual structural change taking place in order to maintain the organization of the living organism stable. By combining various nuclei that are constitutive of sense (patterns of attachment, modes of organizing the emotional domain, the relationship between immediate experience and the image of the Self, levels of integration of the different forms of experience and so on), it is possible to identify different forms of organization of the Self, which correspond to different global configurations of the flow of experience (four forms of self-organization and the combinations that occur).

The therapist who adopts this perspective in order to understand how Robert organizes meaning must put Robert's habitual attitude within brackets and shift the focus from the what of experience to the how of experience. This change in viewpoint, which Guidano calls internally-bound attitude, is the result of reflecting on the patient's real experience and leads to the identification of the invariant principles that explain the experience being analysed. The therapist and the patient agree on a frame of sense (so to speak), which is derived from having reflected analytically on the concrete experience of the patient. That is, therapist and patient identify the regularities, starting from the way in which the patient attributes meaning to his experience.

In this approach, although the experiential data of another person's experience are taken as being valid, they are taken as being accounted for by the organizational principles which guide the patient's cognitive system. In other words, subjective experience (the first-person I) is viewed through the second person (you) and the methodology consists of the suspension of real experience in order to grasp the organizational invariants. In this way, the patient is transformed into a stable and lasting portrait of himself, 'cleansed' of all 'business' with the external world. In Robert's case, the invariants can be hypothesized as being: a vague and oscillating sense of Self, a definition of the Self based on external sources, a tendency to perfectionism, attribution of cause to external entities, a defective perception of others and so forth.

But has this portrait brought the solution to Robert's case closer, or has it simply built a certain connection between invariants, a sort of psychic DNA, without actually making us take a single step forward in finding a solution? And if the latter is the case, what direction should we take at this point? Might the singularity of the experience, that business with external reality, not constitute the key to the problem?

1.6 The continuity of the sense of self

Before tackling these issues seriously, we must first analyse briefly a problem which is closely connected to multiplicity and unity: continuity – the fact, that is, that the multiplicity of experiences and the variety of our experiences take shape over time.

From this standpoint, being a Self seems to imply a continuity in sense, a permanence of the Self across past, present and future experience. The setups both of nonlinear systems and of closed systems offer two solutions to the problem. These two solutions are both based on the same explicative principle: self-organization.

In the case of nonlinear systems, connectivity is governed by both local and global rules. That is to say, it is the way in which connectivity is built up over time that constitutes the invariant which underlies changes in the system.

In the case of closed systems, what remains invariant in relation to current changes is the organization of the system understood as the configuration of static or dynamic relations between its component parts.

In both cases, continuity corresponds to the dynamic nature of the system.

From the experiential standpoint, this would mean that any form of discontinuity that is perceived by the person can simply be attributed to a sense of continuity in the Self. In nonlinear systems this would be attributed to connectivity, while in closed systems it would be attributed to organization itself as an invariant. From this viewpoint, continuity is always located in the Self, in the Self as a coherent flow.

But does reducing experience to the flow not lead to the loss of the characteristics of experience? Does it not mean that we are still viewing consciousness as a thing which exists by itself, as a self-sufficient object, while concurrently considering the world as something separated from it by a fracture?

Let us think for a moment of how Robert perceives himself. Periods of commitment in which he feels his life is meaningful alternate with periods during which he falls into a void in which his sense of Self disappears completely. States of void mean for Robert the lack of an anchor point, of a wavelength which allows him to tune in to himself. He deals with these states of emptiness through technical means which produce experiential spheres capable of absorbing his attention. Sarah's presence, especially at the initial stages, is a human source which can serve as the point through which he can define himself. Then Sarah becomes part of his relationship with the technical means he deploys to handle emptiness. When, at the end of the relationship, Sarah finally disappears, Robert no longer has points of reference, he no longer perceives himself as a Self.

Naturally, it can be said that although Robert experiences void as the disappearance of the Self, this is nevertheless part of Robert's personality system. We can combine, for instance, high novelty seeking with low self-directness with the event of Robert's separation from Sarah. Alternatively, we can thematize the unitary structure of his personality, the way it is organized, and consequently focus on the features denoting the vagueness of his sense of Self, the way he defines himself through the other, his touchiness to comparison and so on. In other words, we can reduce experience to the status of the object of reflection in order to highlight the organizational invariants. By operating in this way, however, we fail to capture experience *qua* experience, life as experienced directly by the subject himself. What we grasp, instead, is the objectivity of subjectivity – the flesh and blood subject slips through our hands. We not only omit a point which is relevant to the patient – that is, that the world in which Robert experiences the Self is discontinuous – but we also fail to engage with the fundamental question of ipseity . . . and starting from that question, the issue of personal identity.

1.7 The return of the world and the question 'Who?'

In a target article of great interest entitled 'The Self', Galen Strawson (1999)[12] deals with the theme of the continuity of the Self over time in relation to character. In so doing, he introduces a difference, as indicated by his words: 'Some people live deeply in narrative mode . . . Some merely go from one thing to another. They live life in a picaresque or episodic fashion' (Strawson, 1999: 15). Two different ways of living, of experiencing, of imagining and of talking about oneself. If we examine these two modes in the light of continuity, however, then the second mode is defective.

If continuity were tacitly or theoretically assumed as the definitional criterion of the normal sense of Self, just think of how many therapists would have the formula of a cure in the palm of their hands! They would only have to help their clients tell their life stories in a different way, or convince them of how unreasonable their picaresque way of life was; or it might be necessary to construct a more adequate frame of meanings, a more appropriate portrait by which to judge the fragmented nature of their lives. In other words, it would suffice to furnish a stable point, perhaps a new story, or perhaps a more precise image of the Self, in order to bring the dispersion of experience back to the sense of personal continuity. For those therapists, normality corresponds to the narrative mode of living. But is being non-narrative really an anomaly? As Strawson

(Strawson, 2007: 86) says: 'one may simply lack any narrative tendency, or one may have a positively anti-narrative tendency'.

This means that caution must be taken when seeking continuity of the Self in a narrative mode, or in an impersonal portrait, as if the narration of a story or the stability of an image were a guarantee of the continuity of the Self. As if bestowing meaning through any story whatsoever were enough to create stability.

Another reason why caution must be exercised is that narration concerning the construction of personal identity is based on, and brings to language, one's own experience of being in the world. The way people narrate themselves differs; not all stories exhibit continuity and go through the stages of beginning, development and end. Some stories consist of variations on a single theme, others consist of a variety of themes, while others still consist simply of variations without a theme (Arciero, 2006). Why?

Although many believe that it is sufficient to tell a story, or to tell oneself a story, to bestow sense on the Self or on others, one must stress the view expressed by MacIntyre (1981) that stories are lived before they are told. Recounting one's life must thus bring to light 'the documents and monuments', the actions carried out and feelings experienced during that life, otherwise the act of recounting is pure fiction. Hence, the problem cannot be solved simply at the level of the story of the Self. Instead, it concerns, first and foremost, being oneself.

Considerations of this nature encourage us to take Zahavi (2003: 62) seriously when he proposes making a terminological distinction to avoid unnecessary confusion: 'When we are dealing with the experiential self, we should stick to the term "self", since we are exactly dealing with a primitive form of self-giveness. But when we are dealing with the narrative model, it would be better to speak not of the self, but of the *person* as a narrative construction.' Zahavi identifies two domains of phenomena that we have not yet encountered, of which one, the experiential Self, is more primitive than the other – the person as narrated.

Thus, before we can start looking for a cure for Robert's discontinuity, the problem Robert's story sets us is to make ipseity manifest: to show that experiential Self which each of us is before any narration. Rendering this phenomenon evident means accounting for the different modes of experiencing continuity-discontinuity, not at the level of narration, but already at the pre-reflexive level; it is in its acting and feeling that this phenomenon must be unveiled.

In order to cast light on ipseity, then, we take a fundamental methodological step – that of taking concrete experience and giving it back the part that is missing, the world, integrating being . . . in-the-world. In other words, we lead consciousness back into direct contact with the world, with daily life, namely with what absorbs us for most of our waking lives without ever requiring reflection.

Instead, taking factual experience not as the object of reflection but as a way of being oneself – that is, as a way of feeling that I exist – has two obvious consequences. The first concerns the Self returning to the world and the second the question of 'who?'. We shall deal with these two issues separately.

Returning to the world

Setting the concrete relationship between subject and world as the main focus of research clearly demolishes the separation between consciousness and the world. In other words, the fundamental presuppositions of modern subjectivity, hence of the theory of nonlinear systems, of closed systems and of cognitive psychology, are left behind: the closure of consciousness,[13] understood as the I think which accompanies all the representations, or as an I that radiates a series of acts (perceptions, actions, images, etc.), to which this same I would return through reflection.

Indeed, if we consider the actual experience of living, such as, for example, feeling hot on this summer afternoon as I sit at this table writing this book, this experience is my very own, but it is not the outcome of an I who first reflects on this experience and then says he is hot. That is, this experience has a meaning even before an I, the centre of all meanings, says 'I am hot' through having reflected on the immediate experience. This experience does not, however, constitute the exception. If we think for a moment of the various events that have occurred during the day – waking up, having breakfast, getting ready to go out, the journey to the office and so forth – the vast majority of these experiences have taken shape without any need for one's cognitive apparatus to come into play.

Rather than going back to reflect on its own acts, the consciousness of Self emerges in its business with the world. We meet ourselves, the Self is present to itself, not in the closed space of an interior room illuminated by introspection, but in doing what we do, in feeling happy at what makes us happy, in thinking what we think of, in loving whom we love, in perceiving what we perceive. Consciousness seems to be rooted in existence, embodied in my body, attuned to a certain emotion.

In recent years, several investigations – above all from new interdisciplinary studies combining philosophy, developmental psychology, primatology and the neurosciences – have all converged in considering self-consciousness as a more primitive, embodied, nonconceptual phenomenon.

Several studies have shown that starting right from early infancy, perceiving movements or objects corresponds to acquiring nonconceptual, pre-linguistic information about oneself (Bermudez, 1998). This type of consciousness is the basis for the earliest processes of imitation which children are already capable of a few hours after birth (Meltzoff and Moore, 1977, 1984). Gallagher and Meltzoff (1996) would thus appear to be correct when they say that the human infant comes already equipped with a minimal Self that is embodied, enactive and ecologically attuned.

The question 'Who?' (Die Werfrage)

The second interesting consequence is the passage to a new ontological perspective in which the difference between what and who is given serious consideration, in which the question that resonates is 'Who is the Self?' rather than 'What is the Self?'.

This standpoint, according to which 'subject' means *what* remains identical throughout the multiplicity of behaviours, or the I which irradiates intentional acts, interprets the being of the subject as a fact, as evidence, as a datum, just like the telephone next to my computer. That is, by means of the very same categories we use to identify things.

Such a perspective does not thematize the different ways of being of the subject which, nevertheless, constitute our uniqueness. It leaves these modes indeterminate and undifferentiated since, We would claim, this perspective does not need to characterize them from an ontological standpoint. In actual fact, it understands the Self as if it were a thing. It understands Robert – to return to our example – as if he were a system in which character traits combine with temperament traits at a certain point in his life; or else as the self-organization of meaning which can be identified by means of a number of invariant characteristics and of certain constitutive elements. This approach guarantees the objectivity of subjectivity, the impersonal portrait of the subject. It might be stated that these categories release us from the need to know *who* we are talking about when, in using them, we refer to a specific individual. These categories refer to a subject who is nobody.

If, however, the being of the subject is not attributed properties the way a product is, but is instead assigned manners of being according to which on each separate occasion the person experiencing the world perceives himself in either this or that other way, then there is an ontological difference between being a star, being a rose, being a monkey and being a man. Man's existence is thus characterized by possible ways of being, by modes of feeling oneself alive: experience is mine, it is always my being that is at stake in my possibilities of being, in my plans, in my expectations, in my encounters, in my choices!

The question 'who?', the *Werfrage*, sets the question of the uniqueness and of the generality of being oneself. Indeed, it asks the question, 'Who am I?', 'Who are you?'. By posing this question, ontology sets out to find, not the real being 'I' or the real being 'you', but being me in the sense in which I, you and everyone else means, each and every time, 'I myself', that is, ipseity.[14] A very peculiar conceptualization, since it attempts to grasp in one fell swoop the generality and the uniqueness of man.

Asking this question, however, also means extending the investigation to a Self that is not already given but which is always under construction. It is no longer a question of grasping the Self by means of an act of reflection, but of understanding how being oneself is there for itself, how it is conscious of Self in its routine activities, in its factual experience.

The question then becomes where does this presence to oneself emerge from, what is the origin of this consciousness of Self if reflection has been banished, and with it the interiority of consciousness?

The answer is in existence itself.[15]

I am present to myself while, in my laziness, I turn in bed before getting up, while, still half asleep, I wash my teeth and tie my shoelaces, or while I walk briskly into the office. And if to exist is being in the world for the sake of its own possibilities, a dwelling with the things of our daily concern, and if consciousness is nothing other than man's openness toward the world, then consciousness is not closed (within the head) but is in the world!

Consciousness of Self implies, therefore, a deeper relationship, a primal and more original relationship that is constitutive and that makes consciousness of Self possible: the relationship with the world, the relationship with the other.[16] That means that existing is already being always open to . . ., being in relation to . . ., being with . . .. But such existence is also concurrently being open itself. . ., being open to itself, on each and every occasion.

Consciousness embodied in a body, my body. The body proper is thus 'the place' in which, every time, the appearing of the world and my feeling alive are actualized. This is the extraordinary feature of the body: it masters its own being, it takes hold of it in one grasp while it reflects itself from the things present in the surrounding world. It is the current way of my being in the world. From this perspective, every sensation, every act of perception, every emotion is concurrently an emergence and a disappearance: it has already dissolved the moment it occurs. As the poet Rilke (Rilke,1939: II, 18 ff.) says:

> For we, when we feel, evaporate; oh, we
> breathe ourselves out and away; from ember to ember
> yielding a fainter scent.

Thus, if ipseity reveals itself and takes shape in daily life in the encounter with what it is not – the world and others – if it encounters and is present to itself in acting and feeling, in doing and undergoing, if it is commensurate to a world which unfolds as it lives its daily life, this is because it recognizes itself to the extent that it recognizes itself every time from things and from others existing in the world.

If being oneself takes shape in the itineraries which each one of us follows in the world each day, in the actions and passions of which those itineraries are made up, this is because the presence to itself opens up, it reveals itself by mirroring itself at each event from the world and from others.

1.8 Finding itself in things and with others

What does it mean when we say ipseity is reflected by things? What does reflection mean here? Through referring to reflection, have we not walked again into the trap of falling back on a person's own interiority, of relating the subject to his acts, which was the foundation of the consciousness of the Self posited by the modern age?

In Heidegger's words, 'The self is there for the Dasein itself without reflection and without inner perception, before all reflection. Reflection, in the sense of a turning back (*Ruckwendung*) is only a mode of self-*apprehension*, but not the mode of primary self-disclosure. The way in which the self is unveiled to itself in the factical *Dasein* can nevertheless be fittingly called reflection (*Reflexion*), except that we must not take this expression to mean what is commonly meant by it – the ego bent around backward and staring at itself – but an interconnection (*Zusammenhang*) such as is manifested in the optical meaning of the term "reflection". To reflect means, in the optical context, to break at something, to radiate back from there, to show itself in a reflection from something' (Heidegger, 1988: 226).

The mode in which oneself is there for itself, the fundamental mode in which it is open, is through refraction, through reflecting oneself from things, just as a beam of light is refracted on the surface it encounters. Ipseity reflects itself from things as if they were a mirror, and in so doing, each time it returns to itself, it is its own. Through what we busy ourselves with and through what worries us, through what we do and through whom we meet, through everyday life, ipseity discovers and understands itself. In this sense, consciousness of Self is founded on factual existence, on concrete life, inasmuch as it is emotionally situated through my business with the world and with others on each and every occasion.

This means that existing does not correspond exclusively to being at all times toward ... but that existing is, on every occasion, also determination of oneself.[17] I may be enthralled, furious, indifferent, impassioned, lost in those events and things surrounding me, in the facts that strike my imagination. Feeling that I am alive constitutes the way in which my existence is consigned to the sentiment of the situation in which I *find myself*.

This accounts for Heidegger's (2001: Section 29, page 176) affirmation that 'A mood assails us. It comes neither from "outside" nor from "inside", but arises out of Being-in-the-World, as a way of such Being'. An emotional state is not closed in an interiority; it is, on the contrary, the mode of being together, of being in the world; at the same time it is the mode in which being here, existence, is mine.

These different ways of being toward things point to an equal number of modalities of the presence of oneself, of the understanding of Self.

Seen in this light, intentionality is not a structure of experience which irradiates from the I, but appears as ipseity itself opening on to the world; it therefore acquires ontological value. It is the essential structure which underlies living experience – as the possibility to gain access to the world and as the fundamental determination of the existence of oneself.

1.9 Reflection

The problem of reflection brings up another issue: how can one reflect oneself from something if one is not already there for itself prior to that act of reflection (Raffoul, 2004)?

Being itself comes about by way of a possibility of being, from anticipations, projects and so on, from a constitutive opening corresponding to a totality of possibilities of being in the world. Hence, the anticipation of Self on itself constitutes a structural component of ipseity. We always live in hope, in expectation, in fear, in desire, being wary of something, relating to something, having something before oneself, for the sake of something.[18]

Consciousness, as embodied consciousness, as Merleau-Ponty states, taking up Husserl's unpublished manuscripts, is not an 'I think that' but an 'I can' (Merleau-Ponty, 1962). Looking for the switch with one's eyes, grasping the lamp and its wire visually and placing it in the foreground with respect to the other objects which 'animate' this office already means looking at these objects as being 'able to be used'. That is, the body proper appears as a correlate of a world which the body is always one step ahead of by means of its different modes of accessing the world, a world on which it acts and which acts on it. 'In reality the body is nothing but the manner in which we gain access to the world and, at the same time, or correlatively, a certain mode of appearance of the world itself ... The body is the ensemble of concrete conditions under which an existential project actualizes itself and becomes, by actualizing itself, properly mine' (De Waelhens, 1951: 109). A number of studies in the neurosciences reveal how this anticipatory capacity is structured in the sensorimotor system (Rizzolatti *et al.*, 1996; Gallese *et al.*, 1996; Noe, 2004; Berthoz, 2000; Jeannerod, 2006).

It can be said that being itself exceeds itself, it is 'overabundant'; in one way or another, it is always ahead of itself, 'in advance' of anything we have to do, for it already exists in a world, 'it has already been born'. In his 1922 winter semester lectures, Heidegger (2001: 72) says 'I encounter myself in the world, in that which I live and in that which engages me, in my successes and failures, in my environment, in my surrounding world, in my shared world. I encounter myself from my own self, but in which the Self "is" not there *qua* Self, and where the "from my own Self" is neither reflectively given nor explicitly placed on state within this reflection'. As often happens in Heidegger, it is evident that the ways in which he employs language and the singularity of experience that these ways evoke do not provide easy access to meaning.

What does the philosopher mean by these enigmatic words? We always find ourselves amongst things and with others in a sort of concerned absorption in the world.

In the world, ipseity is always related to things and to others, and these relationships determine the way it acts or behaves in certain ways, according to certain emotional tones. It is precisely through the different ways in which it encounters the world and the other that ipseity reveals what is significant and concurrently discovers its own modality of being. In this sense, the Self 'is not reflectively present', it is not present to itself through a reflection generated by an interior space. Reflection springs 'outside itself', from things themselves.

And this being 'outside itself' immersed in a background of men and things which reflection presupposes as the very condition for a return to the Self (but not as an I, which is already given and which comes out of the Self in order to meet the world and the other to then return to the Self). It may be said that relating oneself (*Verhalthen*) is situated against the background that is 'already revealed', hence familiar for us, by way of encountering the things we have to deal with in our daily lives. That is, before caring or worrying about this or that, I already presuppose a world that I first take for granted, that I do not take into consideration, because it is obvious.[19] As Zaner (1971: 184) states, 'to belong-to-the-world is to inhabit it as a being who is already familiar with it, its typical course and style, because he is embodied in a body which is "at home" therein'.

Ipseity, understood as my mode of being intentionally directed toward this or that on each and every occasion, co-belongs to the world. It is the continuity of relating to the world that gives every single one of us the sense of the continuity of Self.[20] Heidegger leaves no doubts on this point: '"Who" I am now can be said only throughout this sojourn, and always at the same time in the sojourn lies that with which and with whom I sojourn, and how I comport myself toward [them]' (Heidegger, 2001a: 260). The continuity of relating cannot be anything but discontinuous inasmuch as my relating with this or that is different every time.

Hence, it is precisely because oneself is already always 'outside itself', open to the world and, therefore, emotionally situated, that it can reflect itself from things and thence return to itself. And it is precisely because the things from which oneself reflects itself refer back to that background, to the world, that they can mirror oneself. In his final semester at Marburg, Heidegger returned to the subject, affirming that 'The world is the free counter-hold of Dasein's for-the-sake-of' (Heidegger, 2001: 192). When worried, when in a hurry, when calm, when detached, when in the for-the-sake-of its own being, the world provides or withholds support to a possible play of opportunities

1.10 Meaning

Through what means does ipseity grasp itself in reflecting? 'From the things we have to deal with', those things that are urgent, feasible, indispensable, appropriate, those things that breathe down our neck, that we hope for, that we deem necessary. Success or failure, feasibility or impossibility on the one hand, but at the same time the viability, the impracticality of the world on the other hand; and then those things which are unexpected, ambiguous, new, mysterious, obscure, indefinable, vague. These are the things that enable or prevent oneself from returning to itself.

Not a single thing in itself, but that intertwining of things with the praxis of living, whose meaning is replete with, and complicated by, a series of specific references. Not a significativity connected to raw data, connected to the identity of the object, but an object whose luminosity is acquired through the context it refers to; a visibility that emanates from the totality which supports it. It is that contexture of specific references which constitutes the background of comprehension that enables us, at any and every moment, to attribute meaning to an object.

Take the lamp on the desk in my office as an example. The lamp acquires meaning as it enables me to light up the office, which in its turn is part of the department where I work, which in its turn links up to the need for an environment where man can work, and can work there at night too. The final context mentioned does not make connections with a set of specific references but to being-in-the-world itself.[21]

The object acquires meaning because it is referred back to a context, a wider connective sphere: to its possible uses, which in turn refer back to an even wider context, and so forth until the whole range of references finds anchoring in man's being. The whole range of interconnected contexts – which merge into one another, to the point that the widest contexts are visible even in the most limited ones – is immediately before us each time we are about to use the lamp.

According to Heidegger, it is by way of things that we are returned to a set of possible actions, to a contexture of references from which they retrieve sense and by way of which they offer themselves to comprehension, and of which the ultimate referential final point is man.[22] It is the set of possible uses that may be made of it that give meaning to the lamp that I have on my desk. Those uses constitute the last anchor point for man's mode of comprehension, which, as we have seen, is always based on keeping ahead, always . . . for the sake of itself.

'Consequently,' as Raffoul (2004: 180) underlines, 'when the Self moves, changes places or commits itself to certain relations, it is actually its own being that it assigns itself the task of unveiling and understanding . . . Familiarity with the world is familiarity with oneself.'

For instance, when darkness falls, the possibility that I can continue writing 'points' to the need for light that will enable me to see. For the sake of the exigency to continue working even at night, I search for the switch in order to turn on the lamp. I encounter the lamp without thinking about it. In this encounter, my need for light is allowed, is reflected, in the use of the lamp as a source of light. It is precisely the existence of a possible contexture of specific references, in which the thing takes on significance, that makes it possible for ipseity to be reflected as in a mirror. Reflection may take shape inasmuch as the discovery of the specific functionality of things (significance) presupposes a mode of being of discerning preoccupation, a searching after viability, an allowing the world to come to oneself for the sake of . . .. The experience comes to be meaningful for the very reason that the object illuminated (by the possible contexts of reference) meets up with the position of the person looking, listening, touching.

We may understand Merlau-Ponty's concept of body schema from the same stance: 'constituted by means of the concrete task-at-hand and carried out in bodily movements' (Zaner, 1971: 169). The body schema is the result on every single occasion of the organization and coordination of real and possible bodily activities with certain objects, intended as poles of action in the extant situation. A style of behaviour that is reflected in my vital environment which I deem important: my home, my music, my books, my personal effects and so on . . . the traces of our existence!

Those are the things that speak of me. In this sense, ipseity, which deals with things and which worries about things, is reflected in the contexture of references of intraworldly entities.

But this reflection is mute if it is not emotionally situated! My expectations may meet with disappointment, or I might be surprised by the results of the concrete task-at-hand, I may be spurred on, or I may be swept away by the situations which I encounter, and which encounter me. 'Indeed *from the ontological point of view*,' says Heidegger, 'we must as a general principle leave the primary discovery of the world to 'bare mood' (Heidegger, 1988: Section 29, page 177). In this sense, ipseity expects its own possibilities, relying on what 'things give or what they refuse' (Heidegger, 1988: 289),[23] since ipseity comprehends itself by way of those possibilities that the world of praxis and of things are able to reflect. Through understanding the world, through understanding the other, the Self understands itself.

Finally, in this sense, for an ipseity which encounters the world as a contexture of specific references (significance) through the circumspective engagement with the surrounding environment, meaning corresponds to what has been comprehended, grasped, in a single act.

Hence, it is ipseity that is open to the world in terms of a discerning preoccupation, (that is, concerned with this and that), while it encounters something significant, understands itself; while it expressly relates to something and lives off something, at the same time it brings its own world to experience.[24] We might say, in line with a variation on the same theme, that one's body-proper, emotionally situated, cooriginates with things. It is on this side, on my side, and at the same time it is on the other side, on the side of the world, or, as Merleau-Ponty put it, the touched touching.

In this way both the alterity of the world and that of the other, both individuation and openness, can be thought of together, contemporaneously. Meaning seen from this perspective indicates something, or someone, on each occasion and at the same time itself which comes to experience. In this sense, experience is mine.[25] The always being mine of experience indicates existence belonging to itself. It corresponds to my being in this or that emotional tone in the specific situation I am living through each time.

A private world understood as the sphere of internal experience is thus not given. It is, instead, the being mine of a behaviour. 'I can speak,' says Dreyfus (1991: 145), 'of your comportment and my comportment, and the understanding of being in your activities and in my activities, but that should not lead me to think that your comportment is in your world and my comportment is in my world or that you have your understanding of being and I have mine.'

1.11 Inclination

The being mine of experience, the fact that experiencing belongs to me and corresponds each time to my acquiring a meaning, shows how permanence in time is declined as continually a finding of oneself and/or finding each other. And it is each time experience belonging to itself which founds individuation in its undissociability from a sharing of the world with others.

In the winter 1922 lectures, Heidegger spoke of inclinations to indicate a certain historicity of this being in relation to:

> *'In this inclination of the relationality, in proclivity as a mode of the actualization of caring, the world, in which life lives, has weight for life, specifically such that life, in its facticity, admixes constantly new sorts of weight. The realms of significance which are encountered in the course of the maturation of life, and which become different as its world changes, transport life. In its proclivity, life thereby arrives at the mode of being transported. Life abandons itself to a certain pressure exerted by its world' (Heidegger, 1988: 76).*

We must be careful not to interpret this being inclined as a return to a sort of immanent sphere, to that substantial permanence which represented one of the most significant features of modern subjectivity. Inclination is to be understood by way of being each time, by way of discontinuity, by way of the sense of Self which comes to experience each time. It indicates, rather, that coming toward itself each time ipseity finds itself to be the same, inasmuch as it finds itself each time beside the same things with the same emotional tones. In the following chapters we will see the importance that this return to the Self acquires for the study of character and personality.

This tension – between the sedimentation of one's own experience of Self and the happening each time – which is internal to ipseity, which actualizes itself anew each moment of our existence, almost always remains invisible in daily experience. That is, how the history of our lives, which orients us, remains more or less indistinguishable from how we experience this or that thing. Although we do perceive a feeling of stability in ourselves every time we experience something, that feeling is never called upon explicitly in daily life; it is always silently present. As if there existed a sort of overlapping between the sense of continuity of Self, which remains while it unfolds, and the experience I am undergoing. The hidden dialectic between sameness and ipseity only discloses itself with vibrant clarity in the experience of novelty. It throws oneself out of itself; the encounter with the unexpected event produces the result that in the world we no longer find ourselves as being the same beside the same things with the same emotional tones. In experiencing novelty, it is as if ipseity did not have the support of its history: a history sedimented with actions and emotions with others in the world.

Let us now sum up our argument so far, in order to identify what problems remain to be solved, and to define the trajectory of the next chapter. Robert's case has posed a series of questions that have led us to re-examine the modern concept of Self, in both its foundations and implications. We have therefore traced the origins of this concept and outlined its developments as part of an ontology that, from Plato to Husserl, has always envisaged the Self as a thing. This concept, which has been adopted in psychology without any further thematization, has been seen to underlie the systems theory, the various classifications of personality and the different forms of therapeutic approach. By challenging these foundations, we have followed Heidegger in an attempt to define an ontology that grasps the Self as a 'who': not, that is, by means of ontological categories applied to things produced, but through ways of being – a Self marked by ways of 'feeling-in-the-world'. This exercise has inevitably led us to reconsider the three distinguishing elements that modern thought, as well as common sense, have regarded as the essential qualities of the Self: interiority, unity and continuity. Once again, Robert's case served as a test bed.

On the basis of this new perspective, it would seem that Robert's discontinuity, multiplicity, lack of narrative unity and lack of self-centeredness cannot be understood as inadequate terms with respect to the notions of continuity, unity and privacy. In other words, there may be an alternative way of understanding these three traits of Robert's Self. Our enquiry suggests that permanence does not possess a substantial character. The being-oneself is always something discontinuous: ipseity is constructed in each case in relation to the ongoing situation. While this form of discontinuity is always mine, in each case, depending on circumstances, it is simultaneously reflected in things or in others; as such, it is put off-centre. I meet myself in the way the world reflects my everyday business or life projects; I find myself through my relations with others and through others' relations with me. This multiplicity does not necessarily require any narrative unity. It is possible to describe oneself as a romantic hero or as a range of different characters: a kind of polyphony of the Self; a person may also lack any narrative tendency. From this perspective, Robert no longer appears deficient with respect to the normal functioning of the Self; rather, his case may be examined on the basis of different modes of being.

We do not find ourselves, however, in a situation similar to that which Klaus Conrad brought to Biswanger's attention when he polemically posed the question: does not the taking into account of as many unique and unrepeatable world projects as there are schizophrenic patients prevent us from grasping what is specifically schizophrenic? Paraphrasing Conrad, we may ask in turn: why should Robert suffer? After all, his discontinuity, multiplicity and being in each case attuned to others are all structural characteristics of the Self. In reaching ipseity, we have lost psychopathology!

The question 'who?' must still be answered; yet, it has certainly brought a previously concealed issue to the forefront: the meaning of experience, which is always torn between the happening and the sedimented story of the subject. The section on Inclination raises this question almost by surprise, pointing to the need of understanding ipseity in the context of its quasi-invisible dialectic with sameness.

A human being, unlike an animal, can only grasp the sense of Self – ipseity – in the context of the sedimentation of his own experiences. Without sameness we cannot understand the distribution – so to speak – of the multiplicity of Self in time: the context of meaning, that is, in which Robert's experiences in each case take shape. It is for this reason, on account of the decontextualization of experience, that the strenuous attempts of neuroscientists to locate the Self in the human brain are inevitably destined to fail. The network of relations between ipseity, sameness and narrative (or lack of narrative of Self) thus becomes the thematic object of our research. Following this path, in the next chapter we will mark those stages that lead from the pre-reflexive origin of meaning to its articulation through language.

This will enable us to study – in the footsteps of Paul Ricoeur – the relation between feeling and action, and the narrative reconfiguration of the two.

Endnotes

[1] Heidegger (1988: 11).

[2] 'Psychology itself is dead', said Gazzanica (1998) a few years ago.

[3] See Carr (1999) for a discussion of the relationship between the transcendental I and the empirical I in Kant, which constitutes an alternative to the line of argument we are advancing.

[4] A distinction is generally made between first-order cybernetics, which studies observed systems, and second-order cybernetics, which studies observing systems.

[5] Kant calls the knowledge of something (which also includes intuition and thought) a priori if it comes before any empirical experience. A thought (judgement), therefore, may be regarded as a priori if it finds no immediate reference in experience. An a priori judgement is described as synthetic, for it extends the knowledge contained in its subject concept through the predicate. Albeit anterior to any experience, an a priori judgement is not a mere form: it also possesses content; as such, it assigns a determination to intuition in advance. One of the chief problems addressed in Kant's *Critique of Pure Reason* is precisely the unity between pure thought and pure intuition.

An a priori synthetic judgement measures the real experience we have of things.

[6] For a history of the development of the cybernetic movement, see Heims (1991). For a history of self-organization, see Stengers (1985).

[7] Those interested in delving further into the subject may consult Dupuy (2000) and Heims (1991).

[8] Temperament and character traits are correlated with each other in a nonlinear manner: this means that the ways they are related are neither inevitable nor necessary. That is to say, one temperament trait may be related to different character configurations, and a given character configuration may be the outcome of different temperament structures.

[9] Cloninger and his colleagues also introduce into the model the developmental perspective in the form of 15 steps corresponding to an ideal pathway which leads to full character development. This pathway is consistent with the qualitative descriptions of development provided by Piaget, Freud and Erikson. At each step, it is possible to measure the relationship between the current state of character development and the preceding stage, as well as with the temperament traits and with the pressures exerted by the environment.

[10] Heidegger expressly states that 'the basic problems of Phenomenology' represent 'a new elaboration of the third section of the first part of *Sein und Zeit*'.

[11] This mode of conceiving of self-consciousness corresponds to what Zahavi (2003) calls 'intransitive consciousness'.

[12] Strawson's point of departure is that of a reflective description of the Self, which leads to conclusions that differ from ours.

[13] Closure here means: anything I am conscious of is in my consciousness.

[14] Contrariwise, I-ness does not mean the factical ego distinguished from the thou; egoicity means, rather, the I-ness also at the basis of the thou, which prevents an understanding of the thou factically as an alter ego. But why is thou not simply a second ego? Because being an ego, in contradistinction to being a thou, does not at all pertain to the essence of Dasein, that is, because a thou is what it is, only *qua* itself, and likewise for the I. Therefore I usually use the expression 'ipseity' [Selbstheit] for metaphysical I-ness, for egoicity. For the 'ipse' can be said equally of the I and the thou: 'I-myself', 'you-yourself', but not 'thou-I'. (Heidegger, 1984: 188).

[15] As Raffoul (2004: 118) states, 'consciousness is a mode of being, a particular realization of the presence to oneself'.

[16] But also, as we may glean from the title of one of the great works of Ricoeur (1990), the relationship of *Oneself as Another*.

[17] Heidegger employs an unusual lexeme to define my being as always: *die Jemeinigkeit*. The term indicates a universal concept (what it is that renders possible the existence of all the Is and all the Yous), but at the same time it indicates that experience belongs to me, it is my property.

[18] Even the impossibility of all possibilities, as in clinical depression, consists of living in expectation of . . ..

[19] Dreyfus (1991) speaks of familiarity with a background of shared practices. This familiarity corresponds to common sense (Arciero, 1989).

[20] Continuity is interrupted by death. The importance of being-for-death in the architecture of *Being and Time* is well known.

[21] But this lamp was once on my father's desk, my father having received it as a gift from my grandmother on a certain occasion, together with a paperweight which had belonged to her grandfather. Now, for whoever is unfamiliar with these facts or for whoever does not reflect about the history of this lamp, this object is a mere lamp: access to the lamp is opened up by the use made of it.

[22] In understanding itself by way of things, the *Dasein* understands itself as being-in-the-world by way of its world' (Heidegger, 1988: 171).

[23] Shortly afterwards, Heidegger (1988: 289) explicates the phenomenon of expecting, awaiting as a mode of re-coming toward itself: 'Only because the Dasein is expectant of its can-be in the sense described, as coming from the things it attends to and cares for – only because of this expecting can it anticipate, await something from the things or wait for the way they run off'.

[24] 'The "oneself" in *comporting oneself* and the "my" in "my Dasein" must never be understood as a relationship to a subject or to a substance. Rather, the "oneself" must be seen in a purely phenomenological sense, that is, in the way I comport myself now. In each case the *Who* exhausts itself precisely in the comportments in which I am [it is] involved just now' (Heidegger, 2001a: 159).

[25] This is why *Jemeiningkeit* cannot be considered an empty universal which is separable from the individual event of experience, but it must also not be confused with concrete individuality. As Raffoul (2004: 206) writes, 'Being always mine is the internal, constitutive and undissociable possibility of concrete individuality.'

2 Ipseity and Language

What is alone true is that our open and personal existence rests on a primary basis of acquired and congealed existence.[1]

2.1 Traces of the other

How do we read another person's mind? The question regarding the comprehension of the other was first set, from a developmental standpoint, at the end of the 1970s in the domain of primatology. And it is in this domain of the natural sciences that, since then, this research area has gained ever increasing interest, even in a variety of disciplines that border upon primatology, such as developmental psychology, cognitive neurosciences, the philosophy of mind and psychopathology. The question set by Premack and Woodruff (1978) was, 'Does the chimpanzee have a theory of mind?' and the new field of study opened up by that question was baptized with the name of the question: 'theory of mind'.[2]

The problem of social comprehension, reformulated in the terms set by the theory of mind, runs thus: an organism has a theory of mind if this organism is capable of explaining the behaviours, or the actions, of others in terms of the mental states that generate those behaviours and those actions. Stated differently, one understands observed behaviour by theorizing about it. The ability to attribute mental states to others – which requires a capacity to produce metarepresentations – also provides the power of prediction. Put simply, if I can explain the behaviour of another organism in terms of desires, plans or intentions, I can also understand and anticipate that organism's subsequent course of action. The literature on deception and on social manipulation in the field of primatology has furnished arguments in support of the theory of mind, adding rhetorical force to scientific explanations (Goodall, 1971; deWaal, 1982; Byrne and Whiten, 1988).

On the other hand, the capacity to attribute mental states to others implies that the nonhuman primate is capable of conceiving of itself as possessing mental states and, more generically, is capable of recognizing itself as a Self. This presupposition underlies what can be defined as the argument by analogy: starting from (a) how I access my own mind and (b) the relationship between my mind and my body, I can infer that a body

Selfhood, identity and personality styles Giampiero Arciero and Guido Bondolfi

analogous to mine will be connected to a mind through modalities similar to mine. This is why I can start from another's behaviour and infer the mental states of that other related to such behaviour, either on the basis of innate mechanisms – TOMM[3] – or on the basis of theories – TT.[4] The studies which later provided strong support for this argument, and which enabled the problem of whether primates had a mind to be posed, concern mirror self-recognition. It was with a famous article by Gordon Gallup published in 1970 on the recognition of the Self by the chimpanzee that a rich line of research opened up which, almost 40 years later, still produces solid insights and reasons for reflection.

The most paradoxical aspect of this perspective is that, despite the fact that it developed in the field of evolutionary studies, instead of deriving man's mode of acquiring knowledge from the ape, it derives the ape's mode of comprehending from that of man. The ape is understood, that is, by deploying those very same categories of interiority which modern thought has adopted to understand man; it is attributed to those internal states which take shape in the closure of interior space.

But what happens if we try to change the question and ask ourselves how we encounter the other?

What happens, in other words, if we change the context of our research from the laboratories of primatology to everyday life, to the concrete situations of our daily existence? The problem then becomes: how do we understand the other immediately, when we meet him on the stairs, or at work or in the street – that is, before we attribute to him any mental states?

We have already analysed how oneself always lives ahead of itself, in a concerned absorption in the world, in a range of actions which goes from the simplest to highly intricate life plans. The experiential Self (oneself, namely everyone), encounters the other by way of how it feels, in the context of what it is doing, on the basis of what it needs, what it desires, what it expects or what it does not expect. On the other hand, we meet the other who is working, who is sad, who is in a great hurry, who is taking a walk, who is sitting in silence.

We do not encounter the other as men confined within their reciprocal interiorities – men who employ a theory of mind to attribute mental states to other men through an analogy with their own states – but in a world which we share with other human beings, in which we are already always open, on which we act and which acts on us. We meet the other first and foremost in his corporeity, in his style of conduct, in his actions and passions, which are made manifest in the environment of daily situations, in those contexts of ordinary, everyday life in which actions, passions or traces of the other are comprehended immediately without requiring any mental operations whatsoever.

In the wake of the discovery of mirror neurons (Gallese *et al.*, 1996; Rizzolatti *et al.*, 1996), many of those working in the neurosciences claim that this type of immediate comprehension of the other is founded on the automatic activation of a neural mechanism shared by the person who carries out a certain intentional act and the person who observes him doing so. That is, the act that is perceived elicits in the observer the activation of the same neural code as that of the act executed, thereby generating an unmediated resonance (Gallese, 2001, 2003) between the motor system of the person carrying out the action and the motor system of the observer. This mechanism, which Gallese calls 'embodied simulation', is claimed to underpin the comprehension of the meaning of action and the ascription of intentions.

What does all this mean in concrete terms? Let us return to the lamp on my table. It is getting dark, I am beginning to find it difficult to read, and without thinking about it I switch on the light. My body almost automatically performs a movement whose goal is to find the light switch in order to turn on the light. The action I perform is thus directed toward the achievement of some goal: it has an intention.

Now let us suppose that my wife comes into the study at that every moment and notes my action. How does my wife understand that I am seeking the switch in order to turn on the light? How does that movement manage to be meaningful to my wife? How does my wife manage to anticipate my intentions? Whether she wants to or not, my wife understands that I am about to switch on the light. Why?

2.2 Shared meaning

In order to furnish an answer to that question, Iacoboni *et al.* (2005) designed an experiment whose aim was to evaluate the importance of context in comprehending the intention of an agent. Twenty-three subjects observe three types of stimuli: (a) the action of grasping devoid of context, (b) only the context (that is, no action is taking place), (c) the action located in two different contexts – a table laid out for tea, suggesting the intention to drink, and a table after tea has been taken, suggesting the intention to clear the table.

Let us then suppose we are observing Mary taking hold of a teacup in a context suggesting a table about to be cleared. Through the mirror system I instantly recognize not only the action of taking hold of the teacup, but I also anticipate the immediate goal connected to the accomplishment of that action. Is it possible to say I have anticipated Mary's intention? Yes and no. Yes, because Mary really did want to take hold of the cup. No, because what meaning grasping the cup has for Mary remains obscure.

The data obtained through functional magnetic resonance imaging (fMRI) indicate that the mirror neurons of the premotor area appear to be involved in the attribution of intentions, in the sense of automatically anticipating the goal of a chain of actions, the connection between those actions evidently being suggested by the context. In the case of Mary taking a cup from a table laid out for serving tea, for example, the sequence anticipated is made up of that set of actions which comes to a conclusion with the carrying of the cup to Mary's mouth. It is as if the typicality of the context were automatically interpreted through the unconscious activation of a chain of motor acts connected to the discharge of neurons which are 'logically correlated'. Merleau-Ponty's (1962: 197) words return to mind: 'Already motility, in its pure state, is equipped with the power to attribute meaning'. That is, my body generates each time, and maintains, a meaning starting from its use in a space of shared actions.[5]

Does this explanation, which undoubtedly demonstrates the anticipation of the goal in a chain of actions in a typical context, really account for the comprehension of Mary's action? This poses a problem that does not concern the explanation as to why Mary took the cup (Jacob and Jeannerod, 2005). Mary actually took the cup in one case to clear the table and in the other case to drink. The question at issue is, rather, to understand why, on the one hand, Mary's action is manifestly comprehensible, so much so that we immediately understand its meaning and we anticipate its consequences, and why, on the other hand, what escapes us is the meaning that Mary assigns to her action. That is to say, that while the meaning of the action is obvious, especially when the action is related to the context in which it was carried out, what remains hidden is the co-original link of the action with the person who carries out that action. This is the aspect about Mary that I cannot fathom. And perhaps this also corresponds to the limits to comprehending the other, as well as to the source of the regeneration of meaning.

In order to render those limits manifest, let us transfer the experimental situation into real life. Let us imagine that Mary has invited a friend, Linda, whose acquaintance she made only recently, to her country house for the weekend.

Let us suppose that Linda is still sitting at the table, because she was late in coming down to breakfast, while Mary begins clearing up. While she is conversing with Linda about this or that matter, Mary's face is calm, betraying absolutely no emotion. As soon as Mary makes to clear the table Linda immediately grasps her intentions. This means that, from the sensorimotor standpoint, Linda's mirror system (her mirror neurons generating shared activations) resonates with Mary's anticipating the goal of the chain of actions.

But that chain of actions, clearing away the table, can be understood by Linda as a gesture of courtesy in her regard, or as a sign of impatience at her having arrived late for breakfast, or it may be attributed to Mary's routine habits, or it may even pass unobserved.

On the other hand, Mary may want to clear up because she likes a tidy kitchen, or because she has nothing better to do, or perhaps because she wants to take Linda out on a trip, or because she wants to make Linda feel at home. That is to say, that action, whose meaning is shared inasmuch as it is carried out by Mary and simulated by Linda, is concurrently personal to the who that carries that action out and to the who that simulates it. And it is precisely this second aspect, the mineness of the action in terms of significance, which opens a hiatus of meaning between Mary and Linda, between me and the other – as a result of which the other may surprise me, he may disorient me, he may make me think! 'If the other is really another,' writes Merleau-Ponty (1962: 198), 'then at a certain point I will be surprised, disoriented, and we will meet again, no longer with what we have that is similar, but with what we have that is different, and that presupposes a transformation of myself and of the other too: our differences will have to cease being opaque, they must become meaningful'.

Vittorio Gallese (2005: 43) contends that 'an important component of this similarity resides in the common experience of action'; nevertheless, a further equally important component resides in the difference in the way the shared experience has been perceived by each single individual. This begs the question of how and why experiencing one and the same act can give rise to a range of meanings which, for instance, in the case of Linda may vary from pleasure to indifference. We will explore this matter in greater depth in the following chapter.

Let us now, instead, analyse the immediately comprehensible aspect of action, that part that may be called public, almost objective, so to speak: we will call it the intentional content of the action. Mary begins to clear the table. Linda perceives Mary's action and, after about 30–100 ms, her motor system begins to tune in to the action she has perceived Mary carrying out. Linda's motor system is reflected in Mary's motor system through the simulation of the action observed. At the neural level, this corresponds to the activation of a series of mirror-matching neural circuits. Nevertheless, the activation of Linda's mirror neuron system (MNS) simulates the intention expressed in Mary's action, not Mary's being mine of the action. We could say that the MNS simulates the intentional content of the action, the action as such, but not the agent that accomplishes the action, not the who that acts.[6]

In fact, resonance systems are activated both by one's own actions and by observations of those actions accomplished by others, constituting a sort of neutral (that is, neither first-person nor third-person) common code for perception and action. 'As soon as we see someone carrying out an act or a chain of actions,' write Rizzolatti and Sinigaglia (2006: 127), 'then whether that someone likes it or not, his movements immediately acquire significance for us. Obviously, the same applies to the opposite situation: every one of our actions immediately takes on meaning for those observing those actions. Possession of the MNS and the selectivity of their response thus determine a space of shared action, within which each act, each chain of actions, whether they be executed by us or by others, immediately appear to be inscribed and comprehended without such operations requiring an explicit and deliberate cognitive operation' (Gallese, 2005; see also Hurley, 2006). Stated differently, the experiential Self which perceives an action carried out by a conspecific is actively reflected in the action perceived, thereby generating a similar action (or 'simulation').[7]

Nevertheless, whoever simulates action by means of this process of reflection in the other, concurrently experiences his own mode of comprehending that action: this may range from indifference to active and meticulous participation, to complete absorption. This means that while Linda's motor system comprehends Mary's action by simulating it, that action may go unnoticed by Linda herself, or it may awaken her interest, or it may even become the sole focus of her attention. The being mine of the act corresponds to the personal sphere of experience. It does not need to be internal in order to be private.[8]

From this perspective, the activation of the MNS helps explain how the Self attributes meaning to its encounter with the other, despite the fact that this encounter does not exhaust the comprehension of alterity. These systems are probably part of the neural substratum of that social being which is constitutive of being oneself. 'Constitutive' is not intended here only in its oblique sense, as in Heidegger, namely that we already always encounter the other through things, through artefacts, as if objects alluded to their users, their traders. It is intended, instead, as sociality experienced directly, face on, without it being dazzled by the reflection of the horizon, without leaning on the context for support, inasmuch as it is only through the sharing of meaningful acts anchored in our living bodies that the how I grasp myself through such sharing, the how I reflect myself in it, emerges to experience concurrently with the comprehension of the other. Such sharing is constitutive of being oneself; comprehending oneself is contemporaneously comprehending others.

Unlike the solipsism, where the other corresponds to a datum furnished by reflection, in this perspective we encounter the other starting from his being with us in the world, as if the other were, at one and the same time, text and context, image and background. This is evident right from the first few hours of a baby's life.

2.3 *Finding* oneself in the world: suggestions from phenomenology

'For unto us a child is born' (Isaiah 9:6). With these simple and powerful words, the Holy Bible announces the 'glad tidings'.[9]

A new life enters the world, a voice never heard before breaks into shared space, disrupting it; the face of another, who has never appeared before, stages its entry into existence. It is the epiphany of the face, a presence which shines with its own light, which signifies by way of itself, exteriority which does not require a context, evidence which instantly expresses itself. 'The face speaks. The manifestation of the face is already discourse' (Levinas, 1961: 64).

When we think of childhood, the inexhaustible theme of Levinas' work is blatantly clear. Not the face of the widow, the orphan, the stranger, but a face which is even more naked, that of a son of man, whose naked gaze conveys vulnerability and supplication, expression and injunction, manifestation and commandment.

Levinas' strong words befit this face, almost as if the insistent use of the trope of hyperbole no longer corresponds to the systematic practice of excess – which nevertheless is a major feature of Levinas' style of philosophical argumentation – but constitutes the only adequate measure. As if there really were no other means bar hyperbole to describe a child's bursting into the world at birth, his 'subversive' entry, which is independent of any significance.

It is the entry of that body into the world, its visible vulnerability, its absolute alterity, that moves me into taking on responsibility. Even more important, his fragility questions my being to the very last of the cells of my flesh, it obsesses me, it haunts me, it expels me from myself, it makes a hostage of me, 'it inflicts on me a wound of love' – only the exaggerated words of Levinas can explain that manifestation which is so acute and so serious, and which represents the 'expressive violence' brought about by the fragility of a child's body. His being alive demands my time, my care, my dedication, my concern . . . my desire. I have to make room for him in the world where I exist, I have to build a warm home, one which is safe, I have to protect him growing up, I have to provide him with everything that is necessary for him to develop his own story. His being in life calls on me to respond, his body is the commandment which obliges me to take on responsibility.

My son's injunction, which is made even more 'visible' by my son 'breaking into' my existence, corresponds to being affected by him, and my being affected by him constitutes the manifestation of that passivity which is specific to ipseity.

'In actual fact, at the phenomenological level,' says Ricoeur (1995: 432), 'the many modes in which the other affects the comprehension of the Self for itself indicate, to be precise, the difference between the ego which asserts itself and the Self which recognizes itself only through the ways in which it has been affected'. And in actual fact, ipseity is characterized by openness and by its revelatory function and is, therefore, very different from an I falling back on its own interiority and separate from the world and from others. It is by virtue of this constitutive trait of openness, which is structured according to the various modalities in which ipseity *finds* itself in the world and with others, that alterity is an integral part of ipseity. In the structure of ipseity itself, a structure which is continually decentred and open to the other, action and passion intertwine, as do feeling and being affected, accepting and being called upon, giving and receiving, listening and speaking or, as Ricoeur puts it, attesting and being injuncted. Thus, alterity, which from a phenomenological standpoint is matched by the experience of the passivity of oneself affected by the other, is constitutive of ipseity: it is part of ipseity, as we shall see, in different ways, each of which has different origins and plays its part to different degrees. Passivity and agency are inseparably intertwined at the heart of intersubjectivity.

2.4 Body-to-body

The dialectics of action and of being affected that permeates the adult's interaction with the child is present and obvious from the very start, and it occurs with different modalities and on different levels.

Right from birth it is the body-to-body relationship with the caregiver that constitutes the privileged site of communication and, more generally, of the synchronization of cycles of intimacy which correspond, from a physiological viewpoint, to phases of mutual activation and deactivation. It is in the body proper that openness to the other is based. It is in inter-corporeal space that the child encounters and tunes in to the other, thereby achieving mutual comprehension. On account of this 'tuning in', the adult offers himself, not only as a source of caregiving, but also as a partner of combined resonance, as the source of consent and shared meaning. For the child, the caregiver thus represents the opportunity for him to contemporaneously gain access both to oneself and to shared human meaning. Hence, right from birth, understanding the other also involves understanding oneself through the meaningful signs that irradiate from the child's body to meet the other man in a common world.

The gradual constitution of one's mind, like that of other minds, thus becomes possible only through the combined construction of 'sensed' events, through the sharing of 'regulated' expressive states, which happen (affections) or which are produced (actions) initially by the body-to-body interaction with the caregiver. It is initially in this context that the child externalizes the rudiments of sense by coordinating his actions and passions with those of his caregiver.

The structuring of intersubjective processes thus goes well beyond the behavioural and motivational aspects to which the classic studies on attachment refer. Intersubjectivity thus assumes an ontological importance that can hardly be reduced to instinctive behaviours triggered by parental care. 'The expressive behaviours in affectionate chat and play,' write Trevarthen and Aitken (2001: 6), 'have no immediate role in the regulation of the neonate's physiological state, comfort or survival. They are distinct from maternal breast-feeding, stroking, holding, rocking, vocal comforting and the like'. That is to say, communication cannot be explained exclusively by instinctual behaviour or biological needs. Rather, it takes shape by way of the very existence of the child. Coming into the world corresponds, first and foremost, to openness to the being of the other . . . to being with the other.[10]

This openness is based on the child's body proper and comes about thanks to the capacity of the two bodies – one adult, the other infant – to coordinate their reciprocal comprehension. In other words, the expression produced by one body must count as a sign for another body, so that the perceiver may take his bearings, just as raising one's hand in a classroom indicates to the others the actor's desire to come into the discussion. This process leads to the interactants becoming familiar with a shared 'proto-language', a process which in its turn corresponds to the sedimentation of a communicative code and, at the same time, to the development of an inclination for a certain mode of feeling. Evidence of this is the so-called 'fear of strangers'. At about the age of six months, when a child manifests fear in the presence of an unknown person, what he is actually expressing is the distress created by the fact that the coordination constructed with his caregiver, which normally enables him to feel situated, 'doesn't work' with the stranger. Like an alien, the stranger is unable to coordinate his own expressions in the sequences and in the contexts which the child recognizes as being shared and understood (Trevarthen, 2004).

The first synchronization of exchanges – which Locke (1993) argues could be considered as being a developmental precursor of vocal turn-taking – which begins to emerge during breastfeeding as a contingent alternation of the caregiver's jiggling and the infant's sucking, clearly highlights the fact that this capacity for social interaction is bred of bodily mediation. That communication as tuning – a process which presupposes that the adult possesses the sensibility to respond to the appeals made by the neonate – becomes even more evident from the first vocal turn-taking exchanges, which begin at about the seventh to eighth week of life (Papousek and Papousek, 1989). The quality of these proto-conversations depends on the contingency of the response provided by the caregiver, since from the very outset of language development it appears obvious that communication refers to the contingency of the position of thc hearer and that of the speaker, to the way they find they are related to each other.

For example, in a study of 48 infant males, Masataka (1993) shows that 'the child in the absence of response changes flexibly the intervals between two consecutive vocalizations according to his recent experience of turn-taking with the adult'; that is, in relation to a pattern exhibiting communicative harmony which was developed in the relationship with the caregiver. Reciprocal adjustment, the brunt of which is borne by the caregiver,[11] allows the child to reflect himself by means of a human source of reference (who reflects himself in the child) and to grasp himself through the continuous flow of experience. This joint participation is already present during gestation (Fernald, 2004; Fifer, Monk and Grose-Fifer, 2004).

Moreover, it also seems that the passage that occurs around the age of three months, from a production of 'vocalic sounds' with greater nasal resonance to one of 'syllabic sounds' with greater oral resonance, is facilitated by the caregiver's vocal stimulation contingent to the infant's vocal production. At this age, however, for speech sounds to make vocal production easier, they must be quite familiar to the child (Bloom, 1988; Masataka, 1993, 1995). At the root of the special role played by contingency in the early stages of infant vocal behaviour there may well lie a sub-personal mechanism (in addition to other mechanisms), which allows the child – during a calm and enjoyable interaction – to translate the caregiver's vocal and facial expressions of emotional feelings into the infant's own similar bodily gestures.

It would thus appear that proto-linguistic production and reception imply a matching system which enables the child to reflect himself not only in the vocal gesture but also in the facial expression and emotional state of his partner (Warren *et al.*, 2006). The MNS might carry out that function, thereby enabling the construction of an intersubjective code for the comprehension of expressions (Gallese, 2007). The link between perception and production guaranteed by the mirror neurons (see below) could account for both the infant's capacity to imitate sound patterns (Kuhl and Meltzoff, 1996) and his ability to link the mouth movements he sees to the auditory signals he hears (Kuhl and Meltzoff, 1982; Kuhl, 2000).

Seen in this light, even the fundamental phenomenon of imitation takes on a complex meaning. If imitation is considered as a function of interpersonal communication – that is, within a context of recurrent interaction, as constituting a web of shared actions and emotions with the caregivers – then imitational behaviour is inscribed within the sphere of meaningful reciprocal behaviour, which obviously changes over time. The imitational response thus becomes a mode of constructing or accessing a common code, a shared space of actions and emotions which constitute the foundation for the relationship (Gallese, 2005; Decety and Chaminade, 2005), but it concurrently acts as a mode of accessing oneself. And it is precisely the consensual status of imitational response that enables it, at its most advanced stages of development, to act as 'affirmation, acceptance and commentary' in the flow of interactions when the interlocutor provides a more emphatic ostentation of expressiveness. Imitation, in fact, implies the comprehension both of what another individual is doing and of the contexts in which such knowledge is put to use, namely those contexts in which such acts can be replicated (Rizzolatti, 2005). It is by virtue of shared meaning that the imitational act may be attributed a personal meaning, depending on the various environments in which the interlocutors may find themselves, the various contexts in which those acts may be put to use. Or else, the imitational response may be inhibited, as is demonstrated by a recent study by Meltzoff (2007) on the relationship between the child's anticipation of the adult's anger and possible imitative behaviour.

Imitation is thus not simply a means to acquire a certain behaviour pattern (a learning mechanism), but enables the child to regulate those processes of interpersonal involvement which express the different fields of individual motivation (Trevarthen, Kokkinaki and Fiamenghi, 1999).

Both expressive and vocal reciprocal imitation seem to play a very clear role in the use caregivers make of that singular way in which the child talks, often called 'motherese' or baby talk. This infant-directed speech, which has syntactic, semantic and prosodic features that are simpler than speech directed to adults, appears to be specifically designed to facilitate infant imitation (Ferguson, 1964; Kuhl *et al.*, 1997; Fernald, 1984); that is, motherese is based on the spontaneous vocalizations uttered by the infant which the adult matches and models, thereby generating an imitative form that serves as a contingency for infant vocal production (Masataka, 1993).

The typical higher pitch, the better articulation and the slower tempo of infant-directed speech, accompanied by exaggerated facial expressions and bodily movements, make the phonetic units of their native language easier for children to discriminate. On the other hand, exposure to a specific language – their native language – influences infants' phonetic perception, hence their sound production (Kuhl *et al.*, 1992). Recent studies of three-month-old infants deploying fMRI indicate that exposure to one's native language underpins the activation of left-lateralized brain regions comparable to those of adults, including the superior temporal and angular gyri and inferior frontal regions (Broca's area) (Dehaene-Lambertz, Dehaene and Hertz-Pannier, 2002).

The course of a 'felicitous proto-communication' is thus characterized by cooperative communication, which manifests itself in synchronic phrasing in which expressions of one interactant are reflected in those of the other interactant (synchronization), intertwined with phrasing in which the interaction is characterized by each partner alternately producing linguistic expression (alternation). A simple sequence could begin, for instance, with a vocalization expressing joy on the part of the child, to which the caregiver responds first with an expression of concentration, followed immediately afterwards by an amplification of the expression of joy, both at the visual and at the vocal level, with the child then overlapping with a further manifestation of joy accompanied by the clapping of his hands, reaching a sort of climax, to then return to a state of relaxation (Trevarthen, 1979).

2.5 The significativity of expressions and objects

The comprehension of an expression (such as a gesture) implies that the expression be interpreted as significant. But what is the significativity of the expression observed for the child? What does it consist of? And how is that meaning grasped?

We have already seen that one of the most important aspects of communication is that expressions are comprehended through a system of resonances (mirror neuron systems), which enables the child to reflect himself in the acts of the caregiver, thereby grasping himself. We have also underlined the fact that imitation – which implies the activation of the MNS (Rizzolatti, 2005) – has to be considered in the wider context of interpersonal communication, where the central role is played by the contingency of the position of the caregiver and of the infant, inasmuch as communication refers on each and every occasion to the combined situation of who is expressing himself and who is interpreting that expression.

Hence, the range of communicative responses seems to extend between two polarities: one in which one can perceive oneself by means of refraction through the other person's conduct, as in forms of imitation and in interactions expressing joy – which are often combined with non-basic emotions[12] (Trevarthen and Aitken, 2001) – the other in which the infant perceives himself through an activation which frees him completely from sharing, as, for instance, in the case of the triggering of a basic emotion.[13] For example, an episode of anger on the part of the caregiver may generate fear in the infant in as much as it activates a complex, coordinated set of bodily changes, without the activation of the child's fear being mediated by a mutual resonance system with the caregiver. Between these two polar extremes, a set of intermediate stages may be hypothesized which require coordination between the system of basic emotions, that of non-basic emotions and the perceptuo-motor resonance systems.[14]

From the fourth month on, the issue of the significativity of the expression undergoes an important transformation. The child, whose interaction up to that point was limited basically to a body-to-body relationship, begins to exert an initiative directed at the world of things, gradually acquiring control over the use of his arms and hands to reach and grasp objects. At the same time he follows the shifting gaze of the other person manipulating or seeking an object (Muir and Hains, 1999). In other words, the child perceives not only the adult's attention – of which he is emotionally aware – but also the objects at which the adult's attention is directed. This process of opening himself to the world represents a new stage in the development of the child, his progressive capacity to act in a consensual manner (which will reach its apotheosis at approximately nine months in the renowned 'joint attentional frame', to be discussed shortly). This change goes hand in hand with a new stage in the relationship with his caregivers. This transformation is particularly evident in the evolution of the types of game played: person–child games are supplanted by person–child–object games. However, since, at this age, the child is unable to combine acts which orient to the person through the use of objects, he cannot, for instance, connect the fact that a person is observing an object to the fact that that person intends to do something, for instance use the object. It is as if the child's interest in manipulating the object cannot be assimilated to the person.

On the one hand, the child begins to act with objects in an autonomous fashion: his coordination improves continuously and he learns to recognize the progress made in, and the consequences of, his course of action. On the other hand, the caregiver becomes his first teacher and playmate, creating, participating in or varying – in the more advanced phases (seven to eight months) – the consequences of the possible outcomes stemming from the sequences of actions that the child undertakes during the game. Stated differently, the dimension of increasing autonomy, by means of which the child extends his own course of actions and, consequently, the spatial dimension of his world, is regulated by the caregiver's capacity to coordinate his own actions and emotions in a way that is contingent with those of the child.

A six-month-old infant can share with his caregivers a concatenation of routine actions, which interweave with emotions and with communications lasting many seconds. His increasing ability to sequentialize becomes even more transparent in his ability to grasp the temporal development of lullabies, an ability manifested by children of five to six months in different cultures. The musical structure of lullabies is roughly comparable to a classic narrative structure, with a regular rhythmical beginning, an apex that is emphatic to a greater or lesser degree, and a coda. This cycle is repeated several times in the course of the lullaby, and the child seems fascinated by the 'process of prediction and recognition which is usually described as cognitive, but which in this case is certainly accompanied by an emotional evaluation which, in parallel fashion, varies in a predictable fashion' (Trevarthen, 1977: 243).

The importance of the prosodic aspects of language in early infancy are supported by a study (Homae *et al.*, 2006) using infrared spectroscopy in three-month-old infants, which shows that prosodic information is mainly processed by the right hemisphere. Another event-related brain potential (ERP) study (Pannekamp, Weber and Friederici, 2006) indicates that in eight-month-old infants prosodic cues are relevant for sentence structuring.

2.6 Referential communication

The ability to order events sequentially and to predict the goal of a concatenation of events brings about an important change in communication. From approximately the age of nine months, the child is able to combine his sensorimotor and attentional capacities with those of the caregiver, enabling him to enter into a new type of communication characterized by attention-sharing – which is emotionally situated – on an event or on an object. Communicative pointing (but also showing, offering, giving), which often appears at this age, and which is restricted almost exclusively to third-person reference, is an unequivocal demonstration of this (Bates, Camaioni and Volterra, 1975). Joint attention may in fact be such because, in the course of the communicative event, the child can anticipate the adult's possible intention with regard to the action the latter will undertake involving the object. For instance, in pointing to a particular toy (in a given emotional context), the child predicts the possibility that the adult will offer him the toy, or that he will begin a game involving that toy. This implies that the child can understand that a communicative gesture involving an object can orient the goal of the caregiver's action, and vice-versa.

Such comprehension is facilitated by the reproduction on the part of the child of the adult's novel intentional actions on outside objects – as may be inferred from role-reversal imitation (Tomasello, 2003). For example, in the context of a cooperative game involving a toy, after having observed the goal-directed concatenation of actions executed by the adult, combined with contemporaneous expressions of joy, equally harmonious imitation on the part of the child reverses the child–caregiver role relationship (Trevarthen and Hubley, 1978).

The joint attentional frame, which is emotionally situated, and which characterizes the onset of referential communication, creates a condition which multiplies the possibilities the child has of accessing the world to an unimaginable extent. Indeed, the manipulation of objects, just like combined focalization on shared domains of relevance in the course of interactions, enables the child to develop a common space of action, of emotions, of intentions in which he can *grasp* things, situations and behaviours in a new manner: as meaningful. As Gallese (2005) states, 'This space is *we-centric*'.

And in fact, 'from soon after their first birthdays, infants cannot help perceiving Daddy as "trying to clean the table" or "trying to open the drawer" – not simply as making specific bodily motions or producing salient changes of state in the environment – and these intentional actions are what they attempt to reproduce' (Tomasello, 2003: 27). What is more, these intentional actions begin to have a meaning which the child is capable of understanding because he is able to predict the forthcoming goals. If, for instance, an adult comes into the room with the pram, a joint attentional frame emerges that is focused on the (shared) anticipation of going for a walk. That is, the child comprehends the object on which the attention of both interactants is focused in the light of the prediction of a sequence of actions and in the sphere of the emotional context in which the object – as it has been understood – is embedded. Joint attention is possible because grasping adults' intentions corresponds to the infant's emotively situated anticipation of the consequences of actions. Against this common background the pram acquires shared meaning.

In fact, some of the earliest uses of object words refer to the entire organized sequence of actions and emotions in which the object is embedded. Thus the child uttering the single word 'pram' (accompanied by smiles and bodily movements) indicates that the child is producing an expression such as 'Good, it's time for a walk'.

Hence, for an object to become significant, the necessary condition is that the child acquire the ability to comprehend objects and situations starting from possible contexts of actions and emotions. Meaning is, so to speak, connected to a series of anaphoric references scaffolded and sedimented through the child's history of interactions with his caregivers, which constitute the contexts through which objects, situations and people become relevant for the child. This set of references, which the child does not comprehend explicitly and expressly, is the presupposition which enables words to be linked to meanings for the child. As is emphasized by Catherine Nelson (Nelson, 1996: 106), 'from about 12 months to about 36 months the language system is being developed within and in service to communicative contexts already established as social activities'. It is only on the basis of this relationship that the word (which at 12 months has the same value as pointing) can be understood, inasmuch as it indicates something – which does not yet appear in the word – on which speaker and hearer can agree.

Hence the close connection between joint attention and child language acquisition should come as no surprise (Bruner, 1983a, 1983b, 1978; Scaife and Bruner, 1975); nor should the amount of time infants spend in joint engagement with caregivers and the size of infants' vocabulary (Tomasello and Farrar, 1986; Smith, Adamson and Bakeman, 1988), nor the relationship between faster rates of infant vocabulary acquisition and more cooperative parenting (Akhtar, Dunham and Dunham, 1991; Baldwin, 1995).

The emergence of the child's 'first words', which at this age are typically produced in highly specific contexts or are event-bound (Barrett, 1986), is therefore founded on the comprehension of concatenations of actions and emotions occurring in shared everyday situations.[15] Recurring sequences are made up of organized, synchronic patterns which intertwine with the actions and emotions of the child and his caregivers. They are accompanied by signals that the adult repeats over and over again, marking the beginning, the development and the conclusion of the specific pattern. For instance, nappy changing, bathing, getting ready to go out, mammy or daddy coming back into the room, a visit from granny and so on; and even more complex games with objects involving sequences, cooperative activities accompanied by instructions, or statements, or emphatic expressions on the part of the mother, role reversal imitation and so forth.

When the child enters his second year of life, the type of object he wishes to play with gradually changes. Attention is progressively shifted on to the manipulation of things which are part of routine actions in daily family life (telephones, cups, spoons and so on). It is in the context of these situations pertaining to everyday existence that the first words acquire a referent. Words come into existence starting from what the child and adult can mutually agree upon. The comprehension of the child's first words, hence the development of early word meanings, is based on these shared practices which provide the child with the experiential, and also cultural, data that words refer to.

This origin, which hints at the fact that language is grounded in action and emotion, has been demonstrated by a series of studies of adult subjects (Pulvermuller, 2001, 2002).

Studies on the acquisition of personal pronouns (Bates, 1990) provide a complementary observation point on this developmental period. For example, from the onset of proto-linguistic communication up to the first stages of language, communicative pointing and early words are limited to third-person reference. That is to say that in the course of a communicative exchange, the child never points to himself or to the hearer (either with his index finger or by means of a personal pronoun), but to events or objects in the external world. He constitutes the subject, not the object, of his referring activity. This inability to grasp himself reflectively also manifests itself at the level of imitation.

It appears, that is, that before linguistic development has been completed, the child is capable of imitating action only if he refers the sequence to be repeated to himself, reproducing that sequence, becoming the active subject (for instance, feeding-himself, combing-himself). In other words, he repeats sequences of perceived events, and until the age of 18 months the referent of this imitation is himself (Trevarthen and Logotheti, 1989), while, instead, he is not able to grasp himself reflexively as agent. From 18 months on, children begin to combine words into rough sentences that allow them to symbolize highly repetitive scenes in their lives. The most frequent contents of these first utterances concern possession ('my teddy'), location ('car garage'), nonexistence ('no more soup'), recurrence ('tickle again') and actions ('me fall', 'car go') (Camaioni, 2001).

Together with the emergence of the child's first words and a spurt in his vocabulary, the period 18–24 months sees the child begin to recognize himself as the source of his own (shared) actions and emotions, as is shown by the classic studies on 'Me in the mirror recognition' (Berenthal and Fisher, 1978; Johnson, 1983; Lewis and Brooks-Gunn, 1979; Anderson, 1984; Damon and Hart, 1988; Butterworth, 1990).[16] At the level of language, this ability manifests itself in the onset of the use of an identifying referent, which is generally the personal pronoun 'I', or the child's own name, or the co-existence for a certain period of the name and the 'I'.

This new stage of development sets important questions.

First, is there a relationship between the construction of the sentence – which integrates into one single unit the identifying referent (the subject) and the predicating function (the predicate) – and the ability the child has just developed to recognize the reflection in the mirror as his own image? Second, what has generated this new ability to use the predicate (and therefore the verb) within a sentence, namely, of grasping time through the use of language?

2.7 Oneself in the mirror and in the refraction of language

After the child's second birthday, when the caregiver walks into his room and says, 'Ok, let's go to the park', the child understands that those words refer to a concatenation of actions, to an event that will take place shortly afterwards. That event, tinged by shared emotions, is located in a framework jointly built and sedimented over time. But while at 12–18 months the child employed his first words – which appeared to be a vocal gesture connected more or less rigidly to a given event – to recognize himself in a sequence of actions, predicting the sequence and concurrently recognizing its sense, once the child has entered language he 'interprets' the linguistic expression. The foundation of sense conveyed by the expression (which always disappears by dint of being hidden by the discourse) consists precisely in the shared aim toward a concatenation of actions and emotions connected to a background, and this convergence is produced through the joint act of who speaks and who listens.

In order for the child to comprehend the meaning conveyed by the linguistic expression, the words must first be perceived as being significant. That is to say, the child must grasp the expression as constituting a reference to a domain of shared actions and emotions, without it being directly, pragmatically, context-bound. Putting language to use gradually frees the word from the concrete context of use. This is the principal aspect dominating the pre-school years, which culminates in the development of narrative skills. We may state that by way of its use, language employs the voice and the hands (sign language) to reconfigure a sense that was already shared (*viz.* manifest) at a pre-reflective level in the sequence of actions and emotions that occur in the communicative exchange. In other words, it reconstructs the concatenation of events through sound.[17]

Linguistic communication is thus based from the outset – where undoubtedly such roots are more clearly discernible – on an antepredicative dimension which we do not understand explicitly, and which varies continuously for each one of us and on each and every occasion, depending on the circumstances, the richness of the content and its transparency. This is the context in which our actions and passions take shape. Against this background, what the discourse refers to stands out clearly and manifestly. The salience of this or that entity, of this or that situation, of this action or of that emotion which the linguistic expression refers to, depends, that is, on the pre-reflective context which does not appear in the discourse. It is precisely that context which furnishes the opportunity for the making of the assertion.

The other peculiar aspect consists in the fact that the comprehension of the sentence – whose content concerns a situation extant in the world which the speaker is referring to – comes about through the hearer giving it meaning which is, so to speak, private, in as much as it refers to the hearer's own experience of being in the world. That is, while the hearer is grasping what the sentence means, he relates the experience which the discourse is addressing to his own perspective. In so doing he appropriates himself, he includes and understands himself in one way or another according to the directions indicated by the discourse. The process engaged in by the listener is specular to that engaged in by the speaker: just as what the sentence means refers to what the individual subject who produces the utterance does and feels, that same meaning calls into play the listener's experience.

From this perspective, it is thus obvious that language can only be processed in the context of the discourse.[18] Following Benveniste (1966, 1974), by discourse we mean that every utterance presupposes a speaker and a hearer, and the intention in the former to influence the latter in some way. Indeed, the sentence only acquires reference as a function of the context in a given discourse – hence as a function of an agreement between speaker and hearer as to what is to be understood. Such reference pertains to the situation with which the discourse is actually dealing. It is in the context of the current discourse situation that the speaker refers to this or that entity through the use of language. This use combines the sense of the sentence (what the sentence means: reference to the world, predicating something) with a reference to the speaker (what the speaker means). In this way, predicate and logical subject are combined into one unified sentence.

In the discourse, the speaker takes up the position of enunciating subject. He can do so exclusively because he is able to say 'I'. This is possible only through the use of language. It is only in the current discourse situation that the speaker can appropriate the use of the personal pronoun 'I' and have it refer to himself: he is speaking to a 'you', the latter also being capable of saying 'I'.[19]

This is what Benveniste means when he says that in identifying himself as a unique person, the speaker who says 'I' takes upon himself the entire language. 'When an individual appropriates the language to himself, language is transformed into discourse situations, characterized by a system of internal references the key to which is "I", and which define the individual through the special linguistic construction of which he avails himself when he enunciates himself as speaker' (Benveniste, 1966: 305). In language use, then, 'I' alludes each and every time to the person whose experience is being referred to by the sense of the statement uttered.[20]

But what is the origin of the possibility of saying 'I'?

The assertion 'Let's go to the park', with which the caregiver interpellates the child, creating, through the use of language, a reference to the generic experience of that event, may be met by the child with a response conveying disapproval, such as 'I don't want to go to the park'. The I in 'I don't want . . .' indicates a position in relation to a you which is based on the being mine of experience. It is because ipseity experiences itself on each and every occasion as the source of a possible range of actions and emotions that going to the park as a possible mode of conduct of the experiential Self acquires significance. Saying 'I don't want to . . .' is founded on a practical dimension corresponding to the way ipseity understands itself when it is interpellated in the course of the discourse with regard to that possible situation. Seen in this light, meanings are possible ways of being.

But if saying 'I' is structured on the basis of the being mine of experience,[21] and if being mine is declined by way of each and every event, in order for it to be possible to say 'I', a sense of the permanence of the presence of the experiential Self over time must already be organized in the antepredicative dimension. Obviously, this sameness of Self is realized at each and every event. This means that in the antepredicative dimension, the oneself which perceives itself and acts on each and every occasion must find itself each and every time possessing a sense of being the same.[22] This is the perspective implied by those studies in developmental psychology which stress the fact that a basic sense of Self is established in the newborn – well before the onset of mirror self-recognition – through the sensory-motor system, which enables the infant to locate his body with respect to the environment (Butterworth, 1990; Meltzoff, 1990).

The onset of this nonsubstantial permanence of Self,[23] whose specific feature is that of discontinuity, occurs at the age of 18–24 months, both in the domain of the senses and in that of language. When the child looks at himself in the mirror, he recognizes his mirror reflection as identical to himself. In other words, he can understand that, in each and every one of the different situations he encounters in his daily life, he is both different and concurrently the same.[24]

This capacity is also exhibited at the level of language with equally great force. It is what the use of language bears witness to. My experience, which is recounted in the first person, concerns my perceiving myself in this or that situation, and it corresponds contemporaneously to how sameness manifests itself on each and every occasion. Ipseity, which experiences this or that state of affairs while its continuity remains unaltered, is reflected and reconfigured in language through the 'I' which recognizes and talks about a particular episode, a given event. It is thus not attributable to chance that mirror self-recognition is related to the acquisition of personal pronoun use and pretend play, such that, during the second year, children showing mirror self-recognition used more personal pronouns and demonstrated more advanced pretend play than did children not showing self-recognition (Lewis and Ramsay, 2004; Courage, Edison and Howe, 2004).

Why does this ability emerge only at age 18–24 months? What is the relationship between the capacity to say 'I' and the ability to recognize the reflection in the mirror as one's own self-image?

2.8 Recognition of self in the mirror and in language

There is a story (Gallup, 1994; Povinelli, 2000), which it is said goes the rounds among those that work with the three species of anthropoid apes –the gorilla, the chimpanzee and the orangutan – that you can test the intelligence of these primates by leaving a screwdriver in the cage of each animal.

The gorilla looks at it, smells it and then ignores it. The chimpanzee jumps on it, puts it in its mouth and plays with it. The orangutan looks at it, pretends there is nothing there, takes it, hides it and that very night takes the cage apart.

What does this anecdote tell us? Obviously, the three species have different ways of using tools. We also know that while the chimpanzee and the orangutan exhibit a clear ability of self-recognition in the mirror, the gorilla is incapable of such an act. What is the relationship between self-recognition and the ability to use tools?

Povinelli (2000; Povinelli and Cant, 1995; Povinelli and Prince, 1998; see also Barth, Povinelli and Cant, 2004) explains this difference both from the standpoint of the real life of these primates and from the phylogenetic perspective. While the orangutan, which is probably the nearest to our common ancestors, has a lifestyle that is totally arboreal, the chimpanzee lives both on the ground and in trees, and the gorilla has an 'earthly' lifestyle. Unlike other primates, which have stereotyped movements, the orangutan and the chimpanzee manifest a wide range of movements in the trees. In particular, given the relationship between bodily weight (40–80 kg) and the fragility of the branches along which it moves, the orangutan employs a type of movement called 'clambering', which combines the vertical position of the trunk with the use of various supports that it can grab hold of, depending on the type of movement to be executed. Since the orangutan lives several metres above ground level, it cannot afford to fall. Consequently, this characteristic type of movement obliges it to be constantly aware of its actions and its posture. In Povinelli and Prince's (1998) view, this capacity developed in the course of the Miocene age from an ancestor common to humans and to higher primates in order to maintain adaptation to an arboreal lifestyle in relation to a significant increase in bodily weight. The on-line sense of the position and of the movement of one's body is claimed to explain why self-recognition in the mirror is limited to the orangutan and the chimpanzee,[25] since these species still lead a life which requires a system of 'kinaesthetic awareness'. Thus, while these primates look at themselves in the mirror, they establish a relationship of equivalence between the behaviours which they observe of themselves in the mirror and the on-line experience they have of their own daily experiences.

The loss of, or failure to acquire, that capacity in gorillas, due to a difference in their evolutionary history based on ground locomotion, is claimed to explain, similarly, why this species cannot recognize itself in the mirror. According to this interpretation, it should be clear why the more 'arboreal' species exhibit greater ability in manipulating tools. This type of existence is claimed to favour the development of more precise control over behaviour, hence of a more sophisticated body schema.

The hypothesis therefore follows that, in order to maintain their adaptation to a highly variable arboreal environment, which requires frequent evaluation of new information (Povinelli and Cant, 1995), the orangutan, and to a lesser degree the chimpanzee,[26] has developed a more sophisticated visuo-tactile-motor system to manage its actions more effectively and more efficiently. Such a system would therefore ensure a more successful integration of body and peripersonal space in an ongoing global sense of Self. This would seem to indicate that a more sophisticated mode of executing actions corresponds to greater and improved mastery over one's body and a more integrated and clearly-defined body schema. Continuing to follow this hypothesis – albeit in a different direction from that taken by Povinelli – it would appear to be possible that, in anthropoid apes, the MNS is part of the mechanism underlying the workings of a sort of 'matching system' between the potential range of actions and the action actually carried out, the goal of the system being to favour greater motor control in an environment characterized by great flexibility.[27] This could then account for the capacity that these primates exhibit to form a relationship of 'motor equivalence' between the behaviours reflected in the mirror and the actions they carry out, so much so that, after a certain period of exposure to the use of the mirror, they actually begin to recognize their own reflected image. Moreover, the refining of the ability to execute actions could have indirectly aided the ability to recognize congruence between the acts these apes see others perform and their own behaviour, thereby improving the capacity to predict the consequences of the action of their conspecifics.

This hypothesis, which accounts for the necessary connection between the ability of mirror self-recognition and the development of a unitary visual-proprioceptive sense of one's body, might also explain the difference between higher primates and Homo sapiens. Indeed, exactly the same mechanism employed by anthropoid apes to match kinaesthetic and visual information could have been exploited anew (through the mechanism of exaptation) in the course of human evolution as the neural substratum to recognize oneself as an 'I', in the first person, both visually and through language (*viz.* acoustically).

Unlike the great apes, however, in humans it is obviously the face that plays the most significant role in the recognition of Self and in the comprehension of the actions and intentions of others.

In addition to being at the centre of the world of human emotions, it is also, so to speak, the site of language. As is suggested by many studies on the relationship between audiovisual speech perception and the motor activation of areas involved in planning and executing speech production, the dynamics of facial movement and speech perception-production are clearly integrated (Skipper, Nusbaum and Small, 2005; Hall, Fussell and Summerfield, 2005; Pulvermüller *et al.*, 2006).

From an evolutionary standpoint, the social centrality of the face runs parallel to the emergence of more complex intersubjective dimensions (e.g. closer caregivers–infant relationships, bonds with lovers, friends, long-term mates, family members), implying a more sophisticated ability to tune into the face of individual others (Fridlund, 1994; Parkinson, Fischer and Manstead, 2005; Pulvermüller *et al.*, 2006). Areas within the inferior occipital-temporal region have in fact been identified that are selectively involved in the perception of unknown faces (Kanwisher, McDermott and Chun, 1997; McCarthy *et al.*, 1997), while other areas identified are specifically activated by personally familiar faces, and still others are associated with self-face recognition (Platek *et al.*, 2006).

If in humans the face plays the most important part in recognizing the Self, this difference from anthropoid apes would lead us to infer, from an evolutionary standpoint, that self-face recognition involves the same observation/execution action-matching mechanism recruited in primates for recognizing their own actions and those of others. Three recent fMRI studies on self-face recognition have shown that recognizing the image of one's own face is accompanied by activation of the motor system (Platek *et al.*, 2006; Sugiura *et al.*, 2005; Uddin *et al.*, 2005; Uddin *et al.*, 2007). In other words, in humans those very same mechanisms underlying 'kinaesthetic awareness' in primates can support face-representation functions; they can map the image of one's own face on to one's own motor system. These studies indicate that the right frontoparietal areas[28] – which are typically activated when participants are presented with the image of their own face – overlap with areas that belong to the MNS, that is, they belong to a system employed to map perceived action on to one's own motor system. From this perspective, we can readily comprehend why toddlers who pass the mark-test of mirror self-recognition have an equivalence in performance on the task of recognizing their own leg (Nielsen, Suddendorf and Slaughter, 2006). Moreover, confirmation of this type of overlap may be had from studies on the development of body self-awareness in toddlers (Brownell, Zerwas and Geetha, 2007; Moore *et al.* 2007).

What is the relationship between the ability to identify one's own image in the mirror and the capacity to say 'I'?

Obviously, the fact that the child begins to deploy language through the use of phrases during more or less the same period in which he acquires the capacity to recognize himself in the mirror (through recognizing his own facial expressions) is not accidental. Up to that point, he could only reflect himself in the behaviour of others, despite the fact that he had developed a sense of the permanence of Self. Put differently, despite the fact that he was able to perceive uninterruptedly the sense of the being mine of experience, he recognized its meaning only through reflection in shared behaviour.

The possibility of reflecting himself in his own actions and emotions, of grasping himself as identical to himself (who feels and acts), generates a new feeling of intimacy with himself and of demarcation from others. The child begins to develop a sense of the privacy of experience – which does not need to be interior – a clear indicator of this development being the monologues with himself.[29] This is accompanied by a sense of the 'property' (*Eigenschaft*) of his modes of being, which is discernible in his change of attitude toward himself and toward others. This reflection without interiority hides a new tension: the reconfiguration of Self enabled by the onset of language use defines not an egoic Self or the closure into the Self, but determines the way in which ipseity becomes its own.

Before we can proceed in our discussion in the direction indicated by the question of 'who?', we must first make a small digression to deal with a topic which psychology has linked closely to the subject of the recognition of the Self in the last few years, namely, self-conscious emotions. A series of observations appear to suggest that these emotions already emerge before the development of reflective consciousness.

2.9 Affective engagements

There is a great deal of literature, above all of a representational nature (Lewis, 1987, 1992a, 1992b, 1993a, 1993b, 1995), which underscores the point that during the child's second year of life there emerge new emotions – the self-conscious emotions – whose genesis is ascribed to a changed level of awareness of Self and of others. The nature of such emotions is hypothesized as being characterized by the fact that they develop in the context of a new relational state: that in which the child is self-conscious. These emotions (pride, embarrassment, shame, guilt, envy) would appear to take shape through the conscious evaluation the child makes of his behaviour in relation to the reference parameters.

Other studies which do not concur with this approach emphasize the fact that interpersonal emotions (pride, embarrassment, shame, guilt, envy, coyness, shyness, teasing, humour, emphatic concern and so forth) were already present in the first few months of life. As Vasudevi Reddy (2003) forcefully points out, if the infant is the focus of the caregiver's attention then the relation between the observing parent and the observed child can be experienced directly by the infant; it does not need to be inferred, as the representational hypothesis argues. Awareness of the attention of the other on the oneself corresponds to a mode of self-perception, an affective consciousness of Self. The link between how the caregiver's attending is perceived and how one's own ipseity is experienced – which is different and specific to each and every one of the self-conscious emotions – is directly felt right from the earliest months of the child's life. How the infant perceives the other's gaze depends not on 'beliefs about others' evaluations', but on how he feels at that moment.

For example, as is reported in the study quoted earlier by Meltzoff (2007), after having observed the irritated reaction of an adult on seeing a third party manipulate new objects, the child imitates his behaviour only if the adult's back is turned. Thus, the infant has a keen awareness of the standard and of the rules that govern a given situation without his having to possess an internal representation of himself, of the other, and of the Self as perceived by the observer (Trevarthen, 1992; Draghi-Lorenz, Reddy and Costall, 2001; Reddy, 2005). It is no intellectual feat to predict that were the adult to suddenly turn round and so catch the child 'with his hand in the cookie jar', the child would be embarrassed. In other words, perceiving adult attention on the child refers the child back to the awareness of the (emotional) significance that the caregiver attributes to the child's behaviour and, at the same time, to the inadequacy of that behaviour in the adult's presence.

The child's embarrassment reflects the incompatibility between the adult's expectations, which the infant has anticipated, and the real ongoing situation. It is this incongruence (which corresponds to being found out) which creates a greater focus on oneself, precisely because the child's conduct becomes the focus of attention of both interactants – caregiver and child.[30] Since embarrassment conveys discomfiture with regard to the current situation, it opens up the possibility of repair (Semin and Manstead, 1982). This type of embarrassment is closer to shame.

In any case, even when embarrassment is viewed as a form of shyness, hence not as a result of having committed a *faux pas*, as, for instance, when children are asked to perform, the focus on oneself is retained by the awareness of being at the centre of the unwanted attention of others.

The interpersonal – rather than the representational – origin of these emotions seems to apply to other social emotions such as jealousy, envy, pride, guilt. Hart (Hart and Carrington, 2002; Hart *et al.*, 1998), for example, showed in two studies how six- and twelve-month-old infants manifested distress – interpreted as jealousy – when their caregivers paid attention to a lifelike baby doll. Draghi-Lorenz, Reddy and Costall (2001) report the observations of parents who described a form of distress – interpreted as envy – when their children wanted something (e.g. a toy) possessed by another infant. Pride may be considered to be an emotion which emerges in concomitance with the positive attention (praise) received following a particular achievement (involving a feeling of mastery), rather than being dependent on beliefs about oneself as worthy (Draghi-Lorenz, Reddy and Costall, 2001). Finally, guilt could emerge as a direct perception of the damage caused by an action produced by the child and detrimental to another child who manifests grief at the wrong done to him, rather than as a result of the appreciation of self-blame in a reflexive space. Indirect confirmation of this hypothesis comes from a recent study, which shows that six- and ten-month-old infants take into account an individual's actions toward others in evaluating that individual as appealing or aversive (Hamlin, Wynn and Bloom, 2007).

Not only is each of these social emotions generated in response to a determinate ongoing situation, but in its turn it opens up new possibilities of actions and relationships. Jealousy is a spur to the reestablishment of a privileged situation, envy redirects the caregiver's attention to a desired object, pride creates an effect on the audience, guilt paves the way to repair (Parkinson, Fischer and Manstead, 2005). The occurrence of these emotions does not involve conceptual thought – rather it lays the foundations for this possibility.

It is obvious from this perspective that, rather than being at the root of self-conscious emotions, as is claimed by the representational standpoint, reflexive consciousness, or more accurately, the way in which reflexive consciousness takes shape, is strongly influenced by how affective interpersonal space has been constituted in the preceding months. The fact, that is, that the child is the centre of attention of others, and that this convergence of social attention creates in him social emotions which position him in interpersonal space, may be hypothesized as constituting the necessary condition for the development of reflexive capacities, rather than being the result of such capacities. As Heidegger (1988) stated (in reply to Natorp, who emphasized the distorting nature of reflexive consciousness), reflecting is only one way of grasping oneself, one way that enables comprehension to intensify, rather than constituting the foundational base of self-comprehension.[31]

2.10 Acting and speaking

What, therefore, is the relationship between the ability to identify one's own image in a mirror and the capacity to say 'I'?

From the beginning of his third year a child is able to recognize that he is identical to himself, namely, that he is one and the same Self in each and every situation, both in his actions and in his language. Thus, while he looks at his face reflected in the mirror, he identifies it as his own. In the same way, he identifies himself linguistically as the subject of a statement, that is, he acquires the capacity to grasp each and every time what the sentence means (shared sense), referring it to his own experiential perspective. Thus, he establishes a relationship of equivalence between experience referred to by the sense of the sentence and his own experience. In this way, he appropriates the sense (which the sentence refers back to) while concurrently recognizing and articulating his experience, which is reflected in the conceptual content of the sentence, and which that content interpellates.

Whereas mutual comprehension was achieved, in the previous stages, through (emotionally situated) action, it now begins to be mediated by language. As is shown by Emily's monologues studied by Nelson (1996), the contents of these first rudimentary ventures into storytelling are real-life experiences, actions and passions, all of which recount daily existence. The (shared) sense of actions and passions is reinscribed in the sentence (Engel, 1986; Dunn, 1988). The structure of action and the structure of language gradually come to be superimposed on one another, inasmuch as both are characterized by a shared sense and contemporaneously by the reference to oneself.

From a neuroscientific standpoint, the hypothesis gains further confirmation from an examination of the organization of Broca's area, formerly considered exclusively a speech production area, but where, it has now been discovered, we also find neurons that are activated both by orofacial acts and by hand gestures. It is interesting to note that, in addition to playing a crucial role in language production, Broca's area also plays an important part in imitation and in action recognition (Binkofski *et al.*, 1999; Iacoboni *et al.*, 1999; Molnar-Szakacs *et al.*, 2002; Iacoboni *et al.*, 2005). This region is known, in fact, to be part of the MNS (Bookheimer, 2002; Rizzolatti and Craighero, 2004; Nishitani *et al.*, 2005; Gallese, 2005). Several works by Gentilucci and his colleagues (Gentilucci, 2003; Gentilucci *et al.*, 2001, 2004a, 2004b, 2006; Bernardis and Gentilucci, 2006) have found a close relationship between speech production and the observation/execution of arm and hand gestures, thereby corroborating the relationship between manual and oral language-related gestures.

Thus, on the one hand, the meaning of a gesture is fixed in sedimented sense structures: intentional content[32] – it is common sense that renders actions familiar and actions shared, such as routines or games. On the other hand, meaning refers to the real experience of a 'who' at a given moment and in a specific situation[33] – this is the meaning that the action has for the person carrying out that very action.

In the same way, the meaning of the sentence (that is, its propositional content), on the one hand, is held constant by what the sentence refers to, and, on the other hand, meaning brings to language the speaker's experience. It is precisely because the speaker and the listener can share sense content that one can convey one's experience to another. It is the sense content that, realized on each occasion by each individual speaker through concrete reference to his own experiential domain, enables us to include and grasp the experience being communicated. 'Communication can succeed,' write Liberman and Whalen (2000), 'only if the two parties have a common understanding about what counts – what counts for the speaker must count for the listener'.

How is this equality concerning 'what counts in communication' established?

It is only possible because there exists, in humans, an echo-neuron system, that is, a system that matches verbal perception with speech production (Rizzolatti and Craighero, 2004).

On the one hand, this system can mediate the imitation of verbal sounds, as in the case of the child repeating words which do not refer back to any of his experiences and which are therefore meaningless. For instance, Levy and Nelson (1994) investigated children's acquisition of causal and temporal words ('because', 'yesterday', 'soon' and so on) and found that children's production of those linguistic items was bound to specific discourse contexts and realized exactly the same discourse functions that their parents used them for, without possessing fully adult-like understanding and flexibility of use. (Any adult learning a second language finds himself in a similar situation, that is, of learning a series of words without understanding what they mean).

On the other hand, this echo-neuron system may also perform a semantic function inasmuch as it enables the hearer to refer the words employed by the speaker to his own experiential domain.

What role does the echo-neuron system play in the process of the meaning of an action being conveyed by the sound of a sentence?

For meanings to end up in words, the articulation of sounds must be bonded with the sense of an action. In other words, there must exist shared neural mechanisms capable of linking up action observation and understanding[34] to language production–perception, hence, a neural substratum that is capable of relating acoustic perception to linguistic production and to a shared sense of action. A number of recent studies indicate that the MNS plays a key role in the articulation of the complex relationship between action, language and communication.

In the course of development – from the child's very first words, but even more clearly with the onset of language – the child gradually learns that during communication the sounds, the words which accompany experience refer to that specific current experience itself, to the point that the child also learns to predict what will happen next. This gradual transformation in the way the child communicates is fostered by the caregivers, who generally grasp, underline and repeat those words most relevant for each individual communicative context. This enables the child to integrate the words that are used and repeated during the execution of shared activities into his pre-reflexive comprehension of experience. 'The early establishment of shared meanings,' writes Nelson (1993: 116), 'thus involves an interaction of the child's preverbal interpretation of events and objects, and the adult's use of those words, and acceptance of the child's uses within jointly constructed and mutually understood activities'. These observations suggest that speech perception probably shares a common neural substrate not only with the regions assigned to (a) speech production – because of the parity between sender and receiver of the message invoked by Liberman – but also with the areas engaged by (b) perception – the execution of action.

With regard to the first point (language production–perception), various studies highlight the role of motor areas capable of *resonating*, of activating themselves, by listening to speech. Two transcranial magnetic stimulation (TMS) studies have reported facilitation of tongue and lip muscles when subjects listened to speech (Fadiga *et al.*, 2002; Watkins *et al.*, 2003). A third study (Meister *et al.*, 2007) showed that the disruption of human premotor cortex impairs speech perception. Other fMRI studies reported (a) the activation of motor areas involved in speech production in passively listening to meaningless monosyllables (Wilson *et al.*, 2004), (b) the recruitment during speech perception of specific motor circuits that reflect distinctive phonetic features of the speech sounds encountered (Pulvermüller *et al.*, 2006), (c) an increase in motor system activation on hearing unfamiliar non-native phenomena, compared to that during the perception of native phenomena (Wilson and Iacoboni, 2006).

The second point, which concerns the relationship between action and language, has been developed in a series of studies on the comprehension of action-related sentences aimed at uncovering, above all, the relationship between action-related sentences and the activation of motor areas related to the actions that one can perform oneself (and to which the senses of those sentences refer) (Buccino *et al.*, 2001, 2005; Hauk, Johnsrude and Pulverm¸ller, 2004; Tettamanti *et al.*, 2005; Gazzola, Aziz-Zadeh and Keysers, 2006). The most recent study in this field, which was carried out by Aziz-Zadeh *et al.* (2006) and which replicates and expands on some of the previous studies, shows that reading phrases describing actions carried out with different effectors (hand, mouth, leg) led to activation of specific motor and premotor areas that are active when an individual observes the same visually-presented actions.

This equivalence in human premotor cortex between areas that respond to both the execution and the observation of actions and areas activated by exposure to their verbal description, indicates that sense is grounded in action and passion, that language is rooted in one's experience of being-in-the-world. It might be said that discourse reconfigures what happens in the domain of acting and feeling in the domain of language, and it is precisely on the basis of this possibility of referring to the world in one way or another that discourse is regulated by each and every individual.[35] It composes what is pre-reflexively manifest but, at the same time, it can do so because it stems from, so to speak, communication with others, and via this channel, from the cultural community to which the communicants belong.

As we have seen, alterity intertwines with ipseity a first time at the prereflexive level; it becomes part of the domain of the meaning of subjectivity a second time simply through the use of language. It is in the reception of a discourse that is already under way, a language that has already been instituted, and in having been initiated into a cultural and historical world that is already there, that the shared sense structures are supplied, enabling one to grasp and recognize one's own experience.

Appropriating shared sense thus corresponds for everyone to the possibility of understanding oneself in this or that manner in the various ongoing situations and thus to *communicate* one's own experience of existing. 'Just as our common belonging to the same world presupposes that my experience, as my own and original experience, is the experience of being,' wrote Merleau Ponty (1969: 194), 'similarly, our belonging to a common language, or even to the common universe of language, presupposes a primordial relationship of me to my word, which bestows on it the value of a dimension of being, in which X may participate'.

But it is precisely language that guarantees the possibility of reconfiguring the experience of living in a unitary connectedness exhibiting the features of narration. And this throws new light on the relationship between agent and action. The action, for instance, of Mary taking hold of the cup, considered from the standpoint of the narration of Self, is influenced by new determinations. The agent–action relationship is no longer treated as if the agent were reabsorbed by the goal of the action, as if he were a function of that particular action. Instead, despite the fact that individual action has common-sense meaning for everyone, such action, which is reconfigured in language, takes on a meaning that is personal by dint of the fact that it is found within a configuring framework, the narration of oneself. Individual action is placed within a referential context by the story that it helps to articulate and develop, both in the case where the event falls within the range of expectations that derive 'naturally' from a narrative, and in the case where it takes 'by surprise' the predictions made regarding the development of the story, thereby generating new expectations. From this standpoint, assimilating experience, hence historicizing it, does not mean instituting a chronological order, simply putting events into a sequence. What must be considered is the importance of a given experience in relation to the economy of the narrative, which confers upon the experience a value that changes with the changing of the story itself. That is to say, the meaning of acting and of feeling goes well beyond its empirical dimension.

Every human being integrates the events he experiences to combine the present with sedimented experience, and with the horizons of his expectations, all at the same time. The special relationship between these different components is realized in the continual reshaping of the narrative of oneself (in its various forms, including those of the fragmentation of the story). The narrative recomposition of the experience of living reconfigures the variety of one's own experience into a signifying totality, while concurrently delineating the person to whom those actions and emotions refer. After Ricoeur, we turn to narrative identity to indicate this dynamic modality of composing personal identity.

Endnotes

[1] Merleau-Ponty (1962: 493).

[2] The empirical tools for this new issue came from the development of the first false belief task, which was to remain paradigmatic, by Wimmer and Perner (1983).

[3] Theory of mind mechanisms.

[4] Theory theory.

[5] In a recent study, Fogassi *et al.* (2005) show that in the inferior parietal lobe of the ape, motor neurons which codify specific acts manifest a different mode of activation when those acts are part of different actions (contexts).

[6] Structuring action in linguistic terms is reflected in the syntactic structure of the clause, as realized by the predicate (the propositional content) and the subject (the identifying referent).

[7] With regard to this topic, a brief analysis of the original meaning of *similis*, *-e* is of interest. According to Semerano (1994), right from the archaic form *semol*, *semul*, which then produced the adverbial form *simul*, this lexical item indicated the concatenation of two simultaneous actions which took place at the same time. Semerano also holds that *similis* expresses only similarity and is originally a calque from *omalos*, united, and on *simul*, whose original meaning is 'united with', 'together with'. The term 'simulation' could thus indicate an action which co-occurs, at the same time as another action, and which is similar to that action.

[8] We grasp the other in his worrying, in his hurrying, in his being disgusted, in his going to work – but what escapes us? What residue is left out of our comprehending the other? What do we fail to consider? The face, says Levinas (1961), to indicate that absolute manifestation of the other, irreducible and unknowable; the face, a trace of infinity.

[9] It is the fact of being born that founds the possibility of initiative, the capacity of giving life to a new action. According to Hannah Arendt (Arendt, 1998: 182), 'the unprecedented originality . . . [of Jesus of Nazareth's comprehension of the capacity to act] can be compared to the Socratic comprehension of the possibilities of thought'.

[10] The ontological role of proto-linguistic communication is also underscored by Bateson, who had the first intuitions which gave rise to the study of this domain. She writes (Bateson, 1979: 74), 'Proto-conversations tend to take place after feeding, caretaking, bathing, dressing – at a moment when the bustle is over and physical needs are met and sleep is not urgent. These are the moments that in many households in our culture are kept almost ritualized for the most intimate converse of parent and child.'

[11] With regard to this point, we could take up Winnicot's (1965: 145) definition of a 'good enough' mother as someone who meets 'the omnipotence of the infant and to some extent makes sense of it'.

[12] Non-basic emotions may be defined as those emotional responses which are not attributable to the activation of affect programmes understood as complex, coordinated and automated sets of bodily changes.

[13] Emotion is the subject of Chapter 4.

[14] This domain is, as yet, virgin territory, no research having been done in the area.

[15] With regard to the close connection of the emergence of words to the context, it is significant that 'disappearance' words (e.g. 'gone') emerge in relation to the capacity that the child develops of looking for a previously visible object which has been placed out of sight (Gopnik, 1984).

[16] Some infants start to show evidence of mirror self-recognition from just 1.5 years old, and by the age of 2, about half of all infants demonstrate that they have acquired the skill.

[17] Language becomes symbolic. *Symbolon* means keeping something together using something else. In a symbol, man keeps himself united with something else (the world in which he lives) and at the same time he comes to an agreement with other men with regard to how that symbol should be interpreted. This allows Heidegger (2001a: 309) to state: 'Words emerge from that *essential agreement* of the human beings with one another, in accordance with which they *are open in their being with one another for the beings around them*, which they can then individually agree about – and this also means fail to agree about. Only on the grounds of this originary, essential agreement is discourse possible in its essential function: [*semainein*], giving that which is understandable to be understood'.

[18] The linguistics of the sentence give precedence to semantics inasmuch as they are immediately concerned with the concept of sense. Thus, Ricoeur (1976: 21) writes, 'the most concrete definition of semantics is the theory that relates the inner or immanent constitution of the sense to the outer or transcendent intention of the reference'. From this perspective, grammar can only derive from discourse.

Deriving grammar and semantics from discourse is underscored in the domain of developmental psychology by studies carried out by Nelson (1986; 1996: 144) 'Discourse is the source of knowledge of language forms and is the context within which meaning and use of language forms is developed and elaborated'.

The results of a recent MRI study (Brauer and Friederici, 2007) on 5–6-year-old children investigating the semantic and syntactic aspects of sentence processing found a large activation overlap for these two language aspects in the superior temporal gyrus (STG) in contrast to adults who exhibit function-specific activation. Such results support the hypothesis that there exists a common neural substratum which underpins the development of semantics and syntax.

[19] This 'I–you' opposition, which lies at the heart of the linguistic theory of person, emerges at about 18–20 months of age, during which time the infant begins to mark a person contrast in some explicit way. Bates (1990) calls this new phase 'contrastive reference'. The linguistic category of 'person' belongs exclusively to the position 'I' and 'you'. 'I' designates the speaker, who is also the person the utterance refers to, while 'you' refers to the hearer, the person whom the 'I' is addressing by means of his current utterance. The third-person 'he', 'she', 'it' is not a specific person or entity – it is impersonal, such that a *thing* is predicated in the third person. 'In actual fact, one of the features of the persons "I" and "you" is their specific uniqueness: both the enunciating "I" and the "you" addressed by the "I" are each and every time unique. But "he-it" may be an infinity of subjects – or no-one?' (Benveniste, 1966: 275).

[20] As Ricoeur (1976: 20) says, 'the sense is traversed by the referring intention of the speaker'.

[21] 'Because Dasein has *in each case mineness [Jemeinigkeit]*, one must always use a *personal* pronoun when one addresses it: "I am", "you are"' (Heidegger, 1962: Section 9, page 68).

[22] From this standpoint, time becomes the principle on which identification is based, inasmuch as that which is my own is assigned to me on each and every occasion.

[23] That is, not connected to a consideration of the mind as immaterial substance.

[24] The perspective being argued here is clearly different from Gallup's (1982) viewpoint, summarized by Platek, Myers and Gallup when they write 'to recognize your own face in the mirror, you have to first have a concept of self (i.e. you have to know who you are to be able to recognize who is being reflected in the mirror). Therefore, the ability to recognize oneself in the mirror appears to represent a cognitive capacity related to a sense of self-awareness' (Platek, Myers and Gallup, 2004: 116). In actual fact, the identification of a mirror reflection as one's own is not a cognitive task dependent on pre-existing self-knowledge. The emphasis we place on the expression 'each and every time' underscores the fact that a relationship of equivalence is set up between the behaviour observed in the mirror and one's own experience every time the event occurs, without requiring conceptualization or representation.

[25] There is strong evidence that the bonobo (or pygmy chimpanzee) is also capable of mirror self-recognition (Hyatt and Hopkins, 1994).

[26] Since it leads a ground–tree existence.

[27] That is, control over actions extended to the domain of potentiality, induced by the specific quality and the spatial location of the targets of such actions (Gallese, personal communication).

[28] Hemispheric lateralization in prefrontal cortex during self-face recognition is still a source of debate (Keenan *et al.*, 2000, 2001, 2003; Turk *et al.*, 2002, 2003).

[29] In his 'inner' speech the child creates a dimension of closure between oneself and himself through changing the roles of both speaker and hearer. For an investigation of crib speech, see Halliday (1975) and Nelson (2006).

[30] This cannot happen in younger infants, because they are incapable of recognizing themselves in their own action and emotions, while they can, however, reflect themselves in those of others. This is why embarrassing situations are characterized by a greater focus on the other (Reddy, 2003).

[31] New studies on the relationship between attention and emotional display in the course of mutual engagement might furnish interesting data on this topic.

[32] If we describe the intentional content of action in terms of a goal that has to be achieved, we can see the neural substratum that discharges during purposeful movements as a sort of motor-embodied vocabulary. This is how Rizzolatti and Gallese (1997) describe the set of different types of goal-directed neurons coding different motor acts related to prehension, discovered in area F5 of the chimpanzee's premotor cortex.

[33] We have seen the role played by the MNS in Mary's case in the construction of shared sense at the level of action.

[34] It should not be forgotten that observing a meaningful action is always already comprehending that action.

[35] 'Not only must a pre-predicative manifestness in general constantly already occur and have occurred, however, if the assertion as pointing out is to be accomplished in whatever way, but this *pre-predicative manifestness* must itself be this *occurrence* in which a particular *letting oneself be bound* occurs. This is the prior relation to that which gives pointing out in assertion its measure: beings as they are. . . . Letting oneself be bound must already bring toward itself in advance, and as something that can be binding, whatever is to provide the measure and be binding in one way or another' (Heidegger, 2001a: 342).

3 Personal Identity

I am different from all of my sensations. I cannot understand how. I cannot even understand who feels them. Furthermore, who is this 'I' at the beginning of the three propositions?[1]

At this point, we have to examine another aspect of experience that has not received any attention so far: its temporal nature. The time of doing, or of not doing; common time woven into interactions, into routines, into practices, into shared experiences and contemporaneously into the passing of the days . . . day and night, yesterday, today and tomorrow: the way in which past, present and future are constructed and interrelated in our daily lives. It is the time of experience, the time of what we do, feeling in one way or another, that makes it possible to give new form to events through narration. The meaning of Ricoeur's (Ricoeur,1980: 165) words emerge forcefully here: 'I take temporality to be that structure of existence that reaches language in narrativity and narrativity to be the language structure that has temporality as its ultimate referent'.

Narrative recomposition presupposes, on the one hand, a prefiguration of the sense which appears to be inscribed in acting, in feeling and in the temporal sequence of experience.[2] At this stage of precomprehension, in addition to the daily 'family play', the child encounters the emotional tonalities which accompany the times of living.[3] On the other hand, it transforms the prefiguration of sense through narrative recomposition. This recompositional process – whose initial structure is provided and guaranteed almost entirely by the parent, the child's role simply being to repeat or conform to narrated events (Bruner, 1983; Nelson, 1985; Hudson, 1990) – furnishes experience with the tools of synthesis, drafting and structuring. In other words, caregivers take care of structuring sense in order to enable the child to recognize and master his own experience.

The gradual acquisition of the capacity to structure experience into a constellation of micro-narratives and, subsequently, into a story, develops concurrently and in parallel fashion with the process of the identification and construction of personal identity. Indeed, the ultimate referent of narrative recomposition is the experience of being oneself, ipseity, from which it cannot be separated as if it were an act of pure cognition!

It thus follows that it is the joint ordering (that is, together with his parents) of the events of his own life in narrative sequences by which the child begins to build, and articulate, his own singularity as a person, to give shape to his own who. In this way, while he differentiates narrated experience from that antepredicative background in which his

Selfhood, identity and personality styles Giampiero Arciero and Guido Bondolfi

story was implicated[4] in some way, he appropriates that experience, he recognizes it as his own. He both recognizes and identifies himself in that story at the same time. To do so, the child requires no social metacognitive skill – identity is constructed in the very act of narration.

These single events begin to be amalgamated into rough narrative structures exhibiting the features of micro-stories in the course of the third and fourth years of life. Through joint narration of his own experience, the child discovers an 'intimate' method of organizing events, and at the same time he gives shape to his own way of feeling he is himself. 'The emotional content of parent-child conversations,' writes Welch-Ross (2001: 98), 'is one type of evaluative framing likely to play a critical role in the development of this subjective orientation toward events that imparts meaning to experience'. It is thus no surprise to find that at this stage children begin to take an interest in emotional and mental states, as is shown by the increase in the percentage of questions asked about internal states, and on 'psychological causality' concerning actions performed by others (Dunn, 1988).

Gradually, in the course of the pre-school years, the scaffolding models by means of which parents initially transmit those forms of narration with which they are familiar, and which are culturally appropriate, become a site of cooperation and negotiation. That is, the child contributes increasingly to the active construction of the story through conversing about past events. The process is characterized by an intermediate stage, where the child begins to report accounts of experiences he has not shared with his parents, which are then structured into a narrative in collaboration with the caregiver, by means of a re-edition of the episodes. But it is only between the age of four and five that the child finally masters narrative structure, to the point that, for example, he can invent a character, showing that he can grasp the character's psychological makeup and can structure his actions into a story.

This process, which, as we have said, takes place in the pre-school years, is characterized by the gradual divorce of the narration from the context of situation, from the context in which the speech event took place. If, at the age of two, saying 'pram' helps to signal the fact that the child wants to go, or is going, to the park with his father, at the age of four or five, the very same word is free, so to speak, from its context of utterance, from the immediate situation of reference. In other words, the child appears to have acquired the capacity to recompose events in a diachronic sequence, instead of simply recounting what is happening in the *hic et nunc* of the context of utterance, the capacity to use words to construct a significant whole out of scattered events.

Complete mastery over configurational capacities, meaning that they can combine the episodic dimension of events that constitute the story with the nonchronological dimension, which connects events into an intelligible whole (Mink, 1972), enables older children to employ language without having to refer exclusively to current experience. Hence, not only can they reflect on, evaluate and comment on a certain configuration of episodes concerning themselves to others, as if the episodes constituted a whole, but they can also understand the reconfiguration of events constructed by others as being different from their own configuration.

All this appears to indicate that the reason why children fail false-belief tasks[5] before the age of four is that they are unable to distinguish their own viewpoint from that of the other, since they have not yet acquired the capacity to integrate their own different experiences over time into a narrative structure. Since they do not possess the ability to reconfigure the variety of different experiences of Self in the past and in the present, and unite them into a single, integrated framework, they predict what another will do on the basis of a false belief (for example on Sally's conviction that she will find her marble in the basket where she had left it) by relating it to what they would do based on their knowledge of the current situation (looking for the marble in the box in which Anne had placed the marble without Sally's knowing it).

The child's new ability to reassemble single events into a narrative structure, hence the ability to distance himself from events, goes hand in hand with a change in language use. In the pre-school years, it is the pragmatic use of language that ensures the primary mimetic link is established between language on the one hand and action and feeling on the other. As has been repeatedly stated, up until that age conversation refers essentially to current, interpersonal situations, to ongoing experiences, to shared activities, as if in some way the sense of words was actualized through the on-line reference to those contexts that are being shared in actual practice.[6]

The actors' involvement in games is an essential part of sense, hence of the decodifiability of the action. After all, the symbolic plot connected underlying the actions can be understood because actors participate in the game. This is why even two-year-olds can change the way in which they formulate their utterances when queried by their mother or by an unfamiliar adult (Tomasello and Todd, 1983). Indeed, Tomasello and associates found that, for an unfamiliar adult, children reformulated their utterance more often than they did for their mothers; with their mothers they tended, instead, to repeat the utterance.

Thus, while the child at two communicates, so to speak, within ongoing activities of which using language from inside socially-shared events is part (Nelson, 1996), older children can communicate on events from an external perspective, as if participating in an event were no longer necessary in order to be able to speak about it.

The capacity to organize coherent narratives concerning past events enables the child, who has mastered this new tool by means of having participated in conversations with more or less mature members of the culture, to establish a kind of identity between what he recounts and his own experiences, to conceive of himself as the protagonist of his own different experiences.

3.1 Speaking of the past

A series of studies on parent–child conversations about the past shows that social interaction is critical to the organization of structured narratives about autobiographical memories, and consequently to the construction of an enduring sense of Self (Fivush, 1991; Hudson, 1990; Nelson, 1993; Nelson and Fivush, 2004; Reese, 2002). Furthermore, several findings indicate that mothers with a highly elaborative reminiscing style facilitate children's development of autobiographical narrative skills (Fivush and Nelson, 2006). It should therefore come as no surprise that highly elaborative mothers focus more on the emotional and evaluative aspects of past events, that is, on experiential aspects, hence on those aspects that are significant in events (Fivush and Haden, 2005; Fivush, 2007).

From the opposite standpoint, failure to achieve total mastery over narrational tools might account for differences in comprehending the temporally-extended Self in two-, three- and four-year-old children, identified through a delayed self-recognition paradigm.

In the series of experiments carried out by Povinelli, Landau and Perilloux (1996; Povinelli *et al.*, 1999), the researchers exposed children of that age range to both live and briefly-delayed visual images of themselves in order to assess children's ability to link past events to the present. Each child was videotaped as he or she played a distinctive and novel game with the experimenter. During the game, the experimenter praised the child, and used this as the opportunity to secretly place a large, brightly-coloured sticker on top of the child's head. Three minutes later, the children were shown the video recording of the events that had just happened, including a clear depiction of the experimenter placing the sticker on their head (Barth, Povinelli and Cant, 2004: 16). They found that none of the two-year-olds reached up to retrieve the sticker, while 25% of three-year-olds and 75% of four-year-olds reached for the sticker. They concluded that while two- and three-year-old children can 'recognize themselves' in delayed video, they are incapable of integrating experience that is three minutes old with ongoing self-identity.

In another study, Welch-Ross (2001) reported empirical evidence showing that maternal elaborative and evaluative reminiscing style interacts with both the child's subjective perspective and his ability to engage in temporal-causal reasoning. Indeed, three-year-old children of highly elaborative mothers who reached for the sticker had a higher ratio of memories of significant past events than children who did not reach for the sticker.

It would thus appear that the capacity to integrate an event which has just taken place into a sense of personal continuity is strongly influenced by the ability developed by the child at the age of three to reconfigure experience through joint verbal remembering. This capacity is a consolidated one in four- and five-year-olds, who exhibit the ability to attribute different importance to episodes which have taken place at precise moments in the past compared to present events (Povinelli and Simon, 1998). Consequently, the different responses to the delayed self-recognition task could be due to the different capacities children have at different ages to integrate temporally-disconnected and causally-related events.

If the reconfiguration of one's experience in a story develops a feeling of stability of the Self over time, the impossibility of reordering the connections between one's experiences through the use of language inevitably alters the capacity to recognize those events as one's own, of identifying oneself in them. This would explain the link between children's delayed self-recognition performance and their autobiographical memory. This would also account for why children aged two to three, who can recognize themselves in a delayed video, do not temporally integrate an action accomplished three minutes earlier. Thus, while they are capable of establishing a relationship of equivalence between the delayed image and themselves, recognizing their own physical features, they cannot, however, organize the action they have just seen into a cohesive unit and cannot, consequently, identify that action as being their own, because they do not possess the narrative means to do so.

3.2 Stories of the future

Although many studies have pointed out that during the pre-school years both past and future events are ordered narratively through conversations with caregivers, the variables connected with maternal style affecting joint reminiscing differ from those characterizing parental–child talk about future events (Hudson, Shapiro and Sosa, 1995; Hudson, 2002, 2006).

This difference is ascribable to a fundamental asymmetry in the way humans experience time, and consequently to the way they reconfigure this domain. Thus, while the space of experience that has been lived through, and which is composed of events, situations and circumstances perceived in one way or another is 'saturated with reality', the same is not true of possible experience: the latter does not contain experienced contents. And although expectations may be accompanied by hope, fear, curiosity or desire, nevertheless they remain 'empty' from an experiential standpoint.

It is this very lack of 'tangible' content that renders parent–child conversations about the future more complicated.[7] In contrast to the shared interpreting of the past, in which the words employed are based on the experience lived through, a conversation anticipating future events can only count on experience in an indirect fashion. What is expected in the future is what has already happened in the past. This is the result obtained from studies on the effects of familiar routines on the development of temporal understanding (Friedman, 1977, 1990; Friedman and Brudos, 1988). Indeed, the child can already configure what happens in typical situations (such as going to McDonald's) as a sequence (Hudson, Shapiro and Sosa, 1995). Other recent studies which show that the very same neural substratum that is activated when imagining the future is needed for remembering the past lead to the same conclusion (Schacter, Addis and Buckner, 2007).

However, not all future events can be predicted from a knowledge of past events. Many things that happen may be unexpected, new, unknown, events that differ from one's expectations.

These two ways of dealing with the future are reflected in parent–child conversations. When mothers speak to children about the future, they use a type of language which takes this fact into account: 'they engaged their children in thinking about the future in different ways depending upon whether the event under discussion was familiar or unknown to the child. When discussing routine events, children were encouraged to provide information about what they could expect to happen, whereas when discussing novel events mothers engaged their children in more hypothetical talk' (Hudson, 2002: 65).[8]

In order for a child to be able to situate an event in time, he must be able to grasp the more or less expected future together with the past from which that future event differs (or does not differ) and with the present in which these two experiences of time intertwine in an asymmetrical manner. Through the use of language, the child learns to move between memory and plan, he learns to navigate through time.

This implies that the alchemy between what Koselleck (2004) calls the space of experience and the horizon of expectations is continually recomposed in current temporal experience, a process which is particularly intense in children. As is suggested by the title of a research report, 'Preschoolers' Current Desires Warp their Choices for the Future' (Atance and Meltzoff, 2006). On the other hand, several studies on young children's planning skills show that planning capacity increases considerably in the age range between three and five (Carlson, Moses and Claxton, 2004; Hudson, Shapiro and Sosa, 1995).

Not only are past and future composed out of ongoing conversation, but the superimposition between these different dimensions, and their reciprocal permeation, produces a continual recomposition between the accumulation of experiences and the creation of expectations. While the event corresponding to more or less routine expectations is predicted, and consequently integrated, without disturbing the coordination between the two ways of perceiving time (that is the accumulation of experience and the creation of expectations), the integration of novel events inevitably generates new expectations. In their turn, new expectations change the significance of experiences that have already been undergone.

Consequently, while the accumulation of experience is accompanied by a continual transformation of the possibilities of meaning – hence of the coordination between expectations and memories – at the same time, through narrative-composition supported by conversation with his caregivers, the child gradually comes to grasp his location in time, he comes to master the coordination between the experience through which he has lived and his own potential for acting and feeling.[9]

3.3 The sense of self in the age of reason

When, starting from the age of five, the child acquires the tools that enable him to compose the various temporal dimensions into a narrative unit, what emerges from an experiential standpoint is precisely a new sense of the permanence of Self over time. That is to say, not only does the child reconfigure acting and feeling through narrative plotting, but he is able to define a horizon within which to fix his own stability over time. This ability constitutes the foundation for the sense of responsibility which characterizes the child entering the 'Age of reason' (White, 1996).

In the West, this transition is signalled above all by phenomena which accompany schooling. The entry into the scholastic system provides the child with his first impact with an extended order (Hayek, 1978), in which his own identity is negotiated in terms of individual competition, rather than being regulated by a socially distributed ethical system, as happens in small communities that share habits, beliefs and knowledge. The shared activities and practices of the school routine structure new fields of interaction – with groups of children of differing ages, and other significant adults – in which the child participates with ever-increasing autonomy with respect to his parent figures. This leads to the development of a sense of independent responsibility, which emerges in an intersubjective context outside the family.

Cross-cultural studies show that this very sense of responsibility lies at the heart of the request, on the part of parents, that children be involved in activities of assistance and support, as well as that they take on domestic tasks. Rogoff *et al.* (1996), for instance, concluded their study of children aged between five and seven in 50 communities scattered all over the world thus:

> *It appears that in the age range of 5 to 7 years, parents assign (and children assume) responsibility for the care of younger children, for tending animals, for carrying out household chores and gathering materials for the upkeep of the family. The children also become responsible for their own social behaviour and the method of punishment for transgression changes. Along with responsibility, there is the expectation that children between 5 and 7 years begin to be teachable. Adults give practical training, expecting children to be able to imitate their example; children are taught social manners and inculcated in cultural traditions. Underlying these changes in teachability is the fact that, at 5–7 years, children are considered to attain common sense or rationality. At this age*

also, the child's character is considered to be fixed and he begins to assume new social and sexual roles. He begins to join with groups of peers and participate in rule games. The children's groups separate by sex at this time (Rogoff et al., 1996: 275).

The emergence of a sense of responsibility thus derives from a new relationship between the child's own actions, emotions and sense of Self, which the narrative order makes possible inasmuch as it combines the various temporal dimensions into one united whole. In other words, being assigned responsibilities in the domains of the school and of the family induces the child to develop the capacities to take on responsibilities in a stable fashion, and to carry out the tasks demanded by those responsibilities. This is only possible because the narrative reconfiguration of experience enables him to navigate through time maintaining his sense of identity.

With the development of narrative ability, experience acquires new determinations of meanings within a cohesive framework of experiences, which interweaves the person and his actions over time. Through the operation of narrative, every single action I carry out is introduced into a plot that constructs a cohesive unit of actions and passions, which concern me in as much as I am the protagonist of that narrative. The integration of experience into a sense of the cohesion of Self enriches it with new meanings and thus extends, as we have seen, the practical domain into the narrative domain. This process, which appears when the child reaches the age of reason, achieves final maturation only with the beginning of adolescence, when awareness begins to dawn on the pre-adolescent that the actor may also be the author of his own story[10] (Arciero, 2002).

While narrative recomposition of events (by means of which a series of heterogeneous elements – actions, emotions, motivations, episodes, agents, means, ends, causes – are recombined into a unitary configuration) holds together the various occurrences which form part of that story, at the same time it constitutes the identity of the person to whom those experiences refer. To be more precise, the capacity to organize and express one's own experience over time in a significant fashion discloses what remains in time: the correlation of identity with one's experiences, with the persistence of Self in the different episodes constituting one's life.

3.4 The modes of identity

We now come up anew against the question of the permanence of time. We have already encountered this issue along our path when, starting from Kant, we traced the lines of continuity between his conception of the Self and that of systems theory. In that perspective, the problem of the permanence of the Self over time was solved by appealing to the order of connectivity, or the invariable organization of the relationships among elements that constitute an autonomous natural system. This enabled change to be conceived of in relation to an invariable, to ascribe manifold changing experiences to an immutable order.[11] We then pointed out that this way of solving the question avoided the issue of who undergoes the experience.

It was while we were analysing experience lived in the first person that we came across the problem of permanence a second time. In this new context, characterized by reflections on ipseity of a Heideggerian nature, the sameness of the Self over time appeared as an inclination that is produced starting from being each and every time. It is in finding oneself as being the same each and every time, in the same things with the same emotional tones, that sameness takes shape. The permanence of Self corresponds here to an almost total overlap between the sedimentation of one's personal experience (sameness) and happening each and every time (ipseity).

One example of this overlap – albeit at a purely motor level – is provided by an fMRI study by Calvo-Merino *et al.* (2006) on the influence of motor familiarity on action observation in expert dancers. Male and female dancers, who were shown video clips of gender-specific male and female ballet moves, activated principally premotor, parietal and cerebellar areas when observing movements from their own motor repertoire, compared to opposite-gender movements that they often saw but were not used to performing. Comprehension of ongoing types of movement, that is, came about through the activation of areas connected to prior motor expertise that had sedimented over time. As Polanyi (1958, 1966) observed, we rely on our tacit awareness of the relation of our body with things for attending to these things.

One remove away from bodily practices, we find the concept of habit understood as a modification of the organism, not only acquired but also contracted, destined to last in time: a transformation in the inclination to encounter the world and others, which persists in the living organism over and beyond the continual or repetitive change that triggered it off, channelling its potential.

Proceeding in the same direction, we meet with the so-called 'interiorization' of ethical conduct.[12] Just like routines and habits, ethical rules sediment in tacit knowledge, which constitutes the foundation for our moral judgements and actions.

We may define the set of peculiarities according to which a person tends to remain the same over time as his character.[13] In fact, it is the perseverance of those stable features which exposes sameness to a double gaze; one gaze enables the person to grasp himself from the standpoint of the first person, the other from the standpoint of objectivity. On the one hand, it is my character that makes me unique. My physiognomy, my voice, my face – these are the fingerprints of my being! It is that character, understood as a unity of perspective, which situates me while directing me in my encounter with the world and with others. On the other hand, however, it is those very same traits which enable character to be observed objectively: as a portrait, we said earlier, as abstract patterns which no longer belong to anyone.

Finally, we have run into the problem of the permanence of Self a third time. When a child who enters the age of reason takes on responsibilities (e.g. gathering materials for the upkeep of the family or doing his homework for the following day) – the same might, however, be said of an adult male or female who, for instance, is struggling to realize their aim in life – the constancy required to achieve the task involves a type of permanence which is different from that as a result of which sameness and ipseity coincide. At this stage in the child's life there emerges a mode of stability over time, a modality of maintaining oneself in relation to the changeability of events which cannot be ascribed to the perseverance of character. Here, ipseity is caught freed from sameness. This form of maintaining the stability of Self over time corresponds to the common experience of more or less relying on the person who has taken on the responsibility, on who has made the promise.[14]

While sameness and ipseity mark the boundaries within which a person's identity over time is composed, the interminable dialectical relationship is built up through the construction of a narrative plot, thereby creating Narrative Identity. After Ricoeur, it has become common to speak of Narrative Identity to refer to the mediation operated by the story enabling the composition and recomposition of the dialectics between the two modes of permanence in time. It this type of mediation that enables the person to transform a purely temporal succession of events into the cohesive whole which constitutes their life story. In this way, the person's identity, understood as the character of the story, is moulded contemporaneously with the plot. And indeed, on the one hand, the temporal unity of the story corresponds to the singularity of the person or, we might say, the 'character' of the narrative, while on the other hand, temporal unity is constantly being challenged by unforeseen events, by ongoing situations. As is stressed by Ricoeur (1995: 231) 'The real nature of narrative identity is revealed, I contend, only in the dialectical relationship between ipseity and sameness.'

In this process, far from character manifesting itself as an immutable structure determined by chromosomes, or by the planets or the stars, it is constantly questioned in the event of being. The story that was contained in it is brought back on to the stage in a narrative of which the person is the creator. On the other hand, ipseity, the event of being-there, which, as Weil (1974) noted, challenges the person every single second, may be reconfigured and integrated narratively without backup of sameness, offering an opportunity of continuity over time that differs from character permanence.

In staging this dialectical relationship between ipseity and sameness in narrative, the person takes possession of his own facts, bestowing upon them a singular connection which reflects the specific connection between the two modalities of permanence over time. Consequently, the narrative of Self cannot but oscillate within these two polarities, a process in which narrative acts as the mediator by varying the relationship between the different forms of stability of Self over time.

Thus, if the experience of being tends more toward sameness, the relationship between unity and discontinuity in the construction of the narrative will have to be matched by the dialectic between the recurrence of stabilized traits – which furnish the protagonist with a sense of permanence in time – and the variety of significant situations – which perturbs that sense of personal continuity. This is the inner dialectic of the protagonist of the story whose identity is focused on one character that admits only minimal transformations. Think of the romantic hero who bends all to his fiery passion. 'How I devoured everything . . .' exclaims the young Werther a second before committing suicide.

If, on the contrary, the experience of living is polarized on ipseity, the result is an identity which needs to maintain its stability without being able to count on sameness. In taking up Heidegger's concept of *Selbst-Standigkeit* (Self-constancy), Ricoeur speaks of *mantien de soi* (maintenance of Self) to indicate this affirmation of the position of the Self with respect to the passing of time. In this case too, the degree of narrative cohesion is matched by the combination of stable and unstable aspects of the protagonist, the difference being, however, that the constitution of one's constancy requires anchorage, something to hold on to, as with promises. And it is this we might say 'decentred' Self which enables the return of that constancy of Self that Ricoeur perceived on a moral level to the narrative plane. Suffice it to think of Raskolnikov in *Crime and Punishment*. The entire development of the character up until almost the very end of this long novel is based on one central dilemma: 'what I needed to find out then, and find out as soon as possible, was whether I was a louse like everybody else or a man' (Dostoevsky, 1953: 402). This is the doubt which acts as the anchor for Raskolnikov's identity. Everything that happens, the tormenting thoughts which precede the ferocious crime which for him is 'almost mechanical', even the impossible punishment, are nothing but minimal variations, which are almost out of focus, of a sense of permanence which owes its stability to that cognition, to that problem. Thus does he anchor his identity.

Raskolnikov tells the man interrogating him: 'I simply intimate that the "extraordinary" man has the right... I don't mean a formal, official right, but he has the right in himself, to permit his conscience to overstep... certain obstacles, but only in the event that his ideas (which may sometimes be salutary for all mankind) require it for their fulfilment' (Dostoevsky, 1953: 249).

In contrast to Self-permanence centred on those aspects of character which are almost substantial, Self-constancy polarized on ipseity opens up unexpected possibilities of variability. Building one's identity then becomes a function of both the way of stabilizing oneself (fixed versus changing) and the type of anchorage one grasps on to (people, contexts, thoughts, images, etc.). This varies the way the story and the character or characters are composed.

Raskolnikov, for example, constructs his stability by taking firm hold of a doubt, of 'that strange thought that seemed to be pecking at his brain, like a chick wanting to get out of its shell'. It is this fixity that makes him a character that is almost predictable.

But if we move toward the discontinuity of anchorage, as does Virginia Woolf in her short story 'The Mark on the Wall', the character becomes a transient aggregate. It is as if a multitude of experiences of Self were ready to compose itself discontinuously, in different forms around new objects, gathering together for a while, thereby making a new and different character emerge each time, only to return to swarm again prior to producing yet another new aggregate. It is interesting to note that, in the very middle of this perennial migration, Virginia Woolf writes, almost as if she had caught sight of some sort of relationship between this mode of being and speed:

> *Why, if one wants to compare life to anything, one must liken it to being dragged through a tunnel by an underground train at fifty miles an hour, landing at the other end without a single hairpin in one's hair! Shot out at the feet of God entirely naked! Tumbling head over heels in the asphodel meadows like brown paper parcels pitched down a chute in the post office! With one's hair flying back like the tail of a race-horse. Yes, that seems to express the rapidity of life, the perpetual waste and repair; all so casual, all so haphazard (Woolf, 2000).*

The more the discontinuity of the anchorage becomes marked, clearly, the more inconsistent does the feeling of stability become, and the more picaresque does personal identity become! It is obvious that the narrative reconfiguration of such an experience will manifest features that are very different from those exhibited by an account of a story with a plot and a character. This explains why Strawson (1999: 15) wrote:

> *I have no sense of my life as a narrative with form, or indeed as a narrative without form. I have little interest in my own past and little concern for the future. My poor personal memory largely impinges on my present consciousness. Even when I am interested in my past, I am not interested in it specifically insofar as it is mine ... for me as I am now, the interest (emotional or otherwise) of my personal memories lies in their experiential content, considered independently of the fact that what is remembered happened to me – i.e. to the me that is now remembering.*

The continual changing of the anchor point is the topic of *Rameau's Nephew*. The central topic of this great work by Diderot is the polymorphism of the protagonist, whose identity is redesigned each and every time, either through adopting the thought or the voice of the other, or by aligning itself to the circumstances or exigencies dictated by the situation. 'Nothing is more unlike him than himself,' writes Diderot (1762). 'Today, in dirty linen and torn trousers, dressed in rags, almost barefoot, he slinks along with his head down . . . Tomorrow, he marches along with his head high, powdered, his hair curled, well dressed, with fine shoes . . . He lives from day to day, sad or happy, according to circumstances'. And one step further on, when every anchor point has been lost, when one no longer possesses, nor can posses, an identity because there is nothing or no one to hold on to, only then do we reach that 'I am nothing' which characterizes Musil's *The Man without Qualities*. Only then can that 'I am nothing' which Ricoeur recognizes as the attestation of the eclipse of identity (and which we explored at the beginning of this book when we examined the problematic aspects of Robert's life) be comprehended as the experience of a person who can no longer manage to decentre himself in a stable fashion, who can no longer recognize himself and retain permanence over time: it is a feeling of emptiness, a sensation of nothingness, the feeling that one is nothing. Musil's words are clearly echoed in that expression with which Robert photographs the end of his relationship with Sarah: 'she was my mirror, so while she was with me, I was there too; then she went away and suddenly I no longer existed'.

3.5 Inclinations

The perseverance of character and the constancy of ipseity thus represent two different modes of constructing identity, which, at a pre-reflexive level, correspond to different perceptions of the feeling of personal stability, to dissimilar forms of the inclination of ipseity. From the very first stages of development, the direction taken by the dialectic between ipseity and sameness (which will later be reconfigured through narrative identity), the way 'the significativities which come toward us as our lives mature . . . drag life along with them' (Heidegger, 2001c) depends on a dialectic that is even more fundamental – one's relationship with others. It is in the domain of one's significant relationships that there emerges for the first time the way each of us discovers himself and discovers himself anew, the way those recurrent modalities of feeling that one is alive take shape. That is to say, the tension toward the other and one's own mode of self-perception come together in affectivity. If ipseity reveals itself through the affection manifested by the other, which thus comes to be part of the 'the intimate constitution of its meaning' (Ricoeur, 1990), the historicity of this being-in-relation is sedimented and contracted into a recurrent perception of Self, which will constitute its sameness.

Hence, the two inclinations, which are reflected in the different directions in which narrative identity may reconfigure experience, lead us back to two polarities of the constitution of our emotions – which actually define a continuum – and at the same time, to two ways in which the relationship with other significativities is being constructed. This is the ontological background that enables us to draw up the guidelines of a psychology of the emotions.

It is thus in the sphere of those significant ties – whose patterns of development in the early years of life are studied by the theory of attachment – that the acquisition and regulation of emotional traits gradually become stable in the course of development. Nevertheless, despite the fact that emotional traits emerge through relational experiences originating in the reciprocity with significant figures, they are not reducible to patterns of attachment. Reciprocity with caregivers – which generates its own specific affective component, which is connected to the child's subjective perception of security or insecurity in relation to the predictability of gaining access to his parents – enables the child to structure emotional tonalities from the very first stages of his life. These tonalities will gradually be organized into more stable emotional features. The common origin of the organization of attachment, and the ordering of the affective domain (sameness), should not induce us into confusing patterns of attachment with the constitution of emotional dispositions, despite the fact that those affections generated in that sphere can contribute to emotional development. While patterns of attachment concern the regularities characterizing the relationship with the caregiver, the constitution of dispositions relates to the configuration of the emotional aspects of sameness. A child can, for instance, form multiple attachments, characterized by different modes of reciprocity, and each of these will affect the ordering of the emotional sphere in its own way. It is the emotions generated within each of these different relationships that will sediment into a unitary and unique affective domain.

The fundamental variable which allows the child to develop different ways of feeling emotion appears to be connected to the types of recurrent stimuli the child is subjected to in the sphere of reciprocity relationships with significant people. The more these relationships generate 'specific' episodes and interactions that the organism is biologically ready to interpret as being relevant to survival, the more the child's response will involve the activation of basic emotions. As a result, forms of reciprocity actualized in recurrent situations eliciting basic emotions induce the child to structure emotional traits, as well as personality configurations focused prevalently on basic emotions. These emotions are said to be hypercognized (Levy, 1973).[15] This will orient the quality of emotional experience, the regulation of emotions and the construction of personal identity. Parallel to this process, the child undergoes a subjective experience of gut emotions 'constraining' him to focus his attention on 'internal' polarization, namely, on the bodily states which have given rise to the emotional states.

Precocious and recurrent activation of basic emotions, in response to a more oriented stimulation on the part of significant adults ('oriented' in the sense of providing stimuli which are specific triggers for basic emotions) guides the child's perception of personal stability according to a frame of reference that employs a predominantly body-centred coordinate system. This allows the child to regulate his relationship both with others and in accordance with the variability of the situation through bringing internal states into focus, thus privileging a body-bounded sense of Self. Recurrent emotional states are gradually integrated in the course of development in the form of complex character traits, perceptions and cognitions, connected to emotions, actions and expressive communications, but also as habits, norms and values (Dougherty, Abe and Izard, 1996; Izard *et al.*, 1993; Magai and McFadden, 1995; Malatesta, 1990).[16] This polarization on the experiential flow centred on the body will produce 'originary predilections' that will orient both character construction and its narrative reconfiguration. This is where the tendency that we have called Inward is formed, a tendency which, as we shall see, characterizes prevalently those people whose common distinguishing trait is the search after stability, assigning priority to the understanding of the gut aspects of emotions in their relationships with others and with the world (Arciero, 2002, 2006; Arciero *et al.*, 2004).

Things seem to move in a different direction if the recurrent stimuli the child is exposed to in his interactions with significant adults do not elicit specific responses. In this case, it is as if evolution had not 'prepared' the organism to produce automatical appraisal of stimuli that are relevant to the maintenance of adaptation. This type of reciprocity – which develops gradually and is based, through the child's relationships with significant caregivers, on a 'mediated' affective engagement, in which sphere the non-basic emotions are hypercognized – gives rise to a predictability which must perforce be anchored in the external source of stimulation. This way of emotioning may be described by using the words employed by Draghi-Lorenz, Reddy and Costall (2001: 295) to describe non-basic emotions: 'They seem to owe their distinct status to being *de facto* always and necessarily socially "aware" emotions'. While this produces a recognition of one's own emotional experiences stemming from an initial focalization on the other, it hinders focusing attention on one's own internal states. Shotter (1998) is quite right to define this mode as a 'knowing from'.

Seen in this perspective, emotions take shape from one's engagement with the other in ongoing situations: without needing to build a representation, the other is perceived as a part of one's own emotional experience in the context of transitory relationships. In this type of case, the child is induced to construct traits and then character configurations which involve, in different ways, a concurrent awareness of both Self and other. These traits will incline the quality of an emotional experience, the regulation of emotion and the construction of personal identity.[17]

Unlike basic emotions, those emotions which emerge through mediated affective engagement, because of their 'limited viscerality', can change more quickly and more easily, since they tax the system's visceral resources less. As we shall see in the next chapter, such changeability favours the development of greater flexibility with regard to the flow of ongoing events. Furthermore, while the element of awareness, which is to be considered an integral part of this form of emotional experience, 'slows down' the speed of a person's reactions to events and 'cools down' his passions, at the same time it enables the person's emotional response to be more individualized. It should therefore come as no surprise that this type of emotional experience may give rise to specific patterns of arousal.

Activating prevalently mediated emotions, in response to the stimuli provided by caregivers, orients the child's perception of his own stability from the very early stages of development, by way of a frame of reference that predominantly employs an externally-anchored coordinated system. Thus, the sense of the permanence of Self will come into being as a result of the orientation deriving from the emotional states and the acts of the other (or from adhering to impersonal contexts). Thus begins the development of that inclination that we have defined as Outward, which mainly characterizes those people who construct constancy of Self through time by anchoring their identity to external reference points, attempting to synchronize their feelings with those points. Focusing on an external frame accounts for the reduced and sometimes aspecific viscerality of the emotional states perceived, bolstering the development of the cognitive dimension of emotion. It also explains the sense of emptiness of the emotional states perceived by the person, or the sensation of 'being nothing' which some of these people, as we have seen, may experience in relation to the loss of reference points that support the sense of their continuity over time.

3.6 Situatedness

A superficial glance would seem to indicate that the difference between the two modes of permanence over time consists in a privileged relationship between sameness and the body. In this view, it is as if we gradually move from the pole in which ipseity coincides with sameness to the pole in which the two modalities are completely independent and at the same time ipseity gradually dissociates itself from the body in parallel fashion.

Examining the range of variation between the two polarities from this standpoint means, however, disregarding a fundamental aspect that keeps cropping up insistently in this book. If language reconfigures the experience of living, and if my feeling myself in this or that way (ipseity) is always mediated by my being flesh and blood, then the entire spectrum of variations reconstituted in the narrative corresponds to different modalities of the being mine of the body, of my feeling alive. It thus follows that what distinguishes these two modes of building identity is how one feels 'inside one's skin', rather than the privileged relationship that one of these two modes entertains with one's body.[18] Even Musil's 'I am nothing' is a way of feeling alive.

In this sense, my body appears each and every time as the range of emotionally-situated sensorimotor possibilities generated in response to who or what captures my attention, interests me, directs me, invites me, strikes me. From this viewpoint, corporeity is a phenomenon: it arises as a being able to perceive something significant coming toward us, interpellating us.[19] It is the '*puissance d'un certain monde*'.[20]

It is through the continual occurring of this encounter, in one way or another, that I come to a perception of myself each and every time, which I would otherwise never have had access to. In this sense, my flesh, which experiences, acts on and is subjected to the world and to the others, is the centre of concrete mediation of my openness to the world, but it is also the 'text' which preserves a record of this openness.

Our corporeity, then, is each and every time the being-in-relation-to who and what interpellates us (which is not always materially graspable), but at the same time it is the place of immediacy to oneself. My feeling myself in this or that situation is always mediated by my being embodied. 'It seems reasonable to say,' writes Gallagher (2007), 'that the body is situated differently in different situations and that this difference may not simply be a difference in the situational content, but a difference in how the body processes being situated precisely because the circumstances are so different. To put it differently, we might say, the question is not just about differences in situations, but differences in situatedness.'

The unity between the nature of openness, owing to which man's existence is ontologically exposed to the solicitations coming from the world and from others, and feeling oneself alive, which man is always already entrusted to, is established by emotional tones. Affectivity, from this standpoint, is concurrently intimacy with oneself and the encounter with the world and with the face of the other. That is to say, feeling oneself in a certain emotional situation ties the way one perceives oneself as living to what addresses one in that situation, thereby evoking affection. This is why the famous adage is quite right in saying 'when you are smiling, the whole world smiles with you'.[21] Each and every time, situational engagement resets the vital space in terms of the possible actions that circumstances require.

The result is that, on the one hand, man is always in the situation of being related to a world and to the other, and on the other hand, he is always already invited to respond to what approaches him in the environment in a way that is significant to him, eliciting a response. The dynamics of affectivity is articulated in living flesh, by means of this essential tension between one's grip on the world and on others and the affections which they procure one.[22]

Thanks to this tension which emanates from the body, the sense of being situated, and consequently the notion of perspective, becomes concrete. It is my acting and feeling which leans toward certain inclinations as a result of which certain aspects of the world acquire some importance for me, a significance which orients my possibilities of existence. 'The body proper itself "knows" and "comprehends"' (Merleau-Ponty, 1945: 167).

It is only when I have mastered language, and through it the capacity to comprehend my identity, that I can develop the freedom to accept my dispositions and act, allowing myself to be influenced by those dispositions. Only later still do I develop a sort of interpretative receptivity of my inclinations to act and to feel, a receptivity which is commensurable with my plans for life, with the horizon of my possibilities (Arciero, 2006).[23] But before the advent of this *knowing myself*, it is my body which employs my affective and sensory-motor structures to keep the origin and the limits of my perspective. In this sense, 'our open and personal existence rests on a first basis of acquired and congealed existence' (Merleau-Ponty, 1945: 493–494).[24] It is thus my being emotionally inclined which guides narrative framing by providing, from the earliest stages of linguistic development, the ground to which my symbolic reconfiguration is anchored.[25]

It would thus appear to follow that the different polarities characterizing the profile of one's identity must correspond to different modes of perceiving oneself, which are reflected in the ways of giving concrete form to one's story and its protagonist – to the relationship with oneself, with the world and with others. If different modes of narrative construction are related to different modes of feeling emotionally situated, the analysis of an individual's story should provide clues as to how that person is 'emotionally inclined'. In other words, analysing a personal narrative enables us to grasp the different inclinations of the person's affective sphere, allowing us to comprehend those stable traits which, as we have seen, expose character to the dual perspective of first and third persons.

It is at this point in our research that the study of experience in the first person begins to interact with the neurosciences, and, as we shall see in the following chapters, with the psychology of emotion and of personality, and with psychopathology. In tracing this interaction, we will be obliged to set aside the in-depth analysis of personal stories, a theme that will be treated in another work.

3.7 The body, pain and others

In order to demonstrate that the two polarities – Inward and Outward inclination – of the affective domain, and of the ordering and semantic coherence of a personal narrative, correspond to different modes of perceiving an analogous stimulus, we have designed an experiment aiming to gauge the effect produced by observing pain in one's partner. Before moving on to examine the results of our study, we must first briefly outline the background against which our research is set.

There are two major works on empathy for pain: one by Singer *et al.* (2004), the other by Avenanti *et al.* (2005). Both studies reach the same conclusion: empathizing with pain in others activates a number of brain circuits that are also elicited when we experience pain in ourselves.

In order to demonstrate this hypothesis, Singer studied the female partner in 16 couples while painful stimulation was applied to their own or to their partner's right hand. While they were in the MRI scanner, they could see their partner's hand through a system of mirrors. In addition, cues were randomly presented indicating whether they or their partner were about to receive painful stimulation.

The analysis of the data obtained showed: (a) the activation of bilateral anterior insula (AI), rostral anterior cingulated cortex (ACC), brainstem and cerebellum, both when subjects experienced pain and when they observed the signal that their partner was being subjected to pain; (b) the specific activation of posterior insula/secondary somatosensory cortex, the sensory-motor cortex (SI/MI) and the cuadal ACC, only when subjects received pain.

The data would seem to indicate that the neural substratum of pain-related empathy does not involve the entire 'pain matrix', since the activation of the sensory components fails to occur. Singer and colleagues thus conclude that empathy for pain is mediated by what they define as the affective components of the pain network: rostal ACC and AI.[26]

The study carried out by Avenati *et al.* (2005) seems to go in the diametrically opposite direction.

In a series of experiments in which subjects observed various types of painful stimuli – for example, a needle in a person's hand, a needle being pushed into a tomato and so on – produced by means of transcranial magnetic stimulation (TMS), the researchers recorded changes in motor excitability of the subjects' hand muscles occurring as a result of observation of the same muscles that were pricked in others. No change occurred when participants observed a needle penetrating a tomato.

The analysis of the data showed strong involvement of the sensory-motor side of the pain matrix.

The cautious conclusions drawn by the researchers stressed the possibility of the existence of a form of empathy based on somatic resonance – which is both simpler and complementary to that based on affective resonance – that maps the sensory features of others' pain on to the observer's motor system.

This stark contrast between the findings obtained in these two studies is ascribed by Singer and Frith (2005) to the different instructions given to the participants. In the study by Singer *et al.*, subjects' attention was drawn to the anticipation of the unpleasantness of the painful stimulus.[27] Instead, in the experiment by Avenati, participants were asked to attend to the part of the body that was about to be pricked and to rate the intensity of the pain the stimulated individual might have felt. Quite correctly, Singer and Frith conclude their article with a warning that when studying empathy for pain, what they dub 'the mental attitudes' of the participants must be taken into consideration.

Four studies have taken this advice seriously. (1) Singer *et al.* (2006), an fMRI study in which empathic responses to pain in others (engaged in an economic game) refered to prior evaluation on the part of the participants of the fairness or unfairness of their conduct during the game. It was found that the moral judgement regulated the neural response. (2) A study by Danziger, Prkachin and Willer (2006) investigated the possible influence of the observer's sensitivity to pain upon his perception of others' pain. The 12 subjects studied were patients with congenital insensitivity to pain who, nothwithstanding this fact, were capable of feeling empathy for others' pain on the basis of facial or acoustic evidence of pain. They found it difficult to evaluate the pain experienced by others without seeing their face or hearing them cry. In this case the perception of pain experienced by others was shown to involve the integrity of the onlooker's nociceptive system. (3) An fMRI study carried out by Cheng *et al.* (2007),[28] which showed that the activation of the pain matrix while participants were observing needles being inserted into different parts of the body varied significantly between subjects divided into two groups prior to the experiment on the basis of their degree of expertise in acupuncture. The first group, which consisted of physicians practicing acupuncture, and exhibited no signal changes in the insula and ACC, was compared with a second group composed of naïve participants, who activated those areas to a significant degree. In this study, it was expertise that modulated neural activation. (4) An fMRI study carried out by Gu and Han (2007) highlighted the fact that neural activities related to pain rating were eliminated when subjects counted the number of hands affected by the painful stimuli in lieu of evaluating the intensity of pain experienced by the model. In this investigation, neural response was modulated by differing attentional demands.

Special mention must be made in this overview of an important study carried out by Jackson *et al.* (2006), part of a line of research which has investigated brain activation similarities and differences in subjects' imagining actions (Ruby and Decety, 2001), beliefs (Ruby and Decety, 2003) and feelings (Ruby and Decety, 2004) from the first- (Self) or the third- (other) person perspective (Jackson *et al.*, 2006). Within this framework, the study shows how imagining another's feelings, or imagining oneself in a painful situation, modulates the neural activity underlying the onlooker's evaluation emphasis, which in turn regulates the activation process related to pain. In this case, differences in imagination regulate activation.

In contrast to the studies we have just examined, our fMRI experiment considers how the participants organize emotional experience, hence how they feel inclined in their body-situatedness. This approach leads us to distinguish between two categories of onlookers – Inward and Outward observers – corresponding therefore to the two polarities of the continuum. The hypothesis is that the observation of pain in one's partner's facial expression elicits different cerebral areas, in relation to the fact that the perception of personal stability is based on a referential framework that predominantly employs either a body-centred coordinate system, as in those subjects who hypercognize basic emotions (Inward inclination), or an externally-anchored coordinate system, as in those subjects who grasp their own emotional experience by the way they engage with others (Outward inclination).

We studied subjects in 30 couples as they observed pictures of facial expressions depicting pain in their own partners and in strangers, or, to obtain a comparison, depicting neutral expressions.

Our 30 participants were previously divided into two groups – Inward and Outward inclination – on the basis of a semi-structured interview (Bertolino *et al.*, 2005) independently conducted by two investigators. Briefly, the interview was structured into three consecutive steps: (1) a detailed account of two episodes (involving fear and/or anger); (2) a description of the emotional experiences of anger and fear, to assess the participants' style (i.e. Inward or Outward) of emotional activation and regulation; (3) an analysis of the onset, manifestations and extinction of the emotional experience. Subjects also completed the personality-meaning questionnaire, evaluating key themes characterizing different emotional styles, and an Inward–Outward scale to assess the way they experienced emotions. They also completed a series of questionnaires identifying different personality features, and the Interpersonal Reactivity Index to evaluate empathy for pain, and two of the five subtests of the Body Perception Questionnaire (BPQ) – the Awareness of Bodily Processes (AWP) and the Autonomic Nervous System Reactivity (ANSR) – both of which are related to the perception of bodily responses.

We compared the two groups, each of 15 people, as they were exposed to highly self-related visual stimuli: images of their partners' faces, in both painful and neutral situations, and of unknown faces, in both painful and neutral situations. The partners' facial expressions of pain were filmed during a nociceptive examination. Two investigators reviewed the videotaped recordings and selected by consensus the picture frames conveying evidence of the intensity of pain experience, based on Ekman and Friesen's Facial Action Coding System. Participants were required during fMRI to perform a discrimination task between known and unknown faces expressing pain or with a neutral expression.

In neuroimaging data analyses, a direct comparison between groups revealed that the signal increase in the left posterior insula/BA13 and right parietal lobe/BA40 was greater in the Inward group, and in the Outward group the signal was greater in the bilateral middle frontal gyrus/BA9, bilateral precuneus/BA7 and left posterior cingulate cortex/BA23 (see Figure 2). To better evaluate the effect of the group factor in the differential activity related to the task, a three-way interaction analysis of the two groups was carried out based on painful facial expressions by known facial expressions. This interaction showed greater activation in the left posterior insula/BA13, while the reverse comparison showed a greater activation in the bilateral cuneus/BA19, left middle occipital gyrus/BA18 and right medial prefrontal cortices/BA10 and left medial prefrontal cortices/BA25. This suggests that the group factor significantly contributed toward the differences among the participants.

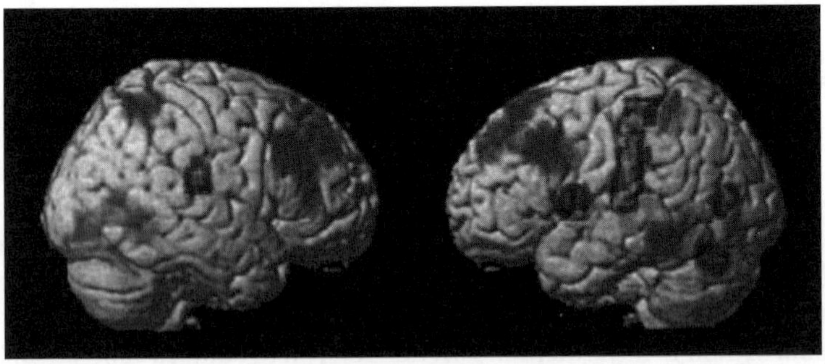

Figure 2

Consistent with our hypothesis, the results seem to indicate that distinct activations are involved in each group. To explain these findings more clearly, it is noteworthy that the regions that the Inward group activated seem to overlap with the neural system of interoceptive awareness, such as the posterior insula and the secondary somatic sensory cortex (SII), in mapping the afferent homeostasic pathway (Craig, 2002). By contrast, the Outward group activated regions functionally involved in self-referential processing like the medial prefrontal cortex (Gusnard *et al.*, 2001), as well as the precuneus and the PCC (Gusnard and Raichle, 2001). We might therefore summarize this point as follows: while activations in the Inward group almost overlapped with the neural system of interoceptive awareness, the Outward group showed activation in those fronto-posterior parietal regions that are engaged in continuously gathering information on the Self and the external world (Cavanna and Trimble, 2006).

By showing how two modes of emotional proneness involve distinct areas in the processing of highly self-related visual stimuli, these data suggest that more than one mode of self-referential processing is available, at least in pain empathy. As illustrated by Northoff *et al.* (2006), self-referential processing concerns stimuli that are experienced as strongly related to one's own person; as such, it implies a focus on subjective aspects, and links different stimuli to the Self. What unifies and categorizes stimuli, in this respect, is the strength of their relation to the Self: here, in a situation where one's partner is shown to be in pain, the strength of the simuli is determined by the way one feels. Emotional proneness, therefore, corresponds to a form of self-reference underpinned by selective neural activations. From this point of view, it is unsurprising that the areas involved in the so-called 'default mode network' (DMN) (Raichle *et al.*, 2001; Fox *et al.*, 2005, 2007; Harrison *et al.*, 2008) show greater activation in those task conditions which have some relevance for the individual, while showing less involvement in attention-demanding tasks; hence, the activation of these areas is modulated by task demands (Greicius *et al.*, 2003). Moreover, our data point to the fact that the DMN areas seem to be a preferential network in those people who continuously gather information about the ongoing external context and the Self as their own mode of feeling, namely the Outward group. Moving toward an understanding of emotion–cognition integration (Pessoa, 2008), it seems that self-referential processing can be related both to cognitive functions and to emotional proneness, that is, the way one is affected.

It would thus seem evident that the different ways in which onlookers structure their feelings of personal stability are reflected in the differences in recruiting the brain circuits elicited when empathizing with the pain felt by their partners.

The most interesting aspect that seems to emerge from this study is that human beings experience the empathy for pain on the basis of a distinct affective engagement with the world, thereby suggesting that an embodied emotional style (emotional phenotype) deeply influences the way we perceive and process information in everyday life. In addition to the numerous points of view on the issue of embodiment, such as embodied cognition (Niedenthal, Barsalou and Winkielman, 2005; Niedenthal 2007), phenomenological embodied experience (Gallagher, 2007), radical embodiment (Thompson and Varela, 2001) and embodied simulation (Gallese, 2007), our results suggest that this issue can be investigated through a new perspective that places the different modality of being emotionally situated at the heart of the problem.

In conclusion, rather than suggesting that humans respond on the basis of automatic response mechanisms to shared pain, the present findings support the notion that humans experience the pain empathy subjectively based on distinct affective engagement with Self and environment, underpinned by distinct neural activations. Therefore, these findings indicate that the empathy's core perception–action mechanism, instead of being a 'superordinate class' (Preston and de Waal, 2002) that includes motor behavior and emotional behavior, relies on emotional phenotype.

As we shall see in Part Two, this perspective will provide us with new paths for understanding psychological disturbances.

Endnotes

[1] Cioran (1998).

[2] Heidegger (1986) called the ontological openness – the opening structure – of ipseity to original preverbal signals *Als (As) Hermeneutical*.
The origin of the structure of an assertion is found in *Als Hermeneutioal*, to name but one. For instance, in saying 'This desk is brown', it is the pre-comprehension of the object as that on which one puts one's plate to eat which precedes the assertion and makes that assertion possible. The predication is structured as an '"insofar as', but this structure is derived, not expressed directly, and it possesses this structure only because it is the predication of an experience' (ibid: 97). Those wishing to pursue the issue may consult Volpi (1996).
If we extend this form of practical pre-comprehension to the temporal dimension we can then affirm that the concatenation of experience has a pre-narrative structure which the story itself brings to light. The search after the possible narrative 'is precisely the search for that personal identity which will ensure continuity between the potential, inchoate story and the story which is actually narrated for which we take responsibility' (Ricoeur, 1984, page 122).

[3] Furthermore, these experiences are inscribed within a wider existential context: the finite time span assigned by fate to every living creature, determining not only that creature's life expectancy but also its experience of time. Just think of how differently a four-year-old child experiences time from a forty-year-old adult.

[4] The way the two planes relate to each other is one of the crucial points of the phenomenology of narration of Wilhelm Schapp, whose main work (Schapp, 1976) develops and articulates the originary phenomenon of the 'emerging' (*Auftauchen*) of stories.

[5] False-belief tasks require the subject to predict where a character (e.g. Sally) will look for an object that has been displaced by another character (Anne) unbeknownst to Sally, the child having witnessed where Anne had placed the object after Sally had left the room.

[6] The specific correspondence of child language to action also appears to constitute the basic framework for the language the child employs to talk about the fictional world.

[7] Around the age of four to five, children show evidence of understanding temporal terms referring to sequence (e.g. 'before', 'after', 'next') (Benson, 1997; Nelson, 1993, 1996, 2001). However, it is only at the age of between eight and ten that they come to understand the conventional time terminology of clocks and calendars accurately (Friedman, 2000).

[8] In the same chapter, Hudson (2001: 62) writes: 'Mothers referred to general event knowledge significantly more often when discussing routine events than when discussing novel events, whereas future plans were mentioned significantly more often when discussing novel events than when discussing routine events'.

[9] In the course of infancy, it is the domain of concrete experience that is reconfigured. Access to written language, accelerated in the West by schooling, facilitates the embedding of categorial thought in the narrative dimension of identity (see Arciero, 2002).

[10] This becomes transparent with the production of the adolescent's earliest plans for his future life or under the imperious drive of his first precocious vocations. The tension toward a possible future, one which is within the adolescent's reach, while he redirects his interpretation of real life, gives the adolescent the sensation that he is master of his own existence. This feeling of authorship is accompanied by the conscious experience of his solitude, which reaches the stages of greatest intensity and frequency in the transition phase from late adolescence to early youth (Perlman and Peplau, 1981).

[11] This topic has obsessed psychotherapists for years, since, by assimilating the identity of their clients to that of a thinking thing, they have wasted vast amounts of energy in attempting to explain the dynamics of change in therapy by seeking the relationship with what remains constant. From a conceptual standpoint, these efforts have not brought us one step closer to a picture of identity than that offered by the account of the Argonauts, which was later taken up

again by Hobbes: the ship *Argo* and the combination of the pieces which make up the ship remain identical despite the fact that the pieces are replaced with new ones.

[12] Polanyi (1969: 148) has clarified this concept with great acumen: 'I have shown how our subsidiary awareness of our body is extended to include a stick, when we feel our way by means of a stick. To use language in speech, reading and writing is to extend our bodily equipment and become intelligent human beings. We may say that when we learn to use language, or a probe, or a tool, and thus make ourselves aware of these things as we are of our body, we *interiorize* these things and *make ourselves dwell in them*. Such extensions of ourselves develop new faculties in us; our whole education operates in this way' (original emphasis).

[13] As Ricoeur (1995: 209, note 5) states, 'character is the sameness in (being) always mine'.

[14] The strong emphasis a civilization as early as that of Mesopotamia placed on the honouring of a sworn bond is a significant indication of the value set on giving one's word right from Antiquity. Even under the last of the great Babylonian kings, Nabucodonosor II (605–562 BC), reciprocal relationships were subject to the swearing of an oath – an insuperable barrier and the foundation stone of the empire. Those who failed to honour their word were blinded and could be denied proper burial, and their male offspring had their throats cut (Arnaud, 2004).

[15] The concepts of hyper- and hypocognized emotions were introduced by Levy in order to underline the greater or lesser importance in communication of specific emotions in different cultural contexts.

[16] A number of studies on the organizational nature of the emotional sphere show that emotional precomprehension renders identifying certain classes of emotive expressions in others (Tomkins and McCarter, 1964) and producing certain classes of emotive expressions (Malatesta, Fiore, Messina, 1987; Malatesta and Wilson, 1988; Malatesta, 1990) both easier and more difficult.

[17] Emotional traits will also influence the way information is interpreted (perception, memory, etc.), intrapsychic and behavioural processes (coping) and interpersonal behaviour. To explore this matter in greater depth, see Magai and McFadden (1995).

[18] These two different modalities of permanence – Inward and Outward – toward which one's own body may tend include, in a wider context, that exclusively perceptual permanence of the body on which de Waelhens reflected in the wake of Merleau-Ponty: 'The permanence of the body is not that of a fixed scene presenting itself in the world, but rather its permanence is that of a sort of lateral factor which accompanies all points of view, yet which is incapable either of being eliminated or of being itself defined as a point of view' (de Waelhens, 1951: 119).

[19] But as Heidegger (Heidegger,2001a: 234) says, 'the decisive point in our context is our insight into the immediate emergence of all of so-called material, bodily nature from the physically intangible capacities for receiving-perceiving and for comporting oneself, in which our Dasein in its unfolding essence consists. This insight allows us to grasp easily how immediately and how limitlessly all bodily nature belongs to the [human] way of existing and how it is, and remains, in this mode of *being* [*Seinsart*]'.

[20] 'The might of a certain world' (Merleau-Ponty, 1945).

[21] For a neuroscientific overview of the embodiment of emotions, see Niedenthal (2007).

[22] Heidegger (1962: Paragraph 29). It is precisely through these three vectors – flesh through living perceives itself, opening to the world, and affection – that what Gallagher calls situatedness and what Heidegger had defined as *Befindlichkeit*, namely, finding one is attuned to the situation (*gestimmtes Sichbefinden*), emerges.

[23] Recent studies highlight the fact that such receptivity is correlated with the development of the frontal lobe, which is not completed before the age of 20. This has extremely important ethical repercussions, such as the age at which an adolescent may be charged with a criminal offence. For an interesting viewpoint on this topic, see Beckman (2004).

[24] Space does not permit an in-depth discussion of the relationship between genetic dispositions and the development of bodily structures, leaving aside the important subject of temperament. Those interested in the topic may consult Arciero (2006).

[25] This implies, first and foremost, the distinction between emotion as experienced and emotion as identified and articulated (feeling articulation) (Arciero and Guidano, 2000: 98); and second, the possibility that the articulation of emotional experiences through different cultural matrixes may generate different emotional phenotypes (cultural articulation) (Parkinson, Fischer and Manstead, 2005).

[26] The magnitude of the subjects' activation correlated with the intensity of the pain observed.

[27] On the relationship between expectations of pain and both subjective experience of pain and activation of pain-related brain regions, see Koyama *et al.* (2005).

[28] See also Prkachin *et al.* (2004).

4 Emotioning

We don't learn how to get angry in the first place by following cultural rules, even if those rules are applied to our anger after the fact.[1]

If being situated is mediated by our body proper, and if the mode in which each of us feels himself in various ongoing situations is established by different emotional tones, it would seem to follow that: (1) there is a correlation between bodily states and emotional states; (2) experiencing an emotion corresponds to perceiving a change in one's bodily state. One of James' most famous observations sums up these two points with great simplicity: 'What kind of an emotion of fear would be left, if the feelings neither of quickened heart-beats nor of shallow breathing, neither of trembling lips nor of weakened limbs, neither of goose-flesh nor of visceral stirrings, were present, it is quite impossible to think' (James, 1884: 193).

But does this perspective really account fully for what actually happens in real life?

4.1 Embodied emotions and judgements of the body

Mary has woken later than usual despite the fact that she has an important appointment at the office, for which she now risks arriving late. She gets up hastily, goes under the shower still half-asleep, she gets dressed and has a hurried breakfast. While she's drinking her coffee she sets about getting a taxi. With her ear glued to the receiver, Mary spends a few minutes waiting for a voice to tell her the number of the taxi that is coming to pick her up, becoming more and more impatient as she listens to the tune playing in the background. Finally, the operator's voice comes on . . . but only to tell her there are no taxis available. Mary feels a sudden tension grip her chest, a kind of weight compressing her breastbone extending to her arms, she feels her breath get shorter and her heart beating more quickly – this is how Mary perceives anxiety.

She rushes out into the street, runs towards a busy crossing so as to increase her chances of finding a taxi. She waits five minutes – in vain – and the weight she feels is becomes heavier and heavier. But now she sees a taxi which is free. She gets in and they travel quickly toward her office without the tension in her breast decreasing one iota. The taxi gets to her office, Mary looks at her watch, she still has a few minutes before her

Selfhood, identity and personality styles Giampiero Arciero and Guido Bondolfi

appointment. The weight which was oppressing her disappears like magic. Mary pulls herself together and gets her ideas straight for the coming interview while she goes toward the meeting room quite sure of herself.

In James' analytical framework, Mary's anxiety corresponds to the perception of her bodily change elicited in this specific case by hearing bad news (no taxis available). Emotion, in this view, is feeling a bodily variation – which for James is 'indubitably psychological' (James, 1884) – that is produced as a consequence of an exciting fact.

The objection that may be made to this method of analysing the episode is that, in actual fact, Mary had already reacted with anxiety – without, however, being conscious of the fact – on waking up, when she realized she was late. In other words, Mary might have already been in an unconscious affective state before actually making the phone call – a state which she failed to perceive, since her attention was focused on getting ready to leave the house with the utmost possible speed.

Conceding the possibility that there may exist emotional states that are not consciously perceived seems to go counter to one of the central tenets of James' position, namely, that experiencing emotion corresponds to perceiving a bodily change. Furthermore, some of those emotions which James himself defines as '*subtler*' (James, 1884) – that is, moral, aesthetic or intellectual – do not involve bodily changes.

The 'Neo-Jamesian' solution offered to these objections by Prinz (2003, 2004a, 2004b) extends the idea of bodily changes to the neural substratum, whereas James limited such changes to the purely physiological. Consequently, an unconscious emotion, or even a 'subtler' emotion, may not be perceived in terms of variations in physiological states, but is nevertheless underpinned by a modification in neural dynamics. In conclusion, every emotion must be embodied.

According to Prinz, whose explanation follows Damasio's (1999) conjectures, there exist two levels of bodily representations associated with different cerebral regions: first-order body representations, which correspond to actual body changes (i.e. visceral organs, skeletal muscle, hormonal changes, etc.), and second-order body representations – which Damasio labels the 'as-if loop' – which re-represent the first-order without, however, being accompanied by any actual bodily change. A certain emotion may, therefore, correspond both to a real body change and to the representation of a body change (the 'as-if loop'). 'If an emotion is a representation of a bodily change,' writes Prinz (2004b: 48), 'then the very brain state that underlies that perception must be able to arise in the absence of a bodily change, acting as if the body had changed'.[2]

Although an affective state may be activated at one of the two levels identified by the Neo-Jamesians, for such a state to be perceived it must become the person's focus of attention. In this sense, 'affective states are like visual states: if attention is focused elsewhere, they are not experienced consciously' (Prinz, 2004a: 218). This could account for the existence of unconscious emotions. That is, an affective state, whether it be connected to a change in current body state or not, might be activated outside the subject's conscious focus of attention.

The Neo-Jamesian approach is countered by the cognitive perspective, whose central tenet is that emotions are evaluative judgements (Solomon, 1976; 2003a, 2003b, 2004). In the cognitive account, Mary's emotional state may be considered as constituting the result of the process of evaluating the stimulus situation. In this view, therefore, anxiety corresponds to the judgement that something distressful could have happened if Mary had missed her appointment.

We might object in this case, too, that Mary reacted with anxiety, without being conscious of doing so, the second she realized, on waking up, that she was late. If emotions may be unconscious while judgements appear to imply the use of higher cognitive abilities, how can this perspective account for the production of unconscious judgements?

The solution proposed by Solomon is to reinstate feelings that have been 'left out' of the cognitive account in a new version in which cognition and judgement are 'properly construed'. This renovated interpretation of cognition, which Solomon defines as *judgements of the body* (Solomon, 2003b), comprises a mix of phenomena which go from autonomic manifestations of action readiness to behavioural tendencies and kinaesthetic feelings. The reintegration of the body into the cognitive sphere allows Solomon to state that 'a judgement is not a detached intellectual act, but a way of cognitively *grappling* with the world' (Solomon, 2004: 77). In Mary's case, it is anxiety understood as body judgement – hence unconscious – that is hypothesized as having a determined set of behaviours aimed at diminishing the amount of time by which she would arrive late at work from the very moment she awoke. After all, Solomon (2003a: 10) states, without intending any irony, that 'animals make all sorts of judgements (e.g. whether something is worth eating, or worth chasing, or worth courting)' without activating conscious thought processes.

In support of this extension of the cognitive to the corporeal, in his later writings Solomon assimilates his expanded vision of judgement to practical knowledge – in a rather hazardous fashion, in our opinion – attributing its origins to Heidegger and Merleau-Ponty, Downing, Dreyfus and Bourdieu.

In commenting on the development of these two approaches, Scarantino (2005) quite correctly identifies their common characteristic as being constituted by the modality of their replies to the criticisms levelled at them, and of their attempts at confuting those criticisms. He defines such methods as 'the placeholder strategy'. If, on the one hand, the Neo-Jamesians have completely distorted the meaning assigned by James to the perception of bodily changes, then the cognitivists have done exactly the same thing with the notion of judgement by transforming it into a placeholder.

Our dissatisfaction with these two perspectives is attributable to a more fundamental cause, for we question the very presuppositions on which research on affect is based.

The presupposition concerning the psychology of emotions upon which both approaches are based is the view that man is separate from the world. In this branch of psychology, such a fracture is continually recomposed through access to ongoing situations guaranteed by somatic or cognitive appraisal. The emotions which thus emerge, which can be assimilated in one case to the perception of bodily change and in the other case to propositional as well as nonpropositional judgements, are claimed to correspond to the modification that the organism generates in the course of its ongoing relationship with the world and with others. In both cases, they are said to furnish information on the stimulus situation contributing to the readjustment of the organism's internal dynamics, or, as Griffiths (2004a, 2004b; Griffiths and Scarantino, 2008) puts it, to the internal psychological economy of the organism.

However, what if instead of examining emotion as information that a body system is capable of generating (though bodily arousal or evaluative judgements) about a given state of the world, we were to think of the body, of being my body and its diverse modes, as that field that is lit up together with what is significant in the world? That is, if, rather than looking at emotions as internal meanings of an external stimulus situation, we were to consider experiencing emotions as a way of perceiving oneself and concurrently a way of manifesting itself of the world? If the significativity of events were to reveal itself contemporaneously with one's way of feeling that which is proper to oneself? If experiencing emotion were to correspond to this incessant encounter between one's own possibilities and the way the world appears? If experiencing e-motion really were that uninterrupted movement from . . . as the etymology of the word (*ex-movere*) suggests?

4.2 E-moting

A series of studies inaugurated by Fridlund (1994, 1997) moves in this direction. In opposition to Ekman's affect programs theory, Fridlund shifts the focus of attention on to the social situatedness of emotions.

As is known, in Ekman's (2003) view basic emotions constitute the mode in which human beings are biologically prepared to respond to specific stimuli ('universal triggers') that are fundamental to remaining alive. They are thus elicited, like a sort of reflex, when the organism encounters environmental stimuli which involve those universal themes that it has always been sensitive to. In order for that to happen, the organism is equipped with mechanisms which Ekman has dubbed 'automatic appraisal mechanisms' and which enable an emotional response to be activated independently of any cognitive evaluation.

On the other hand, according to Fridlund and others (Parkinson, 1995; Parkinson, Fischer and Manstead, 2005; Russell and Fernández-Dols, 1997; Russell *et al.*, 2003), rather than being reflex-like modifications produced by the organism, which may be more or less disguised in daily interaction, emotions are produced and expressed as negotiating signals between organisms in an ongoing social transaction. That is to say, the organism generates expressive emotional behaviours as a way of influencing the conduct of other organisms inasmuch as – Fridlund (1997) argues – vigilance for and comprehension of signals co-evolved with the signals themselves.[3] This different emphasis appears forcefully in two oft-quoted studies by Fernandez-Dols and Ruiz-Belda (1995, 1997) on a gold medallist at the 1992 Barcelona Olympics and on soccer fans watching goals scored by their own team. Both studies showed that instead of being part of the automatic expression of happiness, as argued by Ekman (1972), genuine smiles – the Duchenne smile – occurred almost exclusively when the medallist or the fans interacted with others (namely, smiled to the audience or to another fan). In contrast to Ekman's affective programs, 'happiness per se was not a sufficient cause for smiling' (Fernandez-Dols and Ruiz-Belda, 1997: 269). The authors suggested that while experiencing happiness facilitates smiling, social interaction is the precipitating factor.

An equally frequently-cited study (Kraut and Johnston, 1979, replicated by Ruiz-Belda *et al.*, 2003) on bowlers' behaviour led to the same conclusions: in the course of the game, bowlers' smiles were affected – after rolling the ball – by watching the faces of their bowling companions, rather than by the outcome of the roll.

The correlation between smiling and social interaction is underscored by observation of children (Jones, Collins and Hong, 1991; Schneider and Unzner, 1992; Soussignan and Schaal, 1996). In addition, even facial expressions for pain (Beavin Bavelas *et al.*, 1986), for tastes (Brighton *et al.*, 1977) and for smells (Gilbert, Fridlund and Sabini, 1987) are facilitated by an appropriate social context.

These studies indicate that smiles and other emotional expressions correspond not only to emotional experiences, but also to a communicative gesture of the emoter, produced as a *move* in the ongoing context of occurrence.[4] Fridlund interprets these moves as strategic, that is, as issued to influence the interactant and thus 'serving one's social motives in that context' (Fridlund, 1997: 123). The other side of the coin is that the interactants in turn influence the manifestation of the sender's expressions – Fridlung's audience effect – as if in the course of an ongoing interaction the emoter bore in mind a series of environmental affordances, which allowed or disallowed certain moves in the context of a certain type of social interaction. Hence, the various emotions are shaped in contingent fashion by the interaction itself.

The emphasis on the strategic aspect of the production of emotions, within the framework of an ongoing social interaction, characterizes the further development of the research opened up by Fridlung. This approach, which we shall call *transactionalist* (Scarantino, 2005), interprets emotional signals as being prevalently (though not exclusively) produced for purposes of negotiation or, rather, produced in order to promote the emoter's interests during the course of social transactions (Parkinson, Fischer and Manstead, 2005). The term 'strategic' – which, if truth be told, is misleading, given the connotation of pretence implicit in the term's meaning – indicates precisely this phenomenon of the promotion of one's personal advantage, which the emoter achieves by emotionally influencing those with whom he interacts (Griffiths, 1997, 2004a, 2004b; Griffiths and Scarantino, 2008). Viewed in this light, emotions are considered to be 'more or less effective goal-oriented responses' (Griffiths and Scarantino, 2008) in relation to affordances (opportunities) offered on-line to the emoter, either by the ongoing situation or by the response of the interactant in the context of an evolving mutual transaction. One piece of evidence that is often quoted in support of the strategic hypothesis, and which aims to underscore the goal-directedness of an emotional state, is a study by Stein, Trabasso and Liwag (1993) which shows that the possibility of obtaining compensation produces a response to loss that is not so much sadness as anger.

Clearly, this 'strategic' dimension of affect cannot be taken into account by either the Neo-Jamesian approach or the cognitivist stance, since both focus on a kind of emotional solipsism. The shift in focus from internal to interpersonal processes brings to the fore two aspects of great importance, which are intertwined and which we must examine:

a. the temporal dynamics of the unfolding of emotion, which is implicit in the conceptualization of emotions as social transaction;
b. the *e-motions* of the interactants, the reciprocal *moves* which the transactionalists consider to be goal-oriented responses emitted in the course of the interaction.

We will now analyse the episode concerning Mary once again, but this time in the light of this new approach.

Mary looks at her watch and realizes it's late. The significance of her being late derives from matching Mary's expectations of being on time for the appointment and the fact that she has less time than she had planned to reach the office. It is precisely the realization of being late that changes the possible actions Mary can take. That is, the meaning Mary assigns to being late corresponds to a change in her mode of feeling and, at the same time, to the manifesting of the world to her in terms of possible new actions (and of obstacles to the realization of those novel actions) that will enable her to arrive on time. That is why her behaviour betrays urgency.

The first hitch arises when she cannot find a taxi. Thus, the unavailability of a taxi produces new environmental affordances, obliging Mary to revise the embodied meaning of the ongoing situation, thereby generating a new set of viable options. As the world progressively unfolds itself to Mary in terms of obstacles, Mary reacts by remapping the ongoing context in terms of possible actions, which are even more pressing together, but which are still more uncertain as the possibility of not being able to arrive on time draws nearer. Anxiety would thus appear to prefigure a range of possible actions and perceptions and, at the same time, the possibility that those actions might fail.

It is this new situation – stated differently, anxiety – which drives Mary to leave the house in search of a taxi and which become progressively stronger as Mary's hopes of finding a taxi become weaker and weaker. This emotional state continues throughout her journey to the office, playing, as it were, the role of navigator. Her feeling of oppression disappears only when she looks at her watch on reaching the office. The disappearance of this feeling of oppression is accompanied by the concurrent disappearance of that geography of relevant facts which had characterized the way the world appeared to Mary until just a few seconds earlier. The state of calmness which takes over corresponds to a new range of possible behaviours and, at the same time, to the emergence of a number of different elements that are significant in the ongoing situation and that afford, or fail to afford, new possibilities of meaning.

The analysis of this episode, which involves the presence of other people only indirectly, would seem to indicate that *e-motioning* corresponds, as indicated by the Latin etymology of the word, precisely to the *motion from* a certain context by means of the generation of a new set of possible actions and perceptions – hence, possible new forms of skilful engagement with the environment – which the on-line manifestation of different situations suggests. Emotioning would thus appear to be a continual variation of modes of feeling situated – that is, related – to new possibilities of action, a continual reorientation of oneself in relation to the development of the ongoing context that is remodulated in the practical engagement, rather than coming to an abrupt end as in one-shot reflex-like activation.[5] It would thus seem inappropriate to conceptualize emotions in terms of 'dynamic dispositions of the body (including the nervous system) to action, which specify at every moment the organism's domain of action' (Maturana, 1994). It is the ongoing situation in which one *finds* oneself that determines whether one feels in one way or another. That specific condition (the way we feel at a given moment) represents the starting point from which we see the possibilities that determine the way we feel situated. To return to our example, it is from the moment that Mary learns that no taxis are available that she feels tension in her chest, and it is starting from this condition that she examines with an even greater sense of urgency both those actions that are possible, and the possibilities that each of those actions has of failing. That is how Mary feels situated.

In other words, the fact that one finds oneself in a certain emotional state always depends on finding oneself in a given situation and on the mode in which one is inclined to react to the circumstances. Emotioning cannot be separated from these two aspects as if the original relationship was in no way involved, as if emotion were a condition caused by this or that other and which presents itself as an independent entity. The fundamental feature of emotioning consists precisely in this: a mode of feeling refers to a situation, and the situation reciprocally manifests its significativity revealing itself according to the mode of situated feeling (Arciero, 1988). This is the type of experience that induced Sartre, most probably influenced by Janet's studies on obsession, to speak of emotion as almost being an act of magic which allows one to transform the world. 'The impossibility of finding a solution to the problem objectively apprehended as a quality of the world,' writes Sartre (Sartre,1948: 60), 'serves as motivation for the new unreflective consciousness which now perceives the world otherwise and with a new aspect, and which requires a new behavior – through which this aspect is perceived – and which serves as hyle for the new intention.'

4.3 E-moting with others

Thus, at the level of affectivity we again encounter that dialectic between ipseity and alterity to which we referred in the preceding chapter: feeling oneself in this way or in that intertwines with how oneself is affected by the other.[6] But how exactly is emotional unfolding connected to the way the social context evolves? What happens when the context of emotioning consists of the emotional behaviour of another person?

Let us imagine a row between Joe and Anne which starts over a trifle – Joe has forgotten to buy the milk. Anne brusquely points out that she is the one who will have to do without since she is the first to leave the house in the morning. Joe replies in an irritated fashion that he is sick and tired of continually being reproached. Anne stiffens and, raising her voice, she points out that in addition to going out to work, she also takes care of the household affairs and she cannot go on like that. Banging his fist on the table, Joe shouts that it's about time they separated.

Now let us imagine two endings to this scenario.

Scenario 1. Anne is struck dumb and silently continues doing the cooking with a frown on her face. After a few minutes, Joes goes up to her to make amends with an affectionate gesture, but Anne rejects him abruptly. At table she doesn't say a word. Joe awkwardly tries to beg her pardon. Anne accepts his apologies without putting up any great resistance, but she repeats that they must thrash out new rules for living together because the present situation has brought her to the end of her tether. She is still wearing that frown on her face. Joe admits she is right and says in his defence that his fading interest in the last few months is not due to a change in his feelings toward Anne, but to the tension created by a situation at work which will determine the outcome of his future career and, consequently, their economic future. Anne's frown gradually disappears, her look softens into tenderness and her tone becomes friendly.

Scenario 2. Anne starts crying, and, with tears in her eyes, she shouts that she cannot stand it any longer, so they had better put an end to it. Joe starts insulting her and, with a cry of rage, says he doesn't love her any more. As if hit by a bullet, incredulous, wounded, irate, and with a sombre expression on her face, Anne walks silently off to her study. An hour later she is packing her case to leave. When Joe realizes this, he first tries to dissuade her, unsuccessfully. Then he starts putting the blame on her behaviour, and finally he begs her not to leave him. Anne, totally resolved, her face still frowning, and without saying a word, opens the door and leaves home.

If we go back over the sequence from the beginning, looking at it from Anne's point of view, we will see that the significativity of the episode stems from the mismatch between her expectations and Joe's lack of consideration. The meaning Anne attributes to this situation corresponds to an *alter*ation to her way of feeling – experienced as anger – and at the same time as the emergence of a range of possible actions aiming to modify Joe's conduct. The development, together with the manifestation of the various action tendencies which that emotion of anger allows, depends on the interactant's response, which in turn is connected to the emotive signals as comprehended by the emoter.

If we analyse the first part of the episode, Anne's remonstrations are followed by a series of exchanges which become increasingly more aggressive. Then the situation evolves in different ways, depending on whether the discussion unfolds along the lines of the first scenario or the second. It seems obvious, in fact, that the different ways the two scenes develop both emerge in the very course of the interaction itself, through a continuous and reciprocal readjustment of the possibilities of meaning in relation to the emotive signals received by the other.[7] Seen from this standpoint, reciprocal emotional conduct appears as an indication which everyone uses each and every time to renegotiate his/her relationship with the other, to situate him/herself in relation to the other. The 'strategic' aspect of the expression of emotion, a point which the transactionalists insist on, is thus claimed to be closely connected to the negotiation – in real time – of one's role in the relationship.[8]

In the first scenario, as Griffiths (2004b) says, 'sulking can be seen as a strategy for seeking a better global deal in that particular relationship'. In the second scenario, instead, sulking may be seen as a mode of conduct aiming at bringing the relationship to an end. In both cases, emotion may be accounted for starting from the emoter's aim, which is, of course, to influence the behaviour of other organisms, in an effort to promote the emoter's interests in the course of social transactions (Parkinson, Fischer and Manstead, 2005).

But does this new emphasis on real-time interaction, which allows transactionalists to capture phenomena that other theories were unable to detect – temporal unfolding, the relevance of social context, reciprocal influence in the production and expression of emotions, the opening up of new possibilities of actions and relationships – not bypass the experiential aspect of emotioning? Put differently, does this approach not exclude the very fact that emotion always belongs to someone? The being-mine of emotional experience, which indubitably cannot correspond to 'the internal psychological economy of the organism', cannot even be neutralized by an impersonal description, as if emotioning did not belong to anyone. Stated differently, we cannot assimilate the person to emotion being experienced as if the person were such thanks to the emotion he is experiencing, as if the goal of an emotion provided a complete account of the emoter, as if the experience of an emotion on the part of a human being were not concurrently and inextricably intertwined with a personal life story from which it receives, and to which it gives, directionality.

The episode of Joe and Anne helps to clarify this point. The different ways the stories develop – reconciliation or separation – cannot be attributed simply to the dynamics of goal-oriented negotiation. The dimension of personal experience adds new factors to this type of explanation. These factors derive from the integration of personal experience into a set of actions and passions that is reconfigured into a more or less cohesive totality: the narrative of Self. It is the connection between the ongoing emotional episode within the story of each of the two partners which furnishes the context that makes sense of the two different developments and their respective outcomes. The fact, that is, that the episode is part of the story of a person places that person in a plot, from which the episode receives new determinations of meaning which make that experience unique.

Thus, in order to comprehend why a situation should veer in one direction rather than another, understanding the emotional dynamics of the situation starting from the interactants' goals, the achievement of which determines the reciprocal position the partners take in the course of the negotiation, is not enough. It is also necessary to identify the personal context of meaning in which an episode is set, since this furnishes the determinations of each actor, which make the event intelligible. In the case we are examining, for example, this consists of the state and the history of the relationship as it has been experienced by each of the partners, their level of personal involvement, what is for them the acceptable form of emotional reciprocity, individual and joint planning, and so forth. It is only if we possess this background knowledge that we can understand why the same emotional episode can develop along different lines, why the same manifestation of emotion generated from similar events can lead to different outcomes. Hence, in addition to embodying an emotion every single moment of his life, a person is also the cohesion of a history of emotions which reactualizes itself each and every time in the ongoing emotional condition.

4.4 Emotional inclinations

Being emotionally situated thus corresponds to a tension which is born and which is continually renewed in the sphere of social and practical engagement but which, at the same time, reflects and actualizes the story of the emoter. This encounter enables the emoter to orient himself in the world each and every time, grasping those elements of significavity and the geography of saliences, generating the possibilities of action which are most attuned to the emerging contexts. Viewed in this light, already at a pre-reflective level, e-moting is the embodied meaning of the ongoing situation, perceived as a global mode of feeling and concurrently as a relational domain.

It is on this interpersonal space, marked by the polarity body proper–other, that we must now focus our attention. Depending on the modality of emoting, within this space the emphasis on the body proper, or on the other, changes, hence the inclination of personal stability. In the first case, as we have seen, the hypercognition of basic emotions will shift the gravitational centre of this dialectic on to a referential context which predominantly uses a body-centred coordinate system, thereby a sense of stability that is prevalently centred on 'Inward' states. It is obvious, from this standpoint, that emotional experience is closely connected to the perception of body signals. It is closer to the description provided by James. Moreover, many studies underscore the fact that variations in sensitivity to visceral activity are related to variations in the intensity of subjective emotional experience (Yates *et al.*, 1985; Wiens, Mezzacappa and Katkin, 2000; Wiens and Palmer, 2001; Barrett *et al.*, 2004).

In the other case, the most important activation of non-basic emotions will lead to that space gravitating around a referential frame that uses a system of coordinates which is anchored to alterity, thus giving rise to a sense of permanence oriented principally to 'Outward' referents. What is most evident from this other perspective is that alterity – understood as a type of anchorage used to maintain one's stability over time (people, contexts, images, thoughts, rules, etc.) – becomes the source of information to recognize one's own emotional experience, hence becoming part of that experience.

As we have emphasized a number of times, one perceives alterity and simultaneously co-perceives oneself. This might explain why so-called interdependent Self-construals tend not only to assimilate others to the Self cognitively, emotionally and perceptually (Markus and Kitayama, 1991; Stapel and Koomen, 2001), but also why they tend more to nonconsciously mimic others' habitual movements than do independent Self-construals (Van Baaren *et al.*, 2003; Ashton-James *et al.*, 2007).[9] But it might also account for differences between groups in emotional empathy. In fact, in a study by Sonnby-Borgström (2002), high-empathy subjects were found to exhibit a higher degree of mimicking behaviour than low-empathy subjects when exposed to pictures of angry and happy faces.

With regard to the Outward dimension, therefore, emotional experience appears to be nearer to the descriptions provided of it by the cognitivists and by the social constructionists. For the cognitivists, the anchorage system could be constituted by the evaluative framework, for instance, while for the social constructionists it could be the sociocultural system.

If the Inward–Outward inclinations represent two polar opposites governing the perception of personal stability, from an experimental standpoint the difference in structuring the emotional domain should produce in the two groups the activation of different neural areas in response to exactly the same emotional stimulus. This is the hypothesis behind Bertolino *et al.*'s (2005) fMRI study in which the two groups of testees were presented with a series of images, consisting of three faces (two of which were identical) expressing fear, and were asked to identify which of the three faces were identical (incidental processing). The two groups of subjects were also comparable with regard to the genetic features of the serotonin transporter, which, as demonstrated by Hariri *et al.* (2002), may modify the activity of specific neuroanatomic structures, such as the amygdala, during the implicit processing of faces expressing fear.

In line with Bertolino *et al.*'s hypothesis, subjects manifesting an Inward style personality tending to phobic disorders exhibited greater activation of the amygdala, of the hippocampus and of the mesial prefrontal cortex. On the other hand, Outward style subjects tending to eating disorders exhibited more intensive activation of the fusiform gyrus, of the associative occipital cortex and of the dorsolateral prefrontal cortex.

The analysis of the data obtained from 24 subjects confirmed the initial hypothesis, that is to say that the meaning which the stimulus had for the two groups was different, since the activity in some regions of the neural networks involved was not the same. Phobic-prone (PP) Inward subjects activated neural circuits primarily associated with fear in general and with its visceral correlates (amygdala), which leads one to surmise – in people with that kind of personality – a more pronounced sensitivity to stimuli giving rise to alarm. Outward subjects prone to eating disorders (EDP), instead, activated areas assigned to the recognition of facial features, in addition to those allocated to the integration of emotions and cognitive functions, orienting the subject toward a greater sensitivity to 'cold' facial features.

A subsequent fMRI study (Rubino *et al.*, 2007), whose findings are consistent with ours, showed that the explicit recognition of fearful and angry faces (cognitive labelling) elicited different areas of activation in two groups of 14 subjects each, one consisting of Inward PP, the other made up of Outward EDP. More specifically, PP subjects compared to EDP subjects exhibited far greater engagement of the medial PFC (BA 9), whose activity is associated with cognitive aspects that are closely related to emotional processing.

These differing emotional polarizations – which demarcate a continuum along which the Inward and Outward tendencies combine to different degrees and in different ways in every individual, and which change in the course of one's life[10] – enable one to grasp at a single glance the subjective variety of emotional experience, the modalities of emotional regulation and the roots of personal identity.

In Part Two of this book, we shall see that, starting from these different emotional inclinations, it is possible to develop a theory of personality and of psychopathology.

The different polarizations also help account for the special emphasis placed upon the corporeal aspects which characterizes both the Neo-Jamesian and the affect program theory approaches, albeit to different degrees; for the focalization on cognitive aspects, to which Solomon has paid great attention in his work; and, finally, for the vital importance of sociocultural aspects, which have been investigated in depth by the social constructionists. Emotional experience, whose basic components are visceral or cognitive, or which is connected to social awareness, corresponds, that is, to privileged modalities of engagement, to different ways of perceiving one's own referential centre of gravity. In this sense, the different forms of emotional experience may be understood within the continuum created by the two polarities, Inward and Outward, which refer to the referential coordinates that enable one to feel situated.[11]

To complete the picture, at this point we must briefly examine the constructionist view, which not only furnishes the clearest examples of the Outward mode of constituting the emotional sphere, but which also opens up a new perspective on the mode of emoting which characterizes contemporary Western society.

4.5 Constructionist situatedness

In the constructionists' view, emotion corresponds to a given position of the Self as defined by roles, norms, contexts and discursive practices that a given society generates, which is functional to its maintenance and/or to the stability of the individual who interprets that particular position as being the one he occupies.[12] Emotion arises, that is, as a deliberate attempt to conform to a given social model, which in some cases is perceived as inevitable and beyond individual control. For the subject who lives out that model, as well as for society, such behaviour is absolutely involuntary, whereas for an observer it appears to reflect given rules of the society the person lives in.

If we take the Gururumba, a people of New Guinea, for example, feeling in a particular mood or state called 'being a wild pig' is experienced as producing acts for which the individual cannot be held responsible. In this sense, emotion is seen as socially constructed or, as Averill (1985) puts it, as a transitory social role. This 'illness', which affects young adults between the ages of 25 and 35, is believed to be caused by the bite of the ghost of a member of the tribe who has died recently. Those affected by it run around madly attacking whoever is nearby and throwing objects. Not only does the tribe tolerate the antisocial behaviour of the sick person, but the affected individual is given special consideration. The explanation furnished by the anthropologist, as an external observer, is that the 'wild pig role' seems to emerge when a young man has just got married and is subjected to economic pressures which he cannot face. By interpreting the 'wild pig role', he is accorded the consideration of his tribe members, who recognize that he is in a special condition without, however, denying the legitimacy of the obligations which the young man must at some point come to terms with. Society and the sick man both live the 'wild pig role' as involuntary.

Hacking (1995) believes that an analogous condition in the West is represented by the multiple personality syndrome. The epidemic of cases of this type, which has swamped the West in recent years, is hypothesized as being socially constructed, just as the 'wild pig' malady is a constructed phenomenon. According to Hacking (1995), individuals who suffer from a sense of a fragmented identity are gradually trained by their therapists to channel that malaise into forms which are consistent with current theory. That is to say, they are instructed in how to be multiple personalities and the therapist's diagnosis facilitates their being socially accepted as being ill. This has produced a phenomenon of gigantic proportions, with the birth of support groups, associations, television programmes that have further amplified the production of the symptomatology. Even in the case of the multiple personality syndrome – as with the 'wild pig role' – society and the individual 'cooperate' to define the behaviour that is classified as 'sick' as an action in which the agent has no responsibility inasmuch as it is the consequence of circumstances beyond his control (Hacking, 1995; Griffiths, 1997).

This new function of emotions, almost the watchdog of the values of a certain type of society, perhaps becomes even more evident in contemporary Western society in what we might define as the behaviours of the 'happy consciousness' (Marcuse, 1964). These behaviours correspond to a set of prepackaged possible images of the Self, which a given society recognizes as adequate and which furnish the models to which to anchor oneself in order to give shape to one's identity. 'Being nice' is one eloquent exemplification of these 'modes of conformity'.

'Being nice,' writes Mestrovic (1997: 51), 'is an intricate act that involves the manipulation of self and others in highly predictable and deliberate ways, including one's physical appearance, language, tone, eye contact, choice of clothing, smile, choice and length of conversation, among a myriad of other factors. The average middle-class child today knows the social formula for being "nice" unconsciously . . . and everyone today knows the importance of "having to be nice to everybody" in every profession.'

Consequently, if the emotional order is socially constructed, it reflects the specific conceptions of the particular culture which constructed it. Thus, different cultures manifest different modes of emoting. The constructionists have supplied a host of examples to illustrate this point. One of the most famous, which concerns a sentiment termed *fago*, was described by Catherine Lutz (1988) in a well-known study eloquently entitled 'Unnatural Emotions'. This sentiment, which is characteristic of a population living on the atoll of Ifaluk in the Southwest Pacific, corresponds, from a Western viewpoint, to a kind of contradictory mixture of love, compassion and sadness.

A large part of the argumentative force of the constructionist approach has developed by placing the social and cultural aspects of emotion in the forefront, in open contrast to the naturalist perspective. In the course of this polemic, a few years ago one of the most perspicacious adherents of the constructionist school, Ron Harré, underlined the fact that, instead of concretely studying how people get angry, fall in love, become anxious and suffer in daily situations, philosophers and psychologists generally draw from such situations abstract essences which they call rage, anxiety, sadness and love, and then ask themselves the question 'What is anger?', 'What is love?' and so forth. But perhaps, Harré (1986) asserted, the question should be set in a different way. Perhaps it would be wiser to ask oneself how the word 'anger' has been used in relation to that particular episode and within that culture. There might be natural reactions that accompany anger, such as, for instance, an increase in the heartbeat, but such factors must be considered incidental, 'leakages into consciousness', in Harré's view. 'The dominant contribution to the way in which the emotional sphere develops in the course of our lives derives from our local social world, through the linguistic practices and the moral judgments which characterize that world, and on the basis of which the emotional quality of human encounters are defined' (Harré, 1986: 105).

The most striking aspect of the constructionist perspective, however, is not so much the reproposal in a new light of the old 'nature versus nurture' opposition, which has occupied much of the debate on the social construction of emotions (Parkinson, 1995; Parkinson, Fischer and Manstead, 2005; Griffiths, 1997, 2003), as the possibility that this approach offers of thinking about a phenomenon which is absolutely unique to Western societies: the acceleration in the change of contexts and of the emotional states related to those contexts, an acceleration generated by the impact of technology on human life. The unprecedented expansion of the 'technologies of sociation' – as Kenneth Gergen (1991) has dubbed them – has led to a dramatic increase in the range of significant people and in modes of contact, favouring a plethora of emotional states that are synchronic with the social contexts in which they occur, and that are rapidly modifiable parallel to the speed at which the circumstances change. Such simultaneity accounts for why emoting has become for many a mediated fact; that is to say, emotions have become more volatile and 'less passionate' inasmuch as they are tied to situations which change swiftly. This relative lack of viscerality makes them accessible in a way that is different from the past: they are almost consumer products!

The most clear-cut evidence testifying to this state of affairs concerns the constitution of virtual communities, a reality that is possible thanks to relationships which take shape through the coordination of discursive configurations (chat rooms, for instance) that convey emotional states. Daily participation in situations of pure interrelationships, without individuals being present in flesh and blood, creates a virtual space in which a person may generate several levels of affectivity simultaneously, without their having anything whatsoever to do with the existence of 'real Selves' in the more traditional sense of the concept. The reflection of this mode of being may be captured in the composing of new diaries that are presented to the eyes of the world in the 'blogsphere', to be found on the Web. In these diaries, daily intimacy with Self is exhibited to others without showing oneself; identity is manifested without a face before an enormous, eyeless crowd.

4.6 The impact of technology

The acceleration in the change of the Self generated in relation to technological development has a history. It is presented to Western consciousness in a literary text:

Sentimental Education by Gustave Flaubert (2002). Rapidity penetrates literature almost as if it had been imposed by the radical modifications which technology began to produce in the domain of practical experience. Speed in Flaubert's novel is manifested in the plot as discontinuity between one scene and another, sudden transitions, unexpected changes, 'a white space . . . while the measure of time moves on suddenly from quarters of an hour to years, to decades' (Flaubert, 2002).

It is that 'white space' that Proust (1927) recognized as '*la chose la plus belle*' in *Sentimental Education*. It is that white space which imposes itself in all its ambiguous potential in a crucial part of the text, when Frederic witnesses the killing of Dussardier perpetrated by his old friend Senecal:

> *. . . he fell to the ground, his arms sprawled out.*
>
> *A cry of terror came from the crowd; with a glance the policeman made the crowd give way to him; and Frederic, his mouth wide open, recognized Senecal.*
>
> *He travelled. He became acquainted with the melancholy of boats, cold awakenings under tents, the amazement of landscapes and ruins, the bitterness of interrupted likings (Flaubert, 2002).*
>
> *A brilliant analysis by Carlo Ginzburg (2000) leads us on to the tracks of the white space. Exhibiting all the mastery of a great historian, Ginzburg demonstrates that that broken style which decomposed reality into a sequence of discrete scenes 'brought to light the implications of the new technologies with regard to the perception of reality': of the diorama, of the train, of photography.*
>
> . . .

The impact of technology on the speed of perceptual experience generates new forms of vision that are reflected in narration. Observing the world from a fast means of locomotion, such as, for example, through the window of a train carriage, shatters reality into discrete frames, into photographs which have to be mounted back into their original sequence. It is no coincidence that a critic of the time who failed to grasp the enormous innovatory importance of the work wrote: 'The book is badly written. We see characters, scenes, file by before our eyes, but in a casual manner. The impression is that of being presented with a series of frames or with a set of photographs' (Scherer, quoted in Ginzburg, 2000).

Flaubert is the first to realize what is happening on a wide scale a few decades later, when, with technology penetrating the world of information transmission (telegraph and telephone, and later the radio) and of the reproduction of experience (the cinema), speed silently insinuates itself into daily life, creating previously unknown tensions and eliciting new types of emotions.

For instance, the use of the telephone obliges the user to develop a new capacity to focalize attention that was undoubtedly unknown to those who were used to communicating via letters. A historian of the period noted that 'the use of the telephone has given rise to a new mental habit. Our previous lazy and sluggish attitude has undergone a change . . . life has become more tense, vigilant and vivacious. The brain has been relieved from the anxiety of waiting for a reply . . . it receives that reply instantaneously, and is thus free to consider other matters' (Kern, 1983).

Furthermore, the consequences of the cinema forcing itself into the collective consciousness can be inferred from the reactions of the first inexpert viewers. Kern reports that on seeing a train enter a station on the screen, some of the audience wanted to dive under the chairs in order to avoid being hit by the locomotive. Others complained that creating the continuity of the story by mounting successive scenes made the story incomprehensible. In other words, such people were unable to integrate the sequences into a unified narrative. While the cinema reproduced a given reality according to certain relevance criteria, it imposed a new mode of experiencing.

The number of radio listeners and spectators is a sufficient comment by itself on how much transmission technology and the reproduction of experience – only a few decades following their introduction – saturated everyday life in America. In 1930, 46% of Americans owned a radio, while in 1940 the figure had reached 80%. In 1929, 95 million Americans went to the cinema once a week, whereas in the course of the 1940s – before the advent of television – going to the 'cinema was as much a part of the American way of life as watching television is today' (Singer and Singer, 2001).

The coming on to the scene of television changed this scenario. The 1950s represent the Golden Age of television and of information technology. Millions of people changed the speed and quality of their internal states as a result of television's influence.

4.7 Technological tuning

Trying to be on the same wavelength as external sources, as a means of creating and maintaining one's own identity, constitutes the distinctive feature of the new 'mode of conformity'. The sensitivity required to capture signals coming from others thus becomes the fundamental feature characterizing the shared experience of individuals belonging to certain social classes (mainly the upper-middle class). David Reisman (1961), who analysed this new form of 'social character' at the beginning of the 1950s, labels as 'other-directed' individuals living in that society and as 'hetero-directed' the society in which they live.

In Reisman's view, the emergence of other-directed characters is accompanied by a 'process of the redistribution of words' capable of generating more socialized forms of behaviour. The strong drive toward this modification derives from the impact of information technology on the relationship that contemporary man has with himself, with others and with the world. What changes is that such a relationship, which in the type that Reisman labels 'inner-directed'[13] was structured through a rigid adherence to models conforming to tradition, is now mediated by 'currents of discourses and images' transmitted by the mass media. For the inner-directed man, that is, a large part of the social world coincided with the local community to which he belonged, whose fabric was made up of social relationships founded on reciprocal knowledge and whose limits were clearly defined. As Baumann (2003: 17) writes, 'Within this network of familiar relationships which went from the cradle to the grave, the place each person occupied was so obvious that it needed no evaluation, even less did it need to be negotiated'.

In societies directed by tradition, the construction and maintenance of personal identity aims essentially at maintaining stability, and this reflects the fact that relationships with others are solid, and defined and structured in accordance with the social rules laid down by that society. In fact, it is rare for an individual, even if he is 'maladjusted', to be cast out of the society (understood as *Gemeinschaft*).

In addition, in a context of habit which remained constant for the majority of the population in the course of a lifetime, they could count on a consolidated set of rules and models, and on emotions connected to these rules and models, in order to guarantee the constancy of their personal identity and, concurrently, the stability of their interrelationships. When the control of the primary group responsible for socialization ceases to exist, the 'well-adjusted' individual orients himself in the social world by focusing on sedimented aspects of interiority (cognitive and emotional aspects), by means of that mechanism which Reisman calls the 'psychological gyroscope'. 'Once parents and other authorities have set it in motion, this tool keeps the inner-directed person "on course", even when tradition no longer regulates his movements' (Reisman, 1961: 75).

By contrast, the other-directed individual learns to look at the immense stage of reality represented by the media to find guidelines on which to model his actions and emotions, his images and discourses, to which to adapt himself, and by means of which he can recognize himself (Arciero, 2002). On the one hand, this corresponds to the breakdown of the boundaries of the individual's community and a consequent opening out on to social relationships going beyond those boundaries. On the other hand, in order to feel situated, the individual seeks to tune into significant signals coming from global society (understood as *Gesellschaft*). Yet again, the present-day relevance of Reisman's (1961: 37) words cannot cease to amaze us: 'the goals toward which the other-directed person strives shift with that guidance: it is only the process of striving itself and the process of paying close attention to the signals from others that remain unaltered throughout life'.

This exceptional 'inclination toward people' becomes the individual's primary resource, and in many cases it is the fundamental resource, by means of which to constructs his personal identity. Thus, in other-directed societies, the construction and maintenance of identity, which can no longer count on places of belonging and on the relationships built up historically in those places, sets a new problem: how can an individual maintain a sense of personal stability when sensitivity to others and the need for the definition and confirmation of one's own identity require, instead, an extraordinary capacity for change and variability?

4.8 Mediated affective engagement

The most interesting aspect of the foregoing discussion is that this mode of organizing identity has as its counterpart the emergence of a vast range of 'new' emotions ('new' in the sense of emotions that have been socially transformed), through which the other becomes part of one's own emotional experience. Think, for example, of how, by way of engagement with the other, 'socially aware emotions' come into being, including: ambivalence, ambiguity, indefiniteness, vagueness, complicity, yieldingness, complacency. These emotions have a high percentage content of social awareness insofar as they must be generated in tune with circumstances, and must be relatively *superficial*, since it must be possible to redeploy them (managed or played) in a relatively flexible manner and they must be capable of rapid change. They are therefore less involving because they have been 'cleansed' of their viscerality, but they are also more articulated and individualized. Analogously to the experiment carried out by Schachter and Singer (1962), rather than corresponding to a particular quality of bodily perception, the identity of an emotion is triggered by social cues.

One effect of great interest created by the 'mediation' of feeling is the division between the sphere of emotion and that of action. At the first stage of modern thought, this is what Descartes (1650: 40th Article) had to say: 'For it must be observed that the principal effect of all the passions in men is, they incite and dispose their souls to will the things for which they prepare their bodies so that the resentment of fear incites him to be willing to fly; that of boldness, to be willing to fight, and so of the rest'.

In traditional societies, this definition of the connection between emotion and action implied a sort of concrete commitment to coherence and authenticity, or at the very least the expectation that certain emotions would be followed by appropriate actions – inasmuch as certain emotions led 'naturally' to actions that were congruous with those emotions. This type of expectation is, however, misleading when attempting to comprehend the way of feeling (the social character) of other-directed societies.[14] The 'natural' relationship between emotion and action is severed. Not only is the type of emotion that is to be felt in relation to a given event evaluated strategically – and it also poses problems of authenticity[15] – but the speed of emotional change connected to variations in context dissolves that 'natural' relationship between emotion and action. In other words, it can no longer be expected that the perception of a certain emotion will be followed by a behavioural act consistent with that emotion, in the first place because the emotion may be instrumental to the contingent situation, and furthermore because it may constitute an emotion which is only momentarily in tune with the situation. In this way, reliability becomes one of the sensitive points of contemporary awareness.

In addition, the emotional response and the behavioural action that could ensue are evaluated in the domain of one's own imagination from the standpoint of a possible consideration of others, even when one is physically alone. The need for approval leads to emotion losing its immediacy, inasmuch as it must be rehearsed before it is expressed. In many circumstances, emotional experience is transmuted into a perception of the Self that is lived vicariously.

Thus, inevitably, emotional feelings, just like the expression of emotion, are accompanied by a pervasive sense of inauthenticity which reflects a dual uncertainty: on the one hand, with respect to the fact that the emotional state is really perceived or is only acted out, and on the other hand, in relation to the being one's own (*Eigenschaft*) of that state or to being generated by another. The other side of the coin is the problem of sincerity, and that concerns one's relationship not only with oneself but also with the other.

The notes that follow, taken from our client's diary, clearly summarize some of the aspects which characterize the Outward modality of feeling emotionally situated which the constructionists have helped lay bare.

> *The systematic conformity of how I feel with a reality which is changing constantly, prevents my giving a stable interpretation of the bodily sensations and the emotions I feel, at least in those contexts which do not have a deeply-rooted image of me that can act as an anchor and container for my sensations and my emotions.*

The consequence is that my sensations and emotions have a sense of absolute impermanence in those contexts (that is to say, their meaning is unstable over time). In other words, it is practically impossible for me to remember, both qualitatively and quantitatively, what I really felt in living through an experience which took place even only a few hours earlier (or even a few minutes, if the context has changed in the meantime).

Since, in my case, the quality and the relevance of an experience depend on my level of emotional involvement and on the intensity of the emotions I feel, experience, even the most recent, seems faded. My inability to memorize sensations and emotions produces a profound re-elaboration of those very sensations and emotions, a process which inevitably leads to their being flattened. In other words, their 'bite' is removed and every event is remembered as being more or less ordinary or routine.

I have the impression of never having lived life to the full, of never having really enjoyed myself, of never having really suffered to the point of being unable to bear it any longer, at least compared to the models provided by the external world.

My experiences are thus systematically devalued, deprived of their body and relevance, with the significant consequence that I tend to ask those who shared the same experience with me not how intense that experience was for them, but how intense it was for me!

In actual fact, the memory one has of experiences producing strong involvement does not depend on the sensations and emotions in themselves, but to the evaluations made of them at the time: one remembers, that is, that in that particular situation a certain sensation (or set of sensations), or a certain emotional attitude, had been held to be more or less pleasurable and intense. But how much can we rely on memories of judgements regarding sensations and emotions emitted when the events occurred and which we only vaguely remember?

It is interesting to note that in order to turn that 'impermanent' modality of feeling into a stable experience, our client finds it necessary to seek an image in which to frame and fix it. It is the (culturally-mediated) model of perfection that, while it ensures the permanence of Self, also allows interpersonal relationships to be manipulated 'strategically'. Stated differently, the subject evaluates the situation in the light of a certain image (of perfection) – which may be considered a kind of 'inevitable model' – which determines both personal emotional experience and the ability to manage social interaction.

Again in his words:

. . . All of this exerts a heavy influence over the formation of the sense I have of myself and that is particularly evident – since I have a pronounced tendency to perfectionism – in those contexts where a consolidated image of myself which I have judged positively is missing.

Indeed, in these cases, on the one hand, the comparison between those expectations characterized by perfectionism and reality as experienced each time can easily produce an emotional condition whose major components are a sense of inadequacy and personal incapacity, and making the experience one has just gone through appear disappointing while, on the other hand, the tendency to underestimate the value of the experiences undergone in the course of one's life makes it very difficult to mediate correctly between the importance of the last relevant emotional experience one has gone through, and the significance of the prior events which act as a referential and interpretative framework.

> *In practice, if one feels disappointed by and nullified by what he has just done, felt and experienced in a given situation, he is unable to refer – or can only refer in part – to previous experiences which are much more satisfactory and which therefore bolster one's identity. Hence, when no solid, positive image of the Self is available, one tends to feel, generally and not simply at that particular moment, inadequate or incapable because of the last experience one has just gone through, losing sight completely of one's past successes. That complicates one's relationships with others no end.*

The constructionist position thus presupposes a human being who no longer needs to trace the source of his feelings in the private sphere in order to understand what affective situation he finds himself in. His interior life is constructed 'in full daylight' – and not *in interiore homine*;[16] thanks to its coherence with the constantly-changing context, his emotionality becomes socially constructed.[17] This shifts the emphasis from the organism's physiological states to social practices, bringing to light the fact that some emotions can only emerge in certain relational, social and/or cultural contexts. The most important contribution furnished by the social constructionists to the understanding of the problems set by Western contemporary identity, nevertheless, remains the strong emphasis on the speed of change of emotional situatedness, in tune with the acceleration of the external referential sources through which it takes shape. The speed factor gives rise to a series of new phenomena, which will be dealt with in this book only in part.

Endnotes

[1] Parkinson, Fischer and Manstead (2005: 247).

[2] Unlike Damasio, Prinz also furnishes a perspective with regard to the different intentional contents of emotions which contribute to making them different, thereby rejecting Cannon's argument on the uniformity of the visceral response of the various emotions. As Scarantino (2005: 151) points out when commenting on Prinz's innovation to James' theory, 'the key insight of Prinz's *embodied appraisal theory* is that emotions involve appraisal by virtue of what they represent, and that they represent what they have the function of being reliably caused by . . . Fear is then not, as James would have it under a standard reading, *merely* the perception of a particular suite of bodily changes, but rather the perception of a suite of bodily changes *set up* – by natural selection or by learning – *to be set off by danger*'.

[3] Obviously, this does not imply that there does not and may not exist behaviour whose value is exclusively expressive. Many of the automatic and universal facial expressions studied by Ekman could be considered examples of signals that do not serve negotiating purposes.

[4] For instance, in the three studies (Fernandez-Dols and Ruiz-Belda, 1995, 1997; Kraut and Johnston, 1979) mentioned previously, the smile may be considered as an affiliative signal (Griffiths, 2004a; Griffiths and Scarantino, 2008).

[5] Clearly, this also applies to the production of basic emotions, the study of which must be widened from a photographic view to a dynamic one.

[6] This would also apply even if alterity were that of one's own flesh, as has been pointed out by Ricoeur (1990).

[7] Quite correctly, Griffiths and Scarantino (2008: 20) underline the fact that 'the appraisal which type identifies the emotion does not occur at the beginning of the emotional episode but in the course of it, depending on whether or not the interaction affords the advantageous manifestation of one emotion rather than the other'.

[8] This does not mean, however, that all emotional signals are geared to social transaction. For instance, some manifestations of emotion may be purely expressive, that is lacking in any

negotiating purpose. Hinde (1985a, 1985b, quoted in Griffiths and Scarantino, 2008), who may be considered to be the founding father of this approach, wrote 'Such considerations suggest the view that emotional behavior may lie along a continuum from behavior that is more or less purely expressive to behaviors connected primarily with the process of negotiation between individuals . . . In animals, bird song lies nearer the expressive end, threat postures nearer the negotiation end. In man, spontaneous and solitary laughter are primarily expressive, the ingratiating smile primarily negotiating. However most expressional emotions involve both.'

[9] Interdependent Self-construal is associated with assimilation of others to the Self, whereas independent Self-construal is associated with exclusion of others from the Self (Van Baaren *et al.*, 2003).

[10] Although a certain emotional inclination may predominate in the course of one's life, a range of emotions with these polarities coexists in the same individual and may be activated differently depending on the circumstances.

[11] This perspective enables us to read the studies on field dependence/independence to which Herman A. Witkin (1978) devoted his entire life in a new light – that is, by interpreting them in the light of people's emotional constitutions.

[12] For an interesting analysis of this relationship and for a critical review of the various theories of the social construction of emotion, see Chapter 6 in Griffiths (1997).

[13] From our own standpoint, the differentiation between inner- and other-directed types made by Reisman may be reformulated in terms of a different velocity of change in experience relative to the anchoring contexts. Inner-directed types are anchored to relatively stable contexts while other-directed types are anchored to rapidly changing contexts.

[14] This is the fragmentation that Beck and Beck-Gernsheim (2002: 6) capture from another perspective when they write: 'Social action requires routines for its realization. We might even claim that our thoughts and actions take shape, at a deep level, through something which we are rarely aware of . . . It is this very level of pre-conscious "collective habituation", of facts taken for granted, which is increasingly being dissolved into a cloud of possibilities which must be thought out and negotiated'.

[15] The propriety and authenticity of one's personal experiences becomes uncertain. The title of Robert Musil's novel turns out to be almost prophetic: *The Man without Qualities.*

[16] 'Within the man himself'.

[17] For an in-depth study of the social construction of identity, see Gergen (1991, 2001), Lifton (1993).

Part Two

We are only typical to the extent to which we fail to be fully personal.[1]

The story of Robert that opened this book allowed us to challenge the established view of the Self: that of the Self as an object, thing, *ens creatum*. This story also allowed us to draw light on a way of being characterized by discontinuity, something that could only inadequately be accounted for on the basis of a psychology of the Self rooted in a Kantian perspective. By linking these two themes, we have developed a critique of both Cloninger's model, which introduced the approach of nonlinear systems into psychiatry, and the constructivist one, which introduced a psychology of the Self based on the biology of closed systems. Both these models failed to solve the problem posed by a way of being such as that of Robert – a populated Self, as Ken Gergen would put it – for both inevitably reduced the variability of the experience to the identity of the system: to the permanence of the Self (as an object) in time.

It is at this stage that the discontinuity of Self came to be perceived no longer as a problem, but as the very foundation of research. Seeking to discuss the issue of the Self from a radically different perspective, we addressed the question of ipseity by focusing our enquiry on the actual experience of living existence: on the various ways in which each person is himself each and every time in relation to the world and others. The being oneself reveals and reflects itself in everyday circumstances; in meeting these circumstances, it generates its own unique existential trajectory. Citing Ricoeur (1990), we emphasized that alterity belongs to the ontological construction of ipseity.

The notion of ipseity also led to a different way of understanding the relation between the experience of the Self and the permanence of the Self in time: no longer as the variability of experience in relation to what stays the same, but as finding oneself each time, insofar as the circumstances and emotional tones are the same. The relation between the actual and possible experience of the Self (ipseity) and the inclination of Self (sameness), which varies in the course of one's life, is the other major dialectic (besides that between ipseity and alterity) that characterizes the pre-reflexive ontological structure. Part One of the book was entirely pervaded by this new way of envisaging the experiential Self.

By presenting the problem of the Self in this new light, it was possible to develop the theme of personal identity on a separate level from that of the Self. The person here appears through the narrative reconfiguration of the experience. The entanglement of events in the (more or less cohesive) story of one's life, while uniting feeling and acting by means of a plot (which links them with possible and already-made experiences), is what gives the individual his identity and temporal stability. The character's identity is thus recounted at the same time as the story itself. By not taking the distinction between the experiential Self and personal identity seriously, it was possible to locate the origins of this distinction in the relation between living experience and language. Language was here seen as the ability that, by means of narrative, allows the individual to take possession of his own living experience, to connect and articulate it across time, and thus to construct the identity of the person to which that experience refers. Hence, the expression 'narrative identity' was used.

What all this suggested was that the account a person draws of himself (even in an anti-narrative form) provides a unique reconfiguration of the relation between sameness, ipseity and alterity that ontologically constitutes the pre-reflexive experience. We here considered how a person's character is constantly being challenged by circumstances, in order to emphasize the dialectic between sameness and ipseity that the story establishes and stabilizes over time. According to the direction this dialectic takes, the way in which the person's character and his identity over time are outlined on a narrative level will change. If a person's stability inclines toward sameness, it will be based on what are almost essential traits of his character. By contrast, if stability is maintained through an inclination toward ipseity, which is to say through changeable experience, personal consistency can only be preserved by anchoring variability in a more or less stable way.[2] In this case, an individual's identity will vary in accordance with the form (fixed vs. changeable) and type of anchorage in time (persons, norms, theories, objects, etc.).

These differences in the polarization of identity raised the question of the pre-reflexive origin of identity, and of the various inclinations of the experiential Self that give rise to different accounts of life. It is at this point of the analysis that ipseity acquires affective overtones. Not only is each individual revealed to himself by the way in which he emotionally reacts to others, but his feelings in given circumstances will settle over time and give rise to a recurrent tendency toward self-perception.[3] It is possible, therefore, to distinguish various inclinations toward emotional reaction on the basis of the various polarities of identity. The distinction between Inward and Outward tendencies was seen to be based on whether basic or non-basic emotions are prevalently elicited, as well as on the combination between the two within the continuum they define. The two polarities express different ways of feeling situated: a predominantly body-bound one in the case of the Inward tendency; an externally anchored one in the case of the Outward tendency. As we frequently emphasized, within the framework of these tendencies each individual can then be seen to possess a specific emotional makeup. This makeup may vary across different periods of life and in accordance with contextual factors that can contribute to determining not only what emotional tendency is active at any one time, but also the interplay between established traits and present experience.

If the emotional sphere provides a foundation for the two modes of permanence in time that determine the polarities of personal identity, an analysis of the story and of the identity of the protagonist should allow us to gain access to those emotional inclinations that provide the basis for the account and its narrative reconfiguration. It is the persistence of those inclinations reflected in a person's construction of his own identity that allows them to be identified as established traits, thus making it possible to understand the character of the story in terms of the abstract patterns of living experience. To return to the example of Robert, the combination of a series of traits – a sense of fragility, sensitiveness to the judgements of others, a sense of invasiveness, a feeling of emptiness and so on –

allows one to understand the story and its protagonist in the light of the internal coherence of the narrative. This internal logic establishes coherent connections between the various units of meaning (traits) by removing them from the actual story of Robert and organizing them in an impersonal structure referring to a given inclination in the emotional domain, an inclination that in this case is polarized toward the Outward.

The amphibiology according to which a person's character is both his own and at the same time the organized form of his ways of being allows us to classify one's character according to typology. As we shall see in the course of the following chapters, various categories of identity can be distinguished in relation to the protagonist of the story. These categories point to combinations of recurrent meanings that can be referred to emotional tendencies within a given continuum in the Inward and Outward polarities. As our analysis is based on psychotherapeutic and clinical experience, the definitions we shall adopt to typify personal identity will centre on the propensity shown by a given type of personality – structured in an internally coherent way – toward the development of given disorders (or their persistence after initial recovery). An expression used, therefore, will be 'personalities prone toward. . .'. The various types of personality will moreover be distinguished on the basis of their emotional inclinations within a continuum that extends from the Outward polarity to the Inward (Figure 2). A classification based on affectivity allows us to illustrate the continuity between the study of personality and that of psychopathology. Disorders, on the other hand, find their origin in the relation between the pre-reflexive sphere and its narrative reconfiguration (Arciero, 2006).

The most evident limit of this approach is that it underemphasizes the central aspect of the narrative: the fact that it brings living experience to language. In its search for the objective structures of meaning that allow one to understand the plot, the suggested approach ignores the interpretation of the story as an account of actual experiences. The plot itself is turned into a sort of closed 'object' by emphasizing the inner coherence of its unfolding, which is here abstracted from any living contact with concrete situations. These objects, which we shall be referring to as styles of personality, possess a crucial peculiarity that distinguishes them from psychiatric, but also psychoanalytic, categories: they are constructed, as it were, on the basis of the story itself. The individual story is thus reduced to the structural system needed in order to link the various units of meaning together. This system, which corresponds to a configuration of inner connections, makes it possible to outline, not merely a typology of personalities, but also a criteriology, for each style implies given constitutive rules. On the basis of this, personality styles, not unlike the 'ideal types' of Max Weber (1997), can serve as ideal models.[4]

On the other hand, as the reduction of the story to an ideal model allows one to acquire objective knowledge of a subject's personal story, it opens the field to natural sciences. These can share the aim of discovering the links between experiential and operational invariants through the various ways in which the emotional domain is structured and the semantic coherence of the individual story is ordered (thus providing a new foundation for psychopathology). What a similar approach lacks, however, is an appreciation of the uniqueness of personal experience and individual stories. While objectification here does not involve the expropriation of the subjective character of the experience at the hands of a neutral observer (for it forms the internal matrices of the personal story), it still severs the actual roots of the experience. Once more, it is worth stressing the fact that the reconstruction of narrative logic is not equivalent to the reinterpretation of a life story.

Part Two comprises five chapters devoted to the definition of personality styles. From the perspective of psychopathology, this typification allows one to anchor a range of disorders to a single connective structure (personality style), which in turn makes it possible to identify the causes of a series of symptoms and to reinterpret these within a framework that adequately takes the personal story and emotional inclinations of the subject into account. This procedure will contribute to highlighting the continuity between normality and neurotic psychopathology.

The distinction we shall present – one primarily centred around the pre-reflexive aspects of identity – while falling outside the classification system adopted in a wide range of literature on cognitive styles (Van Den Broeck, Vanderheyden and Cools, 2006), will point these studies in fresh directions by suggesting new areas of potential research in the various fields of psychology, as well as in management practice and industrial and organizational systems.

5 The Eating Disorder-prone Style of Personality

In Chapter 4, we considered how, since the middle of the nineteenth century, the mediation of technology has not only affected the experience of perception by accelerating the change of specific contexts (speed technologies), but has also progressively introduced new sources of meaning, new points of reference that provide the anchoring necessary to create and maintain one's identity (technologies for the transmission of information and the reproduction of experiences). The impact of technological development on human lives has led to a new 'manner of conformity', where the perception of the Self emerges simultaneously and in tune with the perception of a source of meaning. This new style, which we termed eating disorder-prone (EDP), went hand in hand with the spread of technological development and became visible, even in the world of *belles lettres*, in the mid-nineteenth century. It was Flaubert (2003) who most clearly defined its traits through the figure of Emma Bovary – a wife unsatisfied with her husband, a country doctor, and always in search of an identity that might match the fancy life of her dreams – and the protagonists of his posthumously-published work *Bouvard et Pécuchet* (Flaubert, 1954) – who change their identity in a picaresque way to fit their current field of interest (each new field being enthusiastically welcomed initially and then soon replaced at the first sign of disappointment).

The same tension that marks Flaubert's characters can be found, at a later date, in the literature of northern Europe. The protagonists – Nora in Ibsen's *A Doll's House* (Ibsen, 1919), Niels Lyhne in Jacobsen's (2008) novel of the same name, Julia and Laptev in Chekhov's (2004) *Three Years*, Mr M. in Rilke's (2003) *A Character* – all give signs of an uneasiness springing from the laceration of their own identity. If all experiences take shape by way of alterity, and if the other (of his way of being) is the source through which to reach oneself, the underlying dilemma is whether one feels himself to be the author of his own story and/or the episodes of his life, or whether, by contrast, he perceives himself as the actor in a play others have written. Rilke, with all the irony of a poet who is telling a story, touches upon this dilemma in a short novel written in the years 1895–1896, *A Character*. Rilke's novel opens with the funeral of its protagonist on a gloomy, rainy day.

Selfhood, identity and personality styles Giampiero Arciero and Guido Bondolfi

Two men in the funerary procession silently review the life of the deceased and remark that he was 'a man of character'. This moment in the narrative gives the whole novel its title: Rilke's book outlines the life of M., a man of character.

M. was born into a well-to-do family, the son of a salesman and a virtuous woman. Once early childhood had passed, as soon as 'his hands had stopped crawling about on the pavement, preferring to dwell on the mouth and nose', M. grew acquainted with Christmas trees and public meetings. A couple of times a week he would join in his parents' soirées, where their friends would admire, caress and praise him; many on such occasions would utter a solemn prophecy: that M. would soon have proven a brilliant pupil in school. This indeed turned out to be the case: M., who had often heard similar words of clairvoyance spoken, always met people's expectations of him as a student, from elementary school through to university. When M. later joined his father's company, rumours spread that he would be taking over the whole business, as his father was growing old. Not long after, when his father died, this is precisely what happened.

Soon, word reached M.'s ear – by way of friends – that the new head of the company had great plans in store. Surprised by what abilities people believed he possessed, M. actually began to implement the projects he was thought to have in mind, reaping some substantial profit. Years went by and then M. found out that, according to a new rumour, he was engaged to a girl. Almost involuntarily, M. turned his attention toward this very girl, whom he ended up marrying within weeks.

When the well-to-do citizens of M.'s hometown were searching for funds to build a theatre, word suddenly spread – like a storm in spring, Rilke writes – that M. had decided to help. An embassy led by the mayor then came to visit M., in order to thank him for his generosity. Bewildered, M. guessed the reason for this visit, and for a moment considered not paying the large sum required to build the theatre. However, he soon made up his mind, realizing that such a refusal would be detrimental to both his reputation and his business.

The city, in the meantime, was eagerly expecting news of a happy event. Furtive looks were inquisitively directed at M.'s young wife for any sign of pregnancy. M. did his best to meet people's expectations. This time, however, fortune betrayed him: no child was on the way. Suggestions were made among the people that a thermal cure was what was needed. M. followed public opinion, Rilke tells us, and came back from his cure with a pregnant wife.

M.'s reputation spread and so did word of a public award he was about to receive. The award was indeed assigned to him: a public speech was made and M received a badge of honour, along with many compliments.

The following winter, while on a business trip, M. got a cold that later worsened and turned into a lung infection. M.'s health grew worse by the day. One morning, as he was lying prostrated by his illness, he was awakened by some chatter. Confused, he asked his old servant and the sister of charity who was nursing him what was happening. The servant informed him that people were saying he was already dead.

M. stared at the old man in bewilderment. He then reclined on his left side and fell asleep. . .

M. had truly been a man of character, Rilke laconically concludes.

From his first steps as a toddler until his death, the protagonist of Rilke's novel, M., constructs his own experience and identity through the expectations of others. The crucial thing here is that being oneself (ipseity) is characterized by a kind of self-perception that can only be generated through a simultaneous centeredness on alterity. This centeredness takes various forms: alterity may be perceived as a source of expectations one needs to meet, but also as a pole of opposition or a source of emulation. It may also present a mixed form. In all cases, alterity remains the primary coordinate system allowing the person to feel situated: herein lies the problem of authorship of the experience, for the sense of Self is *con-fused* with that of the other.

The fact that the sense of Self is here perceived by focusing on alterity implies that the other represents a central point of reference, which a person must differentiate himself from and at the same time employ in order to grasp his emotional experience. Although this con-fusion also manifests itself in oppositional forms of behaviour, it emerges most evidently in mimetic phenomena: for in these cases, conformity to alterity becomes indistinguishable from the way in which one perceives oneself.[5] So while conformity to the other is a way of co-perceiving oneself, the other also represents that from which a person must distinguish himself. One's relationship with the other thus becomes crucial for the establishment of the dialectic between self-determination and the contemporaneous demarcation of oneself from the other, the modulation of which is renegotiated in every significant circumstance: at every moment, that is, which unsettles the balance between the authorship of one's own experience and its determination at the hands of others. This process is particularly evident in the case of Nora, the female protagonist of Ibsen's *A Doll's House* (Ibsen, 1919).

Ever since marrying Torvald, Nora has been living like a wife-doll, seeking to meet all her husband's expectations. Yet, Nora has a secret she has long been hiding from Torvald: in order to pay for the stay in Italy he needed to recover from a near-fatal illness, Nora has run into debt. For eight years Nora has silently been economizing on her everyday personal expenses and has occasionally been working in order to pay her three-monthly instalment. At the same time, without ever giving herself away, she acts as a spoilt child with Torvald.

When Nora's husband receives a promotion and their financial situation seems likely to improve, so that she may finally extinguish the debt, Krogstad enters the scene. This is the man who had lent Nora the money; he now threatens to inform Torvald not only of the debt, but also of an unlawful act that Nora committed in order to obtain it. Krogstad, who had been a friend of Torvald's in his youth but is now held in low esteem by him, tells Nora that he will be silent if she manages to convince her husband to keep him as one of his workers rather than fire him once the promotion comes into effect. Nora feels lost. Thoughts of death cross her mind, but she also attempts to seduce her husband in order to convince him to help Krogstad. Torvald instead writes him a letter of dismissal. This paves the way for the grand finale, which involves two letters. In the first, which signals a dramatic turning point in the story, Krogstad blackmails Torvald with his wife's misdeed. After discovering Nora's long-guarded secret, a desperate Torvald, feeling helpless in Krogstad's power, attacks his wife: Nora is insulted and confronted with a picture of a future in which she is stripped of her role as mother and wife.

At this point, a maid brings in the second letter. Torvald reads it with a feeling of dread; but after a moment of disbelief, he utters a cry of joy: Krogstad, regretting his actions, is handing back the receipt he had used to blackmail Torvald. Torvald exultingly burns the evidence of his wife's unlawful act, and addresses Nora with words of pardon and understanding.

Something, however, has changed. The person who in the final pages of the play tells Torvald that the incident has brought an end to her love is not the same Nora as before. She is no longer the boisterous and lively bird who in the first two acts was seen to flutter about her husband like a whimsical domestic animal: Nora is now portrayed as a resolute woman who is ready to leave her family and express all the horror she feels for having spent eight years of her life in the company of a stranger who gave her three children:

> *While I was at home with father, he used to tell me all his opinions, and I held the same opinions. If I had others I said nothing about them, because he wouldn't have liked it. . . . I passed from father's hands into yours. You arranged everything according to your taste; and I got the same tastes as you; or I pretended to – I don't know which – both ways, perhaps; sometimes one and sometimes the other. When I look back on it now, I seem to have been living here like a beggar, from hand to mouth. I lived by performing tricks for you, Torvald. But you would have it so. You and father have done me a great wrong. It is your fault that my life has come to nothing (Ibsen, 1919: 143–44).*

It is this way of life that Nora can no longer accept: she can no longer stand being the wife-doll of Torvald, just as she had been the daughter-doll of her father. Nora wishes to be alone.

The crucial turning point that leads to such radical and sudden change at the end of the play is the fact that Nora realizes that Torvald perceives the discovery of the danger threatening her, not as a difficult moment in her life, but as a danger to himself. Nora, in other words, realizes that value is assigned to the meaning she attributes to her own experience only when it conforms to the will, desires and expectations of her husband. If it fails to match the determinations established by her husband, it is no longer assigned an identity. It is this awareness that leads Nora to embrace a different life and allows her to perceive Torvald as a stranger. Nora tells her husband, who is begging her to stay: 'I must stand quite alone if I am ever to know myself and my surroundings . . . I must think things out for myself, and try to get clear about them' (Ibsen, 1919: 146–48).

5.1 Co-perceiving the self and other

As a process, the dialectic between the demarcation and the contemporaneous determination of Self by means of the other finds only a momentary expression, for any event can unsettle the balance brought about by perceiving oneself as the author of one's experiences. The various forms this style of personality can take all revolve around this dialectic.

Oscillation toward an 'excess' of demarcation, which corresponds to a strong sense of being at the root of one's choices without the simultaneous co-perception of a defining alterity, is accompanied by a perception of the reevaluation of the authorship of the experience. The more, that is, a person feels he has acted independently of others, the less sure he will feel about himself. The perception of one's autonomy is here associated with a feeling of inadequacy, unimportance, depreciation and lack of authenticity. The making of even a simple decision, such as buying a pair of shoes, without taking the other as a point of reference, may thus be accompanied by a sense of insecurity with regard to one's own competence, tastes or needs. Paradoxically, the feeling of being the author of one's own actions, emotions and thoughts is here accompanied by a feeling of deficiency, in the form of incapacity, inadequacy, insecurity or insincerity.

The other remains present within the experiential horizon in a negative way, as the lack of validation of one's own experience; hence, it does not allow the complete ownership (*Eigenschaft*) of the experience. It is as if personal experience, deprived of simultaneous reference to the other, were deficient both in value and quality. This engenders a sense of Self that is more changeable and vague, and which is accompanied by a greater fear of self-affirming. A rather common example of this in psychotherapeutic practice is the sense of insecurity felt by young adolescents, particularly in the absence of the important figures they are in need of, but find it difficult or impossible to be in touch with.

One of the ways in which this feeling of personal deficiency can be contained is through the body, which becomes the means to define one's encounter with the other. The body is here employed as an image in tune with other, fashionable images. An example of this is the hyper-seductive adolescent who employs her body as a tool in her search for both independence and forms of approval alternative to those of her family.

We are faced with a more striking paradox when alterity is completely removed from one's referential horizon, as in the case of loneliness. The emotional state in which one's being is perceived as lacking another – which is required to define and demarcate oneself – is described as a feeling of emptiness, bewilderment, loss of meaning, and is often perceived as an affliction: an emptiness in search of alterity at any cost.

Such a paradox was already evident in the case of Robert, the internal coherence of whose experience we can now trace back to a given typology. In the light of the dialectic between the determination of Self and its definition by way of the other, it is possible to understand Robert's 'existential' use of technology, his sense of distance when establishing a more intimate contact with Sarah, the con-fusion of the lives of the two and the end of their relationship, which causes Robert to feel he is vanishing.

Interwoven with Robert's story is that of Sarah. Sarah took possession of Robert's life by concealing herself within it; driven by boredom, or maybe after having been fully accepted, she felt the need to adjust to new sources of meaning. With Sarah seeking to end her coexistence with Robert, we witness the superimposition between the end of a relation and the beginning of a new one.

The same theme of reciprocal determination and definition is articulated, following a different trajectory, in *Three Years*, Chekhov's (2004) novel about the reciprocal transformation of Julia and Laptev. The novel opens with Laptev brimming with love in the moonlight, as Julia decides to marry him in order to leave the provinces; it ends with Julia, arms outstretched, telling Laptev, 'I love you, you know?', while he feels 'as if the two of them had already been married for ten years – and also like having breakfast'. Through the development of their love, Chekhov traces a dividing line that remains unvaried throughout the novel, despite the way in which the positions initially embraced by the two protagonists are later overturned (Arciero, 2002). This line allows Julia and Laptev both to mutually distinguish themselves and for each one to be defined through the other. The stability of these margins makes some kind of intimacy between the two characters possible even in the most difficult moments, whereas the intimacy between Robert and Sarah ends after a short time.

A way of strengthening the dialectic between demarcation (self-centeredness) and the contemporaneous definition of Self by means of alterity (other-centeredness) is to validate one's current experience by reference to an ideal image. This may often be derived from the media,[6] or may reflect a model of excellence in the field of liberal professions, or artistic or sporting careers. Such models, usually close to perfection, represent a shared source a person can con-form to, for they provide stable criteria of self-evaluation. Perceived autonomy is here accompanied by a sense of dissatisfaction punctuated by sporadic moments of fulfilment, rather than by the same feelings of insecurity that characterize the perception of one's own authorship in the absence of validation at the hands of another. It is as if the overall value of the experience had diminished because of awareness of the fact that the experience itself could be perfected. The distance between the perfection of the model and the perfectibility of one's actual experience also ensures a degree of difference between the two, thus fostering competitiveness both within oneself and with others. This constant feeling of being ready to meet a challenge and put oneself to the test, this constant longing for engagement, gives meaning to one's self-centeredness, while also making the contemporaneous definition of the experience at hand possible through a comparison with the model. This is a tension for those at the top of the class!

Conformity to a model (or models) can take various forms, according to the degree of stability, and reach levels of extreme variability in the co-perception of oneself. This picaresque and episodic perception of the Self arises from an ability to adjust to the image required in every context, and, according to Rosen (2001), is the main cause of a chameleon personality.[7] 'In order to adapt successfully to the game of life,' Rosen (2001: 23) writes, 'chameleons must be able to understand intuitively what others think and why they behave as they do. They must recognize the other players' values and adjust to them, or at least conceal disagreement.'

It is interesting to note here that in a study of the differences between people with high and low emotional empathy, high-empathy subjects were found to have a greater degree of mimicking behaviour than low-empathy subjects (Sonnby-Borgström, 2002). Similar conclusions can be drawn from the study conducted by Van Baaren *et al.* (2003), which shows how a higher degree of interdependent Self-construal is associated with more mimicry than an independent Self-construal.

When variations in the dialectic between the definition of the Self and its contemporaneous demarcation are caused by an 'excess' of alterity, this can be seen to correspond to a 'thinning' of the sense of self-determination, to the point that the person may feel he is effectively being led by the other. The feeling an individual has of being the protagonist of more or less significant episodes, that is, coincides with his perception of himself as an actor who is playing the role assigned to him by a director in real life rather than onscreen. No doubt, one can choose to follow the orders of the director and play the assigned role. Alternatively, the excess of perceived alterity can intersect with an autonomous dimension that must necessarily remain secret. This is the case, for instance, with Nora in the first two acts of Ibsen's play: while externally conforming to the script written by her husband, Nora is also guarding a personal secret that concretely informs her everyday experience. Once the secret is revealed, the doll and dollhouse are dissolved. It is clear that the nature of the secret here is only of secondary importance: the matter at stake could equally well have been – as is most commonly the case – an affair.

Frequently, the perception of oneself as the actor, rather than the author, of meaning is accompanied by a feeling of the other's invasiveness and of a more or less temporary – depending on personal circumstances – nullification of the Self, which corresponds to the contemporaneous dissolution of one's own demarcation from the other. The same sense of annihilation may be caused by a negative judgement on the part of a highly significant other.

If a person's perception of himself as the author of his own experience is thus co-regulated through alterity, the need to face a perceived form of invasiveness will increase proportionately to its perceived intensity. This sense of opposition often emerges in the course of a person's adolescence, when it amplifies the physiological need to distance oneself from parental figures that is typical of this stage in human life, thus engendering a variety of phenomena, ranging from manifest conflict to transgression, inability to communicate and indifference. These types of behaviour may continue to manifest themselves in the course of one's adult life in the form of oppositional traits triggered by significant others, for instance, in affective relationships marked by competition and strife.

It is worth considering here a study carried out by Chartrand, Dalton and Fitzsimons (2007) on how individuals with a particularly high degree of nonconscious habitual *reactance*,[8] automatically evoked upon exposure to significant others, are influenced in the pursuit of their goals. The authors of the study suggest that whether or not participants unconsciously comply to their significant other person's wishes (low-reactant) or pursue a goal that directly opposes these wishes (high-reactant) depends on whether they perceive their significant others as a threat to their own autonomy. Low-reactant individuals adopted a subliminally primed goal of their significant others, whereas high-reactant individuals pursued an opposing goal.

The dialectic between conformity to alterity and contemporaneous differentiation from alterity takes various forms associated with a range of emotions, which all emerge in the process of relating oneself to another: a real or imagined other, through which one is both defined and demarcated. A distinguishing feature of 'non-basic emotions' is precisely the fact that, along with the way of being of the other, what is co-perceived is the other's reciprocity with one's own way of being. These emotions thus play a fundamental role in structuring the style of personality we have just been discussing.

Inability, inadequacy, insecurity, deficiency, lack of authenticity, emptiness, dissatisfaction, competitiveness, invasiveness, a tendency toward opposition, self-nullification, but also guilt, boredom, embarrassment, indifference, shame and anxiety are all emotional states that adumbrate the meaning of perceived reciprocity – be it a deficient, lacking, ideal or excessive one.

Perhaps the most revealing emotion of all is ambivalence. This effectively brings together the need for approval and that for independence, involvement and distance, responsibility and avoidance. By making disengagement possible under all circumstances, ambivalence allows one to blur the distinction between reality and fiction, and thus casually and flexibly to redefine bonds and ways out. An obligation will thus only be accepted if it agrees with temporariness or desertion (whether real or imaginary). In such cases, direct engagement will only be accepted if it is nonresolutive. Here too lie the roots of the 'converging love' discussed by Baumann (2003): the kind of love that binds two partners only for as long as both find it convenient; once the interest is gone, the bond is broken.

Flexibility, which is so often praised, is ultimately a product of ambiguity. This is one of the defining traits of a style of personality that in the sphere of love seeks possible intimacy in order simultaneously to safeguard its own independence. This dialectic allows us not only to interpret the dynamics of sentimental relationships in the course of a person's adult life, but also to explain a number of unique phenomena, ranging from a failed sentimental debut, white marriage, disturbances of sexual arousal: erectile impotence and female orgasmic dysfunction (excessive demarcation of oneself from the other) down to 'women who love too much' (Norwood, 1985), unrequited love (Baumeister and Wotman, 1992) and certain forms of ex-partner stalking (excessive self-definition by means of the other). The direction sentimental relations take depends on the modulation of this dialectic, in relation to which the body often plays a central role. The body is here seen as the ultimate source of independence, but also of mergence with the other, as a border that cannot be crossed, but also as a tool to meet the expectations of others, to mimic the desire of the other.

In discussing the complex emotional world that characterizes this style of personality, I have paid particular attention to the non-basic emotions connected to problematic conditions. By contrast, what have not been taken into consideration so far are the 'positive' aspects that emerge thanks to the interpersonal orientation that marks this personality. Sensitivity, delicacy, tolerance, care, compassion, empathic intensity, dedication, consideration, a welcoming attitude, kindness and abnegation are equally fundamental expressions of a type of personality that is centred on a particular relational need, as well as on a unique ability to garner social cues.

Witkin has emphasized how it was precisely thanks to this marked attention to information received from others, and a propensity to share others' points of view, that those he termed 'field-dependent' patients[9] – individuals presenting a wide range of traits that may be assimilated to those of EDP personalities – proved more efficient in situations where there was a need to rely on contextual cues. For instance, under ambiguous conditions, field-dependent subjects made up for the lack of information on which to base their judgement by taking into account the information available to them from other people (Witkin and Goodenough, 1977). These individuals, in other words, not only more easily accepted the point of view of other people, but also took account of this point of view in establishing their own. Clearly, this behaviour can be seen to facilitate mediation in the case of conflict, negotiations and collaborative endeavours. Further confirmation can be found in those empirical studies that emphasize the importance, in the course of social strategic interactions, of a perspective-taking to uncover underlying interests in order to generate creative solutions and to craft more efficient deals (Galinsky *et al.*, 2008), as well as of strategic mimicking to facilitate interpersonal coordination and negotiation outcomes (Maddux, Mullen and Galinsky, 2008).

Another thing observed by Witkin in relation to social interactions is the fact that field-dependent subjects either direct their gaze at or avoid the face of the person with whom they are interacting depending on their ongoing task. 'These opposite behaviours among field-dependent people – avoiding other's faces when engaged in internal processing of difficult cognitive material and looking at faces when they are likely to benefit from the information they may obtain there – both reflect the special tug of faces upon their attention' (Witkin and Goodenough, 1977: 52). According to Witkin, the greater attentiveness to social cues of these individuals is due to their 'looking behaviour'. As we have seen, this trait is particularly evident in more obscure situations that can be clarified on the basis of social cues found in the other's face.

According to the perspective adopted so far, Witkin's observations can be seen to refer to the EDP style of personality, which bases its sense of permanence on a coordinate system (outwardly) anchored to a real or imagined other. An interesting confirmation of this suggestion stems from a comparison between Witkin's observations and the data provided in our studies on the relation between emotional style and the processing of threatening stimuli. Eating disorder-prone subjects who underwent fMRI during the performance of a perceptual task involving exposure to fearful stimuli revealed a greater engagement of the areas of the visual and associative cortex (BA18), of those assigned to facial recognition (BA37), of those connected to cognitive functions (BA46) and of those linked to attention (BA7) (Bertolino *et al.*, 2005). Even the data pertaining to the subjective experience of pain unpleasantness in EDP individuals reveal that the Outward group showed greater activation in the occipital cortex (BA19), the PCC (BA31) and the precuneus (BA7), that is to say, in those regions that are engaged in visuospatial processing and the direction of one's attention (Mazzola *et al.*, submitted).

5.2 Disorders

The EDP style of personality shows a certain inclination toward the development of eating disorders (or their persistence after initial recovery). This definition, however, is hardly rigorous, for eating disorders represent only one part of the symptomatic spectrum that is likely to be associated with the personality in question. The broad range of this personality is reflected in the variety of disorders that mostly affect the body in its various social and private dimensions. The notion of eating disorders in this context is more generally used to refer to an affliction that affects one's body in its relation to the other. A person's relation with his body here represents the means to regulate the dialectic between self-demarcation and the contemporaneous determination of Self by means of the other. The dialectic behind the construction of identity thus also embodies the distinctive core psychopathology shared by a range of disorders, ranging from anorexia nervosa to behavioural addictions.

Anorexia nervosa

From the latter part of the nineteenth century, when anorexia was first identified as a medical problem, this illness was linked to excessive concern on the patient's part for weight and, by extension, food and – only later – the image of himself. It is the media of the 1920s that first gave prominence to the link between one's own body and the image found in fashion, by promoting the model of a woman who is slender, agile and unusually attentive toward her looks (Vandereycken and van Deth, 1990). This is the kind of modern woman Coco Chanel had in mind.

A relation thus came to be established between media models and the image of one's own body (for a review, see Groesz, Levine and Murnen, 2002). New emphasis was placed on the perceptive aspects of one's experience of one's own body: on the body as image. Exposure to media-portrayed 'unrealistic' ideals of beauty is generally regarded today as one of the most important factors behind the high level of bodily dissatisfaction and eating disturbances in Western society. This problem particularly affects women.

But why is it women who, right from the start, have suffered most from the impact of media models? Why is it that, already in the early twentieth century, the image promoted by the media had become the model on the basis of which women in particular constructed their own self-image?[10] An indirect answer to these questions is found in a study on social correlates of the female form of the chameleon syndrome (Rosen and Aneshensel, 1976). According to this study, the chameleon syndrome, as the by-product of long-term gender socialization, aims at preparing females for marriage. One of the central elements of 'chameleonism' is appearance-orientation. This is perhaps where media models come into play.

The images promoted in the media came to be perceived by women as models to be adopted toward the definition of their own physical attractiveness; this element, in conjunction with others, was seen potentially to increase their chances of attracting male interest, including the chances of finding a husband.[11] Female eating behaviour is affected by perceived social and cultural standards and interpersonal expectations, in addition to personal standards of appearance (Mori, Chaiken and Pliner, 1987).

The mass diffusion of television in the 1950s further contributed to consolidating the process of shaping the body in accordance with an established image. These years also witnessed the first large-scale 'epidemic' of eating disorders. Hence, in the 1960s, following the spread of the phenomenon, the alteration of a person's bodily image came to be regarded as the primary cause of the disorder (Bruch, 1962; Selvini Palazzoli, 1963).

But is it really the case that the problem lies in the alteration of one's bodily image, or can the relation between body, food and image be accounted for in a different way?

We previously touched upon the issue of a person's relation with his body by referring to two scenarios: the use of the body as a means to seek consensus, and the use of the body as a way to delimit one's intimacy with the other. In both cases, a person's relation with his body was seen to revolve around the dialectic between self-determination and self-definition by means of the other. Within the framework of this dialectic it makes little sense to consider restricting anorexia as something caused by an alteration of the bodily image. Such an interpretation makes equally little sense from the perspective of those suffering from restricting anorexia. Clear evidence of this stems from a rather self-evident fact: that those suffering from anorexia 'voluntarily' endure starvation.[12] Here the experience of being oneself coincides with the protracted experiencing of hunger. It is the latter experience, therefore, that must be taken as a starting point to examine the condition of anorexia. What is the meaning of self-starvation?

One element many authors have emphasized is the need to distance oneself from an invasive family and to affirm one's independence through strenuous opposition, or by rebelling against demanding parents and their high expectations. References to family strife can already be found in the first two articles on the subject published by Gull and Lasegue (quoted in Vandereycken and van Deth, 1990), who in the latter half of the nineteenth century spoke of the obstinacy and stubbornness of the patients, while recommending a therapy to be adopted outside the family milieu and under the guidance of an authoritative figure. Further emphasis on conflict emerges from the concrete daily struggle between family members, who urge the anorexic subject to resume a normal eating behaviour, and the anorexic subject himself, who perceives his loss of weight as an accomplishment rather than a problem.

An analysis of anorexia in terms of the definition of the Self in opposition to the family, however, does not account for the way in which the anorexic person perceives himself, for his self-experience, and the way in which he constructs a firm sense of Self through hunger.

Starving one's body is a means to perceive the body as different from oneself. What is most significant here is the discovered ability to maintain a sense of radical autonomy without plunging into emptiness, but rather by alertly and constantly fighting against a body – one's own – that is screaming with hunger and/or weariness. The freeing of oneself from determination at the hands of others is no longer perceived in the form of emptiness, for a starved body provides a permanent centre of gravity. Thus the body, simultaneously perceived as one's own and as the other, famished, wearied by excessive physical exercise and exhausted by purging, becomes the privileged interlocutor for the regulation of one's sense of Self – an interlocutor that guides one's imagination, thoughts and actions. Selvini Palazzoli (1963), in describing this condition, spoke of 'delusional alteration' (albeit one centred on the image of the body).

By envisaging his own body as a new centre which he must both differentiate himself from and coincide with, a person is freed from the need to rely on others for the purpose of self-definition. As weight is progressively lost, so does one's interest in others decline, to the point of reaching complete social withdrawal. Herein lie the origins of anorexia, which represents an attempt to escape excessive determination at the hands of others by establishing a relationship with the body as something to which to attune oneself.

Here too lies the origin of that perfectionism which is regarded as a particularly common antecedent of anorexia nervosa (Fairburn and Harrison, 2003; Fairburn *et al.*, 1999). The constant attempt to meet the highest possible standards of behaviour and/or the expectations of significant people, as well as to gain the approval of others by conforming to their expectations, as suggested by Hewitt, Flett and Ediger (1995), is a way of erecting a kind of barrier to buffer – and hence averting – the impact of the critiques and judgements of others on one's own sense of Self. The greater this need, the greater the degree of perfectionism in the subject, as is suggested by those studies that relate the degree of a person's perfectionism to the severity of his eating disorders (Bastiani *et al.*, 1995; Halmi *et al.*, 2000; Pieters *et al.*, 2007).

It is clear from this perspective that weight, shape, and even a simple comment alluding to an increase in weight, will affect the subject's self-esteem. The constant fight against the flesh serves to measure one's own ability, strength and, by extension, worth. The scale is seen to provide an objective confirmation of these values.

For eating-disordered subjects, who structure their own identity by fighting their own famished bodies, thinness – even skeleton-like thinness – can only be seen as a positive thing and a confirmation, even if they are conscious of their unattractiveness.

A study by Jansen *et al.* (2006) has investigated the origin of feelings of unattractiveness among eating-symptomatic subjects, by comparing their body image and control models to the intersubjective evaluations of these bodies given by two panels judging the same slides. Interestingly, normal controls were found to rate themselves as far more attractive than other people rated them, whereas there was consensual validation of the negative body image of eating-disordered subjects. Along much the same lines, a study of 100 female patients suffering from restricting anorexia nervosa, conducted by Probst *et al.* (1998), found that about half of the subjects were accurate in estimating their own body dimensions and only 20% clearly showed overestimation.

Bulimia nervosa

In the 1980s, increasing attention was devoted to a new eating disorder: bulimia nervosa, which was described by Polivy and Herman (1985) as 'the disease of the eighties'. Unlike anorexia, of which it often represents a development[13] (Eddy *et al.*, 2008), bulimia has its roots not in a need to assert one's radical independence from others, but rather in one's actual relation with the other: one's profound awareness of the opinions and judgements of others. In this case, a person measures his own worth on the basis of others' approval or rejection. As several authors have observed, fear of rejection or exclusion is an essential feature of bulimia (e.g. Baumeister and Tice, 1990; Gross and Rosen, 1988; Heatherton and Baumeister, 1991). Bulimic patients learn to cope with this constant fear of judgement by a manipulation of their own physical attractiveness and body shape, which is achieved by regulating bodily parameters on the basis of fashionable images. In a more evident way than anorexics, bulimics can be seen to focus on media models of perfection, which provide a point of reference by which to measure their own degree of desirability, in order to lessen their fear of personal conflict.

Ipseity here is characterized by a constant anxiety with regard to others' judgement,[14] which is nevertheless buffered by the focus on one's attractiveness and body shape. This gives rise to a unique phenomenology, marked by a strange and complex intertwinement between exposure and bodily image. If, on the one hand, acceptance by others is manipulated by a way of presenting oneself that emphasizes physical appearance, thus increasing body-focused attention, on the other hand, any lack of validation is bound to be referred to one's body, thus increasing aversive focus on the body. The crucial relation between one's level of exposure and body-focused attention contributes to explaining one apparently bizarre phenomenon: the fact that lack of validation in any field – something bulimics always perceive as a failure – is automatically transformed into a negative perception of one's body (e.g. the feeling that one's belly is too large or of being overweight), which in turn immediately triggers forms of disordered eating behaviour. It is hardly surprising, therefore, that bulimia is more frequent among high-achieving women, who are more exposed to conflict with others and evaluation, and/or are more specifically concerned with high standards and high expectations for achievement and performance (Barnett, 1986).

Lack of validation – regardless of the contingent situation – is perceived as something all-embracing, which affects the whole life of the subject, greatly amplifying his sense of personal negativity. This form of emotional dysregulation, which radically increases the intensity of the patient's feelings, is also one of the causes for the high incidence of alcohol abuse (Bulik *et al.*, 2004) and substance use (Wiederman and Pryor, 1996) among bulimics.[15]

An idea of how acutely sensitive bulimics are with regard to lack of validation is given by one our patients. This girl, referring to a party she had attended a few days before, explained that because she had not been courted by the most distinguished young man present on that occasion, she had reached the conclusion that she was physically unattractive. In the course of the evening, she kept thinking that no interesting man would ever pay her any attention, and that she was destined to lead a miserable and lonely existence. Feeling desperate, upon returning home she experienced three consecutive bouts of binge eating, followed by purging.

A defining characteristic of bulimia, and something which clearly emerges from our patient's account, is the unique way in which subjects attempt to cope both with emotions pertaining to the outcome of a confrontation or the expectations it engenders – sadness, fear, stress, anger, disappointment – and with feelings related to loneliness (and hence the lack of another through which to define themselves), for instance, emptiness and boredom. In order to cope with these emotions, bulimics manipulate their own perception of the body by means of binge eating and purging, but also dieting and strenuous exercise. This raises a question regarding one of the most enigmatic features of bulimia nervosa: why do these emotions trigger patterns of behaviour that revolve around the ingestion and expulsion of food?

Before suggesting any answers, let us sum up the various steps that have led us to this issue. First, the automatism that underlines bulimia has been seen to derive from a lack of validation that causes a state of intense emotional activation. This profound malaise is referred to one's bodily shape. An emotional activation of a similar degree of intensity may also derive from loneliness or imaginary circumstances. This acutely negative emotional state then acts as a trigger for the unchecked (and more or less immediate) consumption of food, which may be followed by purging, dieting, exercise or a combination of any of these practices.

Baumeister has long addressed the problem of bulimia in the context of his theory of escape (Baumeister, 1989, 1990; Heatherton and Baumeister, 1991). From a cognitivist perspective, he argues that, in order to escape negative feelings, bulimics narrow their attention span down to the immediate present. This allows them to shift to low levels of awareness and hence remove a series of inhibitions against eating that are connected to more articulate levels of self-awareness. As a result, 'the person may become absorbed in the process of eating and may fail to evaluate eating against standards, norms, or guidelines', thus ingesting food in an uncontrolled way (Heatherton and Baumeister, 1991: 95). These events, Baumeister concedes, may also unfold according to an opposite sequence, whereby the process of eating absorbs the person's attention, allowing him to escape from broad self-awareness.

Even if Baumeister's second hypothesis were to prove valid, however, it would still fail to explain why a person needs to create a visceral condition within his own body in order to escape the feeling of suffering caused by an ongoing emotional state. According to the perspective we have adopted so far, in the case of bulimia, like that of anorexia, the subject's relation to his own body can be seen as the means by which the dialectic between self-demarcation and the contemporaneous determination of his Self through others is regulated.

In accordance with what has been argued in relation to anorexia, the creation of visceral states through the ingestion and expulsion of food among bulimics allows the body to emerge as a centre to which to attune oneself in order to free oneself from the negative emotional state engendered by one's relation with others. The stuffing and emptying of one's body, like the filling and later starving of the body and its subjection to physical exertion, is the means by which the bulimic simultaneously perceives his body as his own and as other.

It is precisely the construction of the body as the other that polarizes and narrows the bulimic's attention span, allowing him to escape more articulate levels of self-awareness. In the case of bulimics, however, unlike that of anorexics, what marks the subject's relation with others is not radical separation, but rather an acute need for their approval. In this context, the manipulation of visceral states has the purpose of regulating the lack of validation that emerges in the course of one's relation with others. Episodes of binge eating are the expression of a condition that is characterized by the chronic co-determination of the sense of Self and of acceptance by others. These episodes reflect the acute perception of a negative judgement (be it real or imaginary).

As soon as the binge comes to an end, focus on a given image that serves as a point of reference, or on what is regarded as the ideal weight for one's physical attractiveness, leads to various compensating practices such as self-induced vomiting, the misuse of laxatives, dieting or excessive exercise.[16] As René Girard (2006) observes, 'our modern bulimic is eating for herself, but she is vomiting for others' – and for all those whose opinions matter, we would add. This appears to be the key factor, in which a crucial role is played by the theme of the body as an image and a means to regulate one's encounter with the other by reducing the possible risk of rejection to a minimum. In this light, the sexual promiscuity that is common among bulimics can also be seen as a way of manipulating one's acceptance by others.

Binge-eating disorder

Over the past decade, a rapidly growing literature has documented the clinical significance of a new syndrome, binge-eating disorder (BED), which has been found to be more common than anorexia nervosa and bulimia nervosa (Pope *et al.*, 2006; Striegel-Moore and Franko, 2003; Spitzer *et al.*, 1992). As in the case of bulimia nervosa, the need for frequent binge eating is a core defining feature of BED. This shared feature raises the question of the contiguity/continuity between BED and bulimia, although the form binge eating takes, and the frequency with which it is performed, can be seen to vary within the two disorders. What is necessary is not so much to identify the cut-off point between purging and nonpurging bulimia nervosa/BED (Devlin, Goldfein and Dobrow, 2003), as to understand whether it is the same mechanism that lies at the heart of these two syndromes, which can be seen to radically differ in other respects.

The epidemiological characteristics of BED differ from those of bulimia – BED affects individuals in their forties, frequently occurs in men and is strongly associated with obesity (Walsh and Devlin, 1998; Fairburn and Harrison, 2003; Pope *et al.*, 2006) – as is its inception. As Dingemans, Bruna and van Furth (2002: 301) suggest in their review of BED, 'in the case of bulimia nervosa, most individuals start dieting prior to the onset of binge eating. However, a fairly large subgroup of the individuals with BED start binge eating prior to the onset of dieting (35–54%)'.

Often, bulimics reach the phase of binge eating through dieting; by contrast, those who suffer from BED start with binge eating as their primary symptom. A further difference between the two disorders lies in the fact that, in the case of BED patients, binge eating is not followed by purging or compensative practices, although these distinctions are not always clear-cut. Devlin, Goldfein and Dobrow (2003), for instance, ask whether there may not be a continuum between individuals who binge eat and then immediately fast or exercise to compensate – and who would thus fall into the bracket of nonpurging bulimia nervosa – and individuals who report longer periods of binge eating, alternating with days or weeks of occasionally extreme dieting – these being likely candidates for a BED diagnosis. The issue of the continuity between BED and bulimia nervosa is a matter of debate (Fairburn, Welch and Hay, 1993; Fairburn *et al.*, 1998, 1999; Fichter *et al.*, 1993; Fitzgibbon, Sanchez-Johnsen and Martinovich, 2003; Spitzer *et al.*, 1993).

What do these two disorders have in common? First of all, in both cases, situations that trigger episodes of binge eating are often precipitated by stress and negative affects (Arnow, Kenardy and Agras, 1995; Engelberg *et al.*, 2007; Deaver *et al.*, 2003; Whiteside *et al.*, 2007, Stein *et al.*, 2007). It would thus seem that the rapid ingestion of considerable quantities of food, a process allowing visceral states to emerge, which a person can then focus on in order to escape his ongoing negative sense of Self, is a feature shared by both syndromes. The greatest difference between BED and bulimia emerges once the binge is over: while bulimics are then led to focus once more on a reference point that guides their purging practices, subjects suffering from BED show no signs of compensative behaviour. This difference has two notable consequences.

The first consequence concerns the subject's experience of his body. In the case of BED, the process of rapidly, greatly and uncontrollably filling one's stomach is not followed, as in the case of bulimia, by a more or less sudden (vomiting) or extreme (dieting) change of the visceral condition induced by binge eating. Rather, the subject's perception of the body is connected to the digestive processes brought about by the ingestion of such large quantities of food. The effort of digestion passively captures the subject's attention, giving rise to a unique bodily phenomenology. The body, in other words, manifests its visceral character in what we may regard as an opposite way from that of anorexic hunger: for it is predominantly centred on a feeling of satiety, and is thus similar to that found among obese people. It is thus the case that BED is found among 15–50% of obese individuals seeking treatment (Latner and Clyne, 2008). To get an idea of the physical side of this experience, one may refer to the feelings that follow the consumption of an abundant meal: in the worse cases of BED, the same visceral sensations are reproduced even several times a day. It is certainly surprising how little attention in the literature is devoted to the relation between the digestion of large amounts of food and the perception of one's body.

What are well documented, on the other hand, are the similarities between the concerns for physical shape and weight in non-obese BED and bulimia (obese BED patients reported a significantly lower drive toward thinness) (Crow *et al.*, 2002; Vervaet, van Heeringen and Audenaert, 2004; Santonastaso, Ferrara and Favaro, 1999). This shared concern for physical appearance clearly conceals a form of anxiety for one's relation with others. What is particularly interesting is the fact that BED subjects, while also presenting a high degree of dissatisfaction with their bodies, do not seek to modify their shape and weight in the same way as bulimics: it is as if they passively endure what they perceive as their intolerable appearance.

The second consequence of the aforementioned difference between BED and bulimia, and one that is reflected in the frequent association between BED and co-morbid depression, concerns the feeling of personal negativity that characterizes those suffering from BED, and which increases as episodes of binge eating become more frequent. Striegel-Moore *et al.* (1998), in a population-based survey, found that individuals with full-blown BED syndrome suffered from greater sadness, lower self-esteem and greater stress than subjects with a sub-threshold variant of BED (defined as presenting a minimum of only one episode of binge eating per week). This data would seem to find further confirmation in other studies showing how binge eating not only does not provide any relief, but actually worsens the negative mood of the subject in the period that follows the binge (Stein *et al.*, 2007; Wegner *et al.*, 2002).

To put it another way, the more individuals with BED indulge in binge eating, the more they increase the negative feelings that make them prone to binge eating in the first place. Hence, the frequency of the practice is of crucial importance, both as an indicator of more critical triggering conditions (negative affects and emptiness) and because – through the establishment of a self-contained loop – it fosters and strengthens a range of negative feelings directed against oneself (disgust, guilt, helplessness, anger, sadness, regret and self-loathing).

These two aspects emerge quite clearly in the stories of individuals suffering from BED. On the one hand, the frequency of binge eating appears to be directly related to significant moments in a person's life, which exacerbate his sense of personal negativity. It is as if in order to cope with their perception of themselves, BED subjects were forced to change the frequency of their binge eating, thus affecting the course of their illness. On the other hand, the worsening of the person's feeling of worthlessness, which is caused by repeated episodes of binge eating that often lead to a visible increase in weight, in turn contributes to worsening his disorder. As was the case with anorexia nervosa and bulimia nervosa, the distinctive core psychopathology of BED is the subject's relation with his body, which – through food – becomes the centre to (negatively) attune to in order to regulate the dialectic between self-demarcation and the contemporaneous determination of Self by means of the other.

Disorders connected to male body shape

Only 10% of clinically diagnosed cases of eating disorders occur among male individuals (American Psychiatric Association, 2000). Diagnostic distribution among these subjects is similar to that reported for females, with cases of bulimia estimated to be 5 to 10 times higher than those of anorexia. By contrast, as we have seen, binge-eating disorder is most common among men, but there is no marked difference in distribution between male and female patients (Carlat and Camargo, 1991; Carlat, Camargo and Herzog, 1997; Spitzer *et al.*, 1992; Szmukler *et al.*, 1986). Therefore, how can we explain the congruence of distribution, in the 10% of cases reported among men, with cases reported for females? And what to make of the significant differences in the gender distribution of eating disorders?

It has been suggested that a high proportion of males with eating disorders are homosexual, bisexual or asexual. Gender congruence would thus be accounted for by the sexual inclinations of males who develop the illness (Carlat, Camargo and Herzog, 1997; Herzog *et al.*, 1984; Schneider and Agras, 1987; Fichter and Daser, 1987). Such a conclusion would appear to be supported by the fact that male heterosexual subjects who suffer from these disorders do not differ, in clinical terms, from women with eating disorders (Woodside *et al.*, 2001).

As for diversity in gender distribution, it may be the case that the illness manifests itself differently among male subjects. Eating disorders among men, that is, may be thought to present an aetiology that is similar to that found among female patients, but with a different symptomatology. Besides, if a person regulates his engagement with others by how he relates to his body, differences in the gender distribution of eating disorders are likely to depend on the way in which male individuals use their own bodies in the context of the dialectic between self-definition and acceptance by others. The regulation of this dialectic, in other words, may be seen to revolve around the same factors that lie behind the development of anorexia and bulimia, while taking a specifically male form.

As in the study of eating disorders, most research conducted on male subjects has focused on the issue of body image dissatisfaction, while in addition taking account of a central notion informing the body image of the male population: muscularity.

Unlike women, men not only appear more interested in shape than weight, but their body image dissatisfaction operates in the direction of weight gain (Anderson and Di Domenico, 1992). According to a perspective adopted in several studies of the issue, body image dissatisfaction, and hence the desire to become more muscular and develop a V-shaped figure, justifies rigorous exercise or weight training (Furnham, Badmin and Sneade, 2002). Olivardia *et al.* (2004), for instance, investigated the indices of body image and associated psychological traits among 154 male college students. When asked to choose the body they ideally wanted to have, men chose one with a mean of about 25 pounds more muscle than their actual level of muscularity and about 8 pounds less body fat than their actual level of fat. This preference for a lean and muscular body first arises somewhere between the ages of six and seven years, increases with age, and reaches a peak between early adolescence and the inception of adulthood (Ricciardelli and McCabe, 2004; Spitzer, Henderson and Zivian, 1999). This ideal is intimately tied to cultural views of masculinity.

Pope *et al.* (1999) have studied changes in the ideal image of the male body by measuring the waist, chest and bicep circumference of male action toys – GI Joe, Luke Skywalker and Han Solo – over the past 30 years. They found that action figures over time have grown more muscular and have developed a sharp muscular definition that far exceeds the shape attained by the largest human bodybuilders. In another study conducted by the same team (Leit, Pope and Gray, 2001), a review of 115 male centrefold models featured in issues of *Playgirl* magazine between 1973 and 1997 has shown that the models have grown increasingly 'dense' and more muscular in the course of the years.

So, just as in the case of women, it has been suggested that exposure to media-portrayed 'unrealistic' ideals of beauty may have contributed to the rising prevalence of eating disorders. Cultural ideals of muscularity among men may be seen to contribute to high levels of body dissatisfaction, extreme bodybuilding and abuse of anabolic steroids. In accordance with these suggestions, two disorders can be defined: the first, muscle dysmorphia, may be regarded as a male equivalent of anorexia; the second, the use of anabolic-androgenic steroids, presents some analogies with bulimia.

Muscle dysmorphia, which has been described as 'reverse anorexia nervosa' (Pope, Katz and Hudson, 1993; Pope and Katz, 1994), is a disorder characterized by: (1) a persistent concern for the size of one's musculature, even when this is well developed, to the point of avoiding activities and places where one's body may be seen (beaches, locker rooms, etc.) out of embarrassment for its perceived defects; (2) recurrent thoughts about one's muscular inadequacy; (3) significant distress or impairment in social, occupational or other important areas; (4) lack of control over one's compulsive weightlifting and dieting (Pope, Phillips and Olivardia, 2000; Olivardia, Pope and Hudson, 2000). As Olivardia, Pope and Hudson (2000) suggest in the conclusions to their first controlled study of muscle dysmorphia, 'the pursuit of "bigness" shows remarkable parallels to the pursuit of thinness'.

Like anorexia, muscle dysmorphia does not appear to originate from an alteration of one's perceived body image. Just as the subject's feeling of hunger represents the starting point for an understanding of anorexia, so the perception of one's being in the case of dysmorphia arises from the constant experience of one's muscles. For those subjects who construct their own identity through muscular perception, the pursuit of bigness embodies an absolute value. As in the case of anorexics, this perception of the body frees those suffering from dysmorphia from engaging with others.

A further example of the pursuit of muscularity is the use of anabolic-androgenic steroids. As several studies have illustrated, one of the chief reasons why adolescent males make use of steroids is to improve their physical appearance and attractiveness by conforming to an ideal image (Ricciardelli and McCabe, 2004; Bahrke *et al.*, 2000; Wichstrom and Pedersen, 2001). The adolescent who makes use of steroids to increase his body mass presents a series of traits that liken him to bulimics: low self-esteem and negative affects (Ricciardelli and McCabe, 2001; Irving *et al.*, 2002; Kindlundh *et al.*, 2001), as well as high levels of impulsive behaviour[17] (see the review by Ricciardelli and McCabe, 2004). An increase in the use of steroids, however, has also been found among adolescent boys who are elite athletes, and are thus characterized by a high degree of competitiveness (Bahrke *et al.*, 2000).

As in the case of bulimics, the use of steroids among adolescents and young males would appear to be related to the manipulation of physical attractiveness as a means to lessen anxiety about confrontation with others and others' judgements. Improving physical appearance according to cultural standards of masculinity would thus lead to greater peer acceptance and popularity among both male peers and members of the opposite sex (Eppright *et al.*, 1997; Holland and Andre, 1994). Here too, as in the case of bulimics, the problem revolves around one's fear of validation/lack of validation at the hands of others, something that is buffered by manipulating the shape of one's body. On the other hand, this cure for physical attractiveness is linked to an attunement to the body by means of muscular exercise.

The analogy that can be drawn between steroid use and bulimia is limited to the aspects we have just described. Steroid use lacks any equivalent to some of the crucial features of bulimia, such as the relation between negative emotions and binge eating or the adoption of corrective practices. As current literature, however, lacks any studies of first-hand experiences of subjects suffering from this pathology, it is perhaps too early to attempt to draw any comprehensive outline of the relation between steroid use, exercise and emotional control.

Behavioural addictions (compulsive buying, pathological gambling, kleptomania, internet addiction, impulsive-compulsive sexual behaviour, pyromania)

Analogies with some of the most relevant features of bulimia nervosa – such as binge eating and its relation to negative emotions, or the emergence, in the aftermath of binge eating, of self-evaluative emotions such as guilt, shame and embarrassment – become more evident when we consider disorders connected to behavioural addiction.

Before describing which elements allow us to recognize the same core psychopathological process in these pathologies that marks eating disorders, it is necessary to stress that behavioural addictions can also emerge in other styles of personality. What this implies is that different ways of emotionally perceiving oneself can trigger the same impulsive behaviours.

For instance, while the buying (or stealing) of useless objects may be triggered by a feeling of emptiness (as in the case of Robert, discussed at the beginning of this book), it may also be caused by the idea that resisting a purchase would be to lose out on a bargain.

Likewise, pathological gambling may be triggered by the unbearable weight of boredom – which in the case of certain EDP individuals corresponds to a lack of stimuli

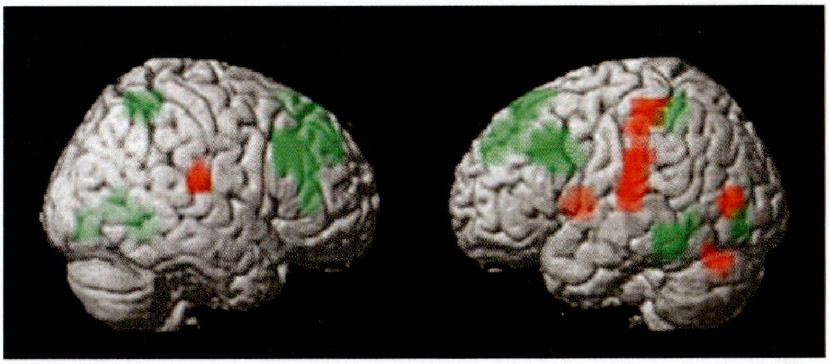

Figure 2

with which to define oneself. This drive to gamble, however, will be quite different from that experienced by the main character in Dostoevsky's (Dostoevsky,2006) novel *The Gambler*, who in the extraordinary epilogue of the novel, after accepting the few coins thrown to him almost in contempt by an old friend, feels that in resisting betting he is missing the chance of his life. 'All it would take would be shrewdness and patience, for once! All it would take would be to show one's character for once, and in one hour I could change my whole fortune!'

The emotional antecedents that trigger the disorder are therefore connected to the story of the patient, whose first-hand experience is needed in order to correctly interpret symptomatic dynamics. The interplay between the first- and third-person perspectives would seem to be an essential epistemological prerequisite for psychopathology.

In the framework of the EDP style of personality, what distinguishes behavioural addictions from eating disorders and disorders connected to male body shape is the fact that the person's perception of his body is focused, not on a visceral aspect (hunger, satiety, weariness, muscularity), but, rather, on a condition of profound arousal, which patients themselves describe as a feeling of euphoria, a high, a rush or even a sexual feeling (as, for instance, is often the case with compulsive buying).[18]

The emotional context in which these behaviours emerge is invariably characterized by emotions that revolve around conditions of loneliness, such as a sense of emptiness or boredom; conditions of lack of validation, which trigger self-critical thoughts or anger; and conditions of exposure anxiety. Although systematic studies of the subject have yet to be carried out, the highly specific nature of the triggers involved suggests that the behaviours (generally perceived as pleasurable) that characterize these various disorders come about as a way of overcoming negative affects (Jacobs, 1989; Faber, 1992). This, at any rate, has clearly been documented in the case of compulsive buying. Scherhorn, Reisch and Raab (1990), Faber and O'Guinn (1992) and Miltenberger *et al.* (2003) all found that negative emotions were the most common antecedents to shopping binges. Depressive states and tension are also often reported as precursors to kleptomania and other kinds of theft (Bradford and Balmaceda, 1983; Goldman, 1991).

The sequence in which these behaviours occur, moreover, is largely the same for all disorders and appears similar to that in binge eating. Driven by an unpleasant situation, the person develops an urge to act, which may be satisfied depending on the circumstances. If the circumstances at hand do not allow the subject to act, he then focuses his attention on the anticipation of a series of actions by preparing himself for their coming into effect. The chronological gap between preparing a given action and implementing it is characterized by an increased arousal that absorbs the subject's attention through the planning of the sequence, thus progressively narrowing his range of self-awareness.

The performance of the actual behaviour, which is characterized by an exacerbation of the person's present condition, is described across different disorders as the most intensely exciting moment of the process; it corresponds to complete absorption in the experience: a kind of tunnel vision accompanied by a loss of context.

One of our patients, for instance, who had already been reported repeatedly to the police for indecent exposure, explained to me that he would start planning to expose his naked body when he perceived he had been judged negatively by his boss at work, and at times even when finding himself alone in the office.

The need of our patient to expose himself, therefore, arose both from situations where he felt annulled by negative judgements, and from circumstances in which the experience of finding himself alone triggered a strong sense of emptiness. In both cases, our patient lost the usual points of reference through which to co-perceive himself. The dynamics of exposure, repeated several times a day, consisted in showing himself naked before groups of students aged 14–18 who attended the female school whose windows overlooked his terrace. As our patient's apartment was not far from his office, and as he could only expose himself to the students during their morning break, he would leave work whenever the circumstances allowed it.

Our patient's level of arousal would thus progressively increase as he was going home, increasing even more once he had entered his apartment, had taken his clothes off and was waiting behind the curtains, his eyes on the windows of the school. As the hour of the morning break approached, he would feel his heart race; his body would stiffen, his breathing grow heavy... until the school bell announced the break. As soon as the windows opened and the students showed themselves, our patient would start running about naked on his terrace. As the girls screamed and laughed at him, he would be pervaded by an extraordinary feeling of satiety: a mix of euphoria and excitement.

A similar sequence has also been described by Black (2007) in relation to compulsive buying. Black identifies four distinct phases: (1) anticipation, (2) preparation, (3) shopping and (4) spending.

A compulsive buyer described a 'binge' episode in terms that suggest a process of activation similar to that experienced by our own patient: 'But it was like, it was almost like my heart palpitating. I couldn't wait to get in to see what was there. It was such a sensation. In the store, the lights, the people; they were playing Christmas music. I was hyperventilating and my hands were starting to sweat, and all of a sudden I was touching sweaters and the whole of it was just beckoning to me' (O'Guinn and Faber, 1989).

The creation of visceral states would thus appear to be the common thread that links the various disorders triggered by this style of personality. From hunger to satiety, vomit to diarrhoea, weariness to physical exertion, excitement to a sexual arousal caused by an urge to buy – focus on one's body experience serves as a way to readjust a sense of Self that has lost its anchoring on the other. As this chapter has repeatedly stressed, a person's relation with his body becomes the means by which he regulates the dialectic with the other he must both conform to and distinguish himself from. By far the most surprising aspect of this problem, and one that offers new research prospects, is the fact that the personality style in question, one that finds stability in focusing on external points of reference (through the co-perception of others), in order to cope with difficult relational situations, can be seen to create visceral states to which to attune. It is as if the creation of these states were the only way in which the person could free himself from the other.

Endnotes

[1] Mounier (1946: 41).

[2] Honouring a commitment, for instance, binds changeable experience to a fixed point of reference.

[3] Affectivity is what allows the ontological relation between sameness, ipseity and alterity to be studied from a psychological perspective.

[4] 'An ideal type is formed by the one-sided accentuation of one or more points of view and by the synthesis of a great many diffuse, discrete, more or less present and occasionally absent concrete

individual phenomena, which are arranged according to those one-sidedly emphasized viewpoints into a unified analytical construct...' (Weber, 1997: 88).

[5] In the case of oppositional behaviour, by contrast, the other acts as a model through which the person can define himself and generate meaning.

[6] In the 1950s, Reisman described the impact of the media representation of reality on education in the following terms: 'With the new models, the peer group – the group formed by individuals of the same age and belonging to the same social class – acquires greater importance for the child, as his parents will reprimand him not so much on account of his violation of internal norms, as for failings connected to his own popularity or relations with others' (Reisman, 1961: 81).

[7] Rosen argues that many members of the Generation X elite possess this type of personality. 'Generation X', a name derived from that of a British punk band, comprises 80 million souls born in the 20-year period between 1965 and 1984.

[8] *Reactance* is here understood as the state that motivates individuals to behave in oppositional ways in order to maintain or acquire autonomy (Brehm and Brehm, 1981).

[9] Witkin used the expression 'field-dependency' to describe the inclination – which we would regard as part of the Outward polarity – that characterized those subjects who orientated their erect posture on the basis of their sensory field rather than bodily indicators (as was the case with 'field-independents'). Witkin's distinction is here provided with an emotional foundation that allows it to be integrated within an ontological view of the body.

[10] The media therefore, while altering perceptions by introducing discontinuity, offered new forms of consistency and new recurrent points of reference.

[11] This would also contribute to explaining why eating disorders usually manifest themselves for the first time during adolescence.

[12] It is possible, no doubt, to follow Janet and interpret the term 'voluntarily' as a fixed idea, thus examining the problem as an obsessive disorder. The case of anorexia, however, differs from that of obsessive disorders, as we shall see in the next chapter.

[13] Various studies suggest that 20–50% of individuals with anorexia nervosa will develop bulimia nervosa over time. Other studies (i.e. Eddy *et al.*, 2008) convincingly suggest that the transition from anorexia nervosa (particularly the binge-eating/purging type) to bulimia nervosa may not represent a change in disorder but a change in stage of illness.

[14] The correlation between chronic anxiety and bulimia has long been documented: see Johnson, Lewis and Hagman (1984), Mizes (1988), Mitchell *et al.* (1985) and Schlesier-Stropp (1984).

[15] Affective instability, along with identity disturbance and impulsiveness, is indicative of a certain degree of contiguity between bulimia and borderline personality disorder (Cooper *et al.*, 1988; Vitousek and Manke, 1994; van Hanswijck de *et al.*, 2003; Wonderlich *et al.*, 2005, 2007).

[16] As bulimia takes a chronic form, the passage from binge eating to purging becomes increasingly automatic. This contributes to explaining why many bulimic patients attribute the same power to purging that others attribute to binge eating.

[17] 'Adolescents who use anabolic steroids have been found to be more likely to drink alcohol, use other licit and illicit drugs, drink and drive, engage in unprotected sex, report truancy and poorer school achievement, become involved in fights and display other aggressive type conduct problems, and possess a gun' (Ricciardelli and McCabe, 2004: 195).

[18] The noradrenergic system, for instance, has been postulated to underlie sensation-seeking behaviours, aspects of which are thought to be abnormal among pathological gamblers (Roy *et al.*, 1988).

6 The Obsessive-Compulsive-prone Style of Personality

The structural characteristic of this style of personality is a stable anchoring to an external system of coordinates, on which to fix the variability of one's experience by providing it with definite and certain meaning. Being oneself, here, corresponds to a form of self-perception generated through the conformity of ongoing experience to an impersonal set of references. Be it law or religion, morals or the scientific method, common sense or mathematics, musical arrangement or bureaucratic structures, philosophical analysis or military hierarchy, social conventions or molecular biology, the structural stability of a person's reference system provides the peculiar alterity – merely a reflection of the actual living other – that the individual must conform to in order to feel stably situated. This mode of co-determination of Self is centred on the constant adherence to a given order. As such, it profoundly differs from the attunement to alterity that characterizes the eating disorder-prone style of personality, although – as we shall see – intermediate forms allow the two styles to share a degree of contiguity within the same Outward polarity.

The greatest difference regards the way in which the dialectic between ipseity and alterity is articulated. Whereas EDP subjects were seen to face the problem of how to differentiate themselves from the other, by means of which they simultaneously define themselves, in the case of obsessive-compulsive subjects the problem is an opposite one. The issue at stake here is how to adhere to an alterity that is abstract, so to speak: one that is independent of people, and thus cannot pose the problem of self-demarcation (from others). In this case, the person's relation to others is itself mediated by abstract reference systems. This process generates a particular form of intimacy between the subject and his dear ones, an intimacy that – as we shall see – is characterized by a strange alchemy of care and distance, solicitude and indifference, severity and dedication. On the other hand, strangers may be perceived as part of a broader order, and thus defined on the basis of the determinations applied to that order, to the point of disregarding their very humanity. The alterity of the other, that is, only becomes relevant in the light of the

Selfhood, identity and personality styles Giampiero Arciero and Guido Bondolfi

set of impersonal references that apply to it. This is something Kafka (1995) illustrates with horrifying lucidity in 'In the Penal Colony'.

The highly heterogeneous phenomenology of the obsessive-compulsive-prone (OCP) style, therefore, can be seen to take shape within the framework of the dialectic between the experience the individual has of himself from time to time on the one hand, and his correspondence, excessive adherence (as in the case of paranoia) or lack of adherence – to the point of disunion – (as in the case of ruin delusion) to the system of co-determination of Self on the other. As we shall see when examining the two literary figures of Kleist's (1997) *Michael Kohlhaas* and Dostoevsky's (1998) *Mr Prokharchin*, shifts in the balance of this dialectic can alter individuals' perception of themselves, their way of generating meaning and being with others, to such an extent that it is often difficult to trace a clear line between reason and loss of reason.

It is precisely this thin line generated by the development of a total and inflexible adhesion to the system of co-determinations of Self that we will be exploring through Kleist's writing.[1]

6.1 *Michael Kohlhaas*

The crux of this extraordinary novel is already embedded in its first page: as clear as a theorem that only awaits development. Right from the start, Kleist gives the protagonist's name and describes his home, job and father; in the very same sentence – as if this were part of the character's immutable identity – he also adds that he was 'one of the most honest and most terrible human beings of his time' (Kleist, 1997: 209).

Such is Michael Kohlhaas, a horse-dealer and an exceptional man: a hard-working, loyal, charitable and righteous man who wants to help others. Toward the end of the first section, while praising the protagonist, Kleist subtly presents the premise to his argument: in one of those valued virtues Kohlhaas had passed the mark. In the next sentence, the theme of the whole novel is cast like a stone: 'His sense of justice turned him into a robber and murderer' (Kleist, 1997: 209).

As a horse-dealer, Michael Kohlhaas leads a herd of young horses across the border into Saxony, to be sold at some fairs. As soon as he has crossed the Elba river by the castle of the feudatory Junker Wenzel von Tronka, Kohlhaas meets an obstacle: accused of lacking transit papers, he is asked not only to pay a tribute, but to leave a pledge later to be redeemed by presenting the required documents. Kohlhaas leaves two blackish horses and a servant to care for them and continues his journey to Leipzig. Once in Dresden, he visits the Secret Chancellery, where his suspicion is confirmed: that the need for transit papers was a lie. Kohlhaas is issued a document certifying his right of transit and gets back on the road home 'with no more bitterness' (Kleist, 1997: 212).

When he reaches the castle, Kohlhaas shows the document and asks for his two horses. Unfortunately, not only does he find that his servant has been dismissed on account of his unseemly behaviour, but instead of his own well-fed and healthy horses, Kohlhaas is presented by the stable boy with two gaunt and rangy ones: for the whole time he was away, his horses were used as draught animals in the Junker's fields. Kohlhaas vehemently protests against this abuse, thus attracting the attention of the steward; but his complaints only elicit threats from the man. Despite a strong urge to cover the steward in dung, 'his sense of justice, delicate as a goldsmith's scales, still wavered'

(Kleist, 1997: 213). As the circumstances in which his servant was dismissed are not clear, instead of venting his rage on the steward, in a low voice Kohlhaas asks him to explain what mistake the servant had committed. After receiving an elusive answer, he leaves his two horses at the castle and sets off toward home, secretly yearning to learn from the servant whether the loss of the horses was really due to a misdeed on his part. Driven by this sense of justice (*richtiges Gefühl*), upon reaching home Kohlhaas questions his servant with the meticulousness of a judge. The man tells him that he had been unjustly accused, beaten and expelled from the castle. Having learnt the truth, Kohlhaas, with the help of a jurist he knows, sues the Junker, asking for the rehabilitation and restitution of his horses, and compensation for the damage wrought to both him and his servant.

Almost one year later, Kohlhaas is informed by his lawyer that the suit was turned down because of the political influence of the Junker's relatives; the lawyer advises him to renounce any further attempt to solve the question. Kohlhaas does not give up and, through an acquaintance, sends a petition to the Elector of Saxony asking for the court of Dresden to reopen the case. Soon, however, he learns from a visiting magistrate that his case has been ignored. The sadness he feels is overwhelming. When he receives a resolution from the Chancellery, advising him to retrieve his horses and settle the question, Kohlhaas is enraged.

It is at this turning point in the narrative that the first transformation of the protagonist occurs: 'in the midst of the pain it gave him to see the world in such monstrous disorder he felt a sudden access of inner satisfaction that at least his own heart was in order now' (Kleist, 1997: 221). As the unity between his own actions and feelings and the order of the world (i.e. justice) is broken, Kohlhaas himself becomes the source of the order to which the disorder of the world must correspond. With a flurry of resolutions that upset both his life and that of his family, Kohlhaas decides to sell his house and possessions and send his wife and children abroad. His desperate wife asks him to 'play a final card': through an acquaintance she might present a petition to the Prince of Saxony. Kohlhaas, moved and proud of his wife, allows her to leave in the company of a servant. This will prove the most unfortunate move of all: when attempting to hand in the petition, the woman is beaten by a guard. A few days later, having been brought home by the servant, she dies in the arms of her husband. After giving his wife a funeral worthy of a princess, Kohlhaas vows revenge.

At dusk, like the 'Avenging Angel' (Kleist, 1997: 226), Kohlhaas breaks into the castle of Junker Wenzel von Trotta with some armed servants and destroys it. The Junker, however, manages to escape. A furious Kohlhaas, 'a man subject to no law of the empire or the world, but only to God's' (Kleist, 1997: 230), spreads terror and death in his search for the Junker.

It is in these circumstances that Martin Luther addresses Michael Kohlhaas with a public notice affixed in all the cities and towns of the principality. The message accuses Kohlhaas of injustice and is signed by Luther himself, 'the name of all the names he knew best loved and fittest to be revered' (Kleist, 1997: 236). Kohlhaas thus leaves his men and hurries to Wittenberg, dressed as a tenant farmer, in order to meet Martin Luther to induce him to change his opinion.

The meeting between the two men constitutes a second turning point in the story and the life of the protagonist. The theme is again that of justice. The step Luther takes is to show Kohlhaas that there was no need for him to disrupt the unity between himself and the state – the conforming of his actions and feelings to the justice of men – for no one had denied him the protection of law. The sovereign, who had not been informed of the quarrel, could not be held responsible for the failings of some officials. By proving the groundlessness of Kohlhaas' desire to seek justice on his own, Luther persuades him to submit once more to the law. Kohlhaas then leaves with a safe conduct, disbands his troop, and tries once more to bring his case to the attention of the law court that had previously dismissed him. Luther, in turn, promises to ask the prince to grant Kohlhaas an amnesty.

Here starts a new section of the novel, which unfolds through the countless intrigues of the court of Saxony (the Junker still being under the protection of his influential family), intrigues which end with the violation of the amnesty and Kohlhaas' arrest. This time the sovereign (the Elector of Saxony) can no longer be said to be unaware of the facts.

At this point, it would seem that the very theme around which the novel was developed has been abandoned. Under armed surveillance, Kohlhaas is led to Berlin to face what the royal family hopes will be an exemplary trial. He loses his battle.

It is in the course of this journey, on the road to Berlin, that Kohlhaas receives a visit, when one night his guards stop for a rest. Only a short distance separates the prisoner's lodging from a merry band of gentlemen and ladies, who are hunting deer in the company of the Elector of Saxony and his wife. As the entire party, under the influence of wine, is busy pursuing a herd of deer, the wife of the prince is driven by curiosity to invite her husband to visit the famous prisoner in disguise. They find Kohlhaas taking care of one of his sons, so in order to strike up a conversation, they ask a series of questions which he answers without pausing in his task. The prince, not knowing what to talk about, notices a capsule attached to a silk thread hanging from Kohlhaas' neck, and asks the prisoner what it contains.

Kohlhaas then tells the prince the story of the capsule and the note it contains.

The note, he explains, had been given to him under strange circumstances by a gypsy woman who read horoscopes. The Elector of Saxony and that of Brandenburg, while on an evening stroll in the city, had stopped to speak to this woman, and had jokingly asked her if she had anything to reveal to them. Kohlhaas had happened upon this scene and had stopped to watch. The woman, while speaking with the princes, had scribbled something on a piece of paper. Suddenly, leaving the princes, she had approached Kohlhaas and handed him the note, telling him to store it, for one day it would save his life.

Kohlhaas has just finished telling this story when the Elector faints. He is taken to the castle, where he faints again twice. In the following days, he continues to feel ill. When questioned by the treasurer, the prince reveals that the cause of his illness is the worthless note in Kohlhaas' possession, which he fervently desires to lay his hands upon. He thus sends a young nobleman to tell Kohlhaas that, in exchange for the note, he will be spared his life and granted freedom. The horse-dealer Michael Kohlhaas gives the following answer:

> *Sir, if your sovereign came and said: I will annihilate myself with all the band of those who help me rule – annihilate himself, do you understand me, which is of course my soul's dearest wish – I would still refuse to give him the paper which matters more to him than his existence, and should say: 'You can bring me to the scaffold, but I can do you injury, and I will' (Kleist, 1997: 267–68).*

What makes this such a powerful comeback is the theme through which the whole novel initially took shape: the striking of an enemy, even at the cost of one's own life, owing to one's sense of justice.

The mystery surrounding the note is solved in the final pages of the novel. On that piece of paper the gypsy, who had impressed the two princes by giving extraordinary proof of her powers as a clairvoyant, had written the name of the last sovereign of the royal house of Saxony, the year in which he would lose his reign and the name of the man who would usurp his throne.

On the scaffold, his eyes fixed on the Prince of Saxony, Kohlhaas takes out the note, reads it, places it in his mouth and swallows it. As the prince faints again, his body shaken by convulsions, Kohlhaas' head rolls under the executioner's axe.

6.2 *Mr Prokharchin*

Of a rather different character from *Michael Kohlhaas* is Dostoevsky's novel *Mr Prokharchin*. Here too the narrative revolves around the relation between the experience an individual has of himself and his adherence to the principles of order of the world, although in this case the relation takes the form of a distance between the determinations of the person and the truths of the world. If it is indeed the case that 'the lofty principles behind the person's worldview are one with the principles behind the most concrete of his personal experiences', as Bakhtin (1984: 103) writes with reference to Dostoevsky's characters, it is important to emphasize that it is particularly the tension emerging from the loss of this coincidence that profoundly disturbs the characters in question. Kohlhaas, when faced with the disruption of this correspondence, personally becomes the source of all lofty principles: like the archangel Michael, he punishes 'the wickedness to which the whole world had succumbed' (Kleist, 1997: 81). Prokharchin, by contrast, is overcome by the end of coincidence he so feared, to the point that his life loses all meaning. It is this change that Dostoevsky explores in his novel.

Semen Ivanovic Prokharchin was getting on in years; a respectable man and a teetotaller, he worked as a humble clerk, earning wages proportionate to his role. He lived at the place of Ustin'ja Fedorovna, occupying the darkest corner of the house, and led a modest and withdrawn life. Although Prokharchin only paid half the rent of other tenants, his meekness made him one of Ustin'ja Fedorovna's favourite lodgers. Prokharchin, however, was not held in the same esteem by the other tenants. Although they regarded him as a decent person, they did not consider him one of theirs.

Most striking of all was Prokharchin's frugality: he always managed to economize on food and he never spent more than 25 kopecks, by contenting himself with just a portion of cabbage or beef. Most of the time, however, in order to economize even on this miserable fare, he would just eat bread with onions, cheese and cucumber. Only when losing his strength would he return to his meagre lunch, for which he had to pay.

Prokharchin was not keen on company and chatter. He could not stand it when those who knew his reserve asked him what it was he kept in the small chest under his bed. Everyone in the house knew that all it contained were old rags, three pairs of worn-out boots and some other junk. Prokharchin, on the other hand, greatly valued his property. When, one day, a fellow lodger dared suggest that Prokharchin was accumulating stuff in that chest he wished to pass on to his heirs, Prokharchin at first muttered insults under his breath, then calmed down; but after getting into bed he started again, this time addressing the man directly. In the following days, joining the other lodgers as they were drinking tea, Prokharchin took up the subject again in order to make it clear that he was a poor man with nothing to save, and that all his wages went on supporting his sister-in-law. After a long and elaborate explanation, which he repeated several times to impress his listeners, Prokharchin fell silent. Three days later, however, he surprised everybody by insulting the young tenant who had had the bad idea of teasing him about his alleged inheritance.

The people in the house found Prokharchin's attitude not only bizarre, but also amusing, to the point where they chose to attack him en masse. As lately Prokharchin had started taking part in the lodgers' conversations at teatime, whenever he arrived the younger ones, exchanging glances, would start telling some new and utterly fabricated tale with the same recurrent theme in mind: Prokharchin's frugality. They would relate stories from the office about how married clerks were better suited to the career than bachelors, how some good manners were going to be taught to those who had none by cutting their wages, or about how a few clerks, particularly elder ones, were going to be asked to sit some exams – the implication here being that these people would need to spend some money in order to train properly.

Prokharchin, who hated all novelty, suddenly and for no apparent reason began to change in character. He became restless, suspicious, alarmed, and particularly concerned with the veracity of the news that reached him. This change became so acute that the behaviour of Prokharchin, absorbed as he was in his own fantasies, proved shocking. Finally, one day, he was gone both from home and his office.

Prokharchin's disappearance threw the house into confusion. Three days later, Ustin'ja Fedorovna, who had always regarded Prokharchin as her favourite lodger, sent the rest of the tenants to search for him. Two of them returned, reporting they had seen him in the company of a rather disreputable person who, a few weeks earlier, had asked Ustin'ja Fedorovna to be accepted as a tenant but had been rejected. Reassured at having found Prokharchin, the lodgers played another trick on him. With an old shawl and the proprietress' bonnet they constructed a manikin; they placed this in Prokharchinn's bed with the intention of telling him, upon his return, that his sister-in-law from the provinces had moved into his room. The lodgers waited most of the night for Prokharchin, but he never arrived. At four in the morning, they were all awoken by a violent knock on the door: a coachman dragged in a drenched Prokharchin, who had passed out and was shaking with convulsions. The tenants looked at him and realized he was not drunk. They laid him down on his bed, where he spent several days, occasionally complaining about his poverty.

Prokharchin was destined never to recover. Incited by the other lodgers, amid fits of delirium and fainting, Prokharchin provided a clear explanation for his condition: '. . .as I am poor, were they to take my job. . . were they to take it just like that. . . for, brother, there is a job for me now, but it might not always be there. . . do you understand?'. A moment before dying, sobbing, Prokharchin repeated once more that he was poor, that they were to give him something to eat and drink, and take care of him.

The other lodgers were moved. Some sobbed, some wished to hold a collection, some regretted having frightened poor Prokharchin so much, some were surprised at how this man could have upset his whole life because of a few words spoken to him in jest.

Prokharchin's small chest was opened and was found to contain rags and various items of junk. His cushion was inspected, and so was his mattress. How surprised the ten lodgers were when a bundle of money fell out of a hole in the mattress! When the whole mattress was opened, a small fortune came to light. Semen Ivanovic Prokharchin lay amid mattress feathers 'like a hardened capitalist of long experience, who even in his coffin would not dream of wasting a single moment in inactivity, he seemed to be wholly immersed in some kind of speculative calculations' (Dostoevsky, 1998: 248).

The two novels by Kleist and Dostoevsky reconfigure what are apparently noncomparable experiences. In the first case, a man, Kohlhaas, after perceiving that the justice governing the world is no longer a righteous one, chooses to place himself above it in order to rectify it. In the name of justice, having been refused any compensation for the two horses that had been ill-treated, Kohlhaas spreads terror and death around him, to the point of preferring to be executed rather than renounce his quest for vengeance.

In the second case, a mounting fear that the present order of things might change induces Prokharchin to lose all sources of meaning. Through a series of jests – which he does not perceive as such – Prokharchin is led to believe that he will lose his job. The poor man then starts to perceive that the correspondence between his possible actions on the world and the principles that regulate his own feeling and acting – a connection based on frugality – is threatened and may well come to an end. Frugality is the meaning system which allows Prokharchin to feel both situated and at one with his experience of the world; yet, at the same time, frugality only represents a source of meaning (and thus situates Prokharchin in the world) provided he is guaranteed a job in the office. Were he to lose that job, his life would break down, for the entire system of coordinates that frugality provided his everyday experience with would also lose all meaning. Significantly, the last sensible sentences Prokharchin utters before abandoning himself to bewailing his poverty and, finally, dying, concern the possible loss of his job.

The crucial difference between the two ways of being of these characters lies precisely in the way in which they perceive the relation between the set of rules governing the world and their own experiences. The issue at stake in the case of Kohlhaas is the overdetermination of one's personal experience: on the basis of this, the character proclaims the failure of justice, here understood as the order of the world, and the need to restore it. In order to understand what is happening in the mind of Kohlhaas, it is useful to refer to the previously-quoted words of Raskolnikov in *Crime and Punishment*: 'I simply intimate that the "extraordinary" man has the right... I don't mean a formal, official right, but he has the right in himself, to permit his conscience to overstep... certain obstacles, but only in the event that his ideas (which may sometimes be salutary for all mankind) require it for their fulfilment' (Dostoevsky, 1953: 249).

It is with dread and anguish that Prokharchin perceives the possibility of a change in the order of the world, for the scenarios described by his fellow lodgers would not allow him to continue acting in conformity to those principles (i.e. frugality) that are meaningful for him: not only would his actions become meaningless, but so would the whole system. Following the collapse of frugality as a meaning system, the experience of Self becomes painful: it is as if the subject were overwhelmed by a world he can no longer order and access through his experience, which thus becomes meaningless.

In between these two poles, marked by opposite perceptions of Self, are a series of intermediate states, which are characterized by an incomplete adherence to the objective system of co-determination of meaning. If in each case ipseity acquires meaning through its correspondence to an impersonal set of references, which at the same time mediates the subject's encounter with the world, then any decrease in the subject's coincidence with that order will entail a degree of distance between experience and sense. For instance: if a subject's actions and emotions become relevant in relation to the righteousness of his behaviour as a father, the fact that he may have had an outburst of anger against his son, merely because the latter disturbed him while he was reading the paper, cannot be reconciled with his sense of being a righteous father. The person's experience of anger, that is, does not fit with the system of co-determinations of meaning that guides his conduct. This gives rise to an inconsistency between experience and sense.

This alteration of the unity between an individual's meaning system and his experience translates into a condition that is defined by a more or less profound feeling of indecisiveness, insecurity and incompleteness (Janet, 1904). This condition engenders a range of heterogeneous and shifting behaviours which are nevertheless aimed at the attainment of stability: a search, that is, for the correspondence between experience and sense. To return to the above example, a father who has just had an outburst of unmotivated anger against his son is likely to ask for his forgiveness, and justify his own reaction on the basis of the sense coordinates of his own system, to which he will conform once again. Alternatively, the individual in question might spend hours thinking about the episode that occurred, questioning his own behaviour as a father, measuring the consequences of his reaction for his son, assessing the possibility that similar actions – and their dangerous consequences – might occur again in the future because of unchecked anger, and so on. The same dialectic between ipseity and an impersonal meaning system (alterity) that underlines the formation of the subject's personality also embodies – as we shall see in the next section – the distinctive core psychopathology common to all obsessive-compulsive disorders.

If the meaning of one's experience is assured by the possibility of corresponding to an impersonal system of sense, and if it is this correspondence that provides a feeling of individual stability, a central role is also played by non-basic emotions. Non-basic emotions originate from the subject's correspondence with the system of sense through which concrete experience is always co-determined. In the case of this style of personality, as opposed to the EDP style, individuals co-perceive their feeling and acting through the values of an impersonal system of sense by means of which they assess their own behaviour. Self-focused emotions like shame or pride – which pertain to the overall evaluation of Self – or guilt – which is connected to the assessment of a given action or the embarrassment stemming from the sharing of one's behaviour – are a prominent feature of this style of personality. Similarly important are other-focused emotions, such as the anger, disgust and contempt related to the violation of the sense coordinates through which the subject regulates his experience and orders the world. Of particular interest, in this context, are disgust and its relation to inter-group attitudes. A study carried out on a group of English Canadians revealed that interpersonal disgust indirectly relates to attitudes toward immigrants, which are channelled through individual differences in ideological orientation (e.g. right-wing authoritarianism), and through dehumanizing perceptions of the out-group (Hodson and Costello, 2007).

The subject's relation to his emotional world has often been regarded as the crucial problem behind this style of personality. It is as if an emotional dimension were incompatible with this way of being, marked by a hypertrophic over-development of cognitive aspects.

This commonly-stated assertion is only partly true, as the complex variety of emotional experiences that characterize this style of personality is co-determined by the systems of sense to which these emotions correspond. The same emotional state, therefore, for example anger, may be regarded as appropriate by the person experiencing it – as in the case of Kohlhaas – or as utterly inappropriate and almost alien – as in the previously mentioned example of the father – depending on whether the emotional condition in question (and its intensity) corresponds to the system through which it is co-perceived. In the absence of any correspondence, the condition is perceived by the subject as a threat to his integrity and hence stability. Unsurprisingly, situations in which affective quality and intensity cannot be foreseen can have a critical impact on the maintenance of personal stability. This is the case, for instance, with adolescent detachment; with the establishment, consolidation and severing of sentimental ties; with bereavement, pregnancy and birth. A clear example of this is the postpartum obsessive-compulsive disorder, in which a prenatal onset is often characterized by fears of contamination, and a postpartum onset by unwanted thoughts of harming one's infant (see Abramowitz *et al.*, 2003).

On the other hand, even the value system on which a person bases his stability can be challenged by events that disprove its truths, to the point of being completely overturned – as is the case with certain forms of conversion.

An analysis of the foundations of the OCP style of personality that did not take account of one of its forms bordering on the EDP would be incomplete. As the line between the two personality styles has long been a matter of debate when it comes to anorexia and bulimia nervosa, it will be worth outlining the characteristics of this unique form in a section devoted to structural disorders.

6.3 Disorders

In the course of the previous section, we repeatedly stressed how at the basis of the OCP style of personality lies an ipseity shaped by an adherence to an impersonal system of meaning that can be configured in various ways. This adherence simultaneously bestows order on the world and meaning on one's experience, thus providing a perception of personal stability. Hence, the alteration (to the point of complete disruption) of the correspondence between one's experience and one's system of meaning, by releasing feelings and actions from the stable set of coordinates used to co-perceive oneself, engenders a feeling of indecisiveness, insecurity and incompleteness. This ontological perception of Self, so to speak, springs from the very heart of ipseity, for it comes about through the loss of that correspondence to impersonal alterity that makes OCP individuals feel situated. As Janet has correctly observed, this feeling – manifested in the spheres of action (e.g. indecision), of the intellect (e.g. doubt), of the emotions (e.g. unease) and of self-perception (e.g. a sense of self-alienation) – is one of the marks of psychasthenia.

Examining this feeling at the end of his first volume – as in so many other sections of his weighty study on obsessions and psychasthenia, Janet asks: '*Ne se pourrait-il pas qu'il (le malade c.m.) ait généralisé à tort et à travers, qu'il ait appliqué à un acte insignifiant un sentiment détermine' par une imperfection psychologique réelle?...c'est vers cette opinion que je tendrais et pour moi le problème des scrupuleux consiste a trouver quelle est cette imperfection psychologique...*'[2] (Janet, 1904: 429).

We can now attempt to answer the above question: *le sentiment d'incompletude* that Janet talks about corresponds to an alteration of the feeling of being situated that arises from the distance between the subject's ongoing experience and his impersonal system of sense. This is the 'psychological imperfection' that 'like a thorn in their side, constantly troubles the subjects' and engenders the characteristic traits of an obsessive personality.

In accordance with this perspective, it is possible to re-examine a series of fMRI findings that suggest that at the basis of the illness lies a dysfunction of the orbitofronto-striatal-thalamic circuits (Saxena *et al.*, 1998; Saxena, Bota and Brody, 2001; Graybiel and Rauch, 2000; Kringelbach and Rolls, 2004) and, less consistently, of the limbic structures (hippocampus, anterior cingolate gyrus, amygdala) connected to the processing of reward (O'Doherty *et al.*, 2001; Murray, O'Doherty and Schoenbaum, 2007; Kalin, Shelton and Davidson, 2007). This alteration may explain the absence of a feeling of goal completion, for instance when a certain action is performed in ways that are perceived as being inconsistent with given meaning principles. The subject's sense of incompleteness would thus be seen as arising from the imbalance between excitatory and inhibitory pathways within the fronto-striatal circuits (Saxena *et al.*, 1998; Saxena, Bota and Brody, 2001). Although a series of studies provide evidence for the recruitment of a distinct neural network for each symptom (Phillips *et al.*, 2000; Saxena *et al.*, 2004; Mataix-Cols *et al.*, 2004), what remains to be defined are the common correlates behind these many and heterogeneous disorders. Only in the light of a shared feature underpinning the sense of insecurity of the subjects can symptomatic variety be accounted for in a coherent way (Mataix-Cols, do Rosario-Campos and Leckman, 2005).

The subject perceives his indecisiveness as a blurring of meaning, for it prevents him from understanding his ongoing experience through the coordinates of an anchoring system. He thus perceives his experience as something that is distant, to the point of being alien. Moreover, just as the certainty of an order to which the individual can conform provides him with a sense of security with respect to his own conduct under all circumstances, and allows him correctly to foresee the consequences of his actions, a condition of insecurity precludes any such possibility.

The sense of incompleteness of Self focuses the subject's attention on the present to such an extent that it limits his sense of initiative. This appears particularly evident in what several authors have described as two distinctive traits of obsessive personality: perfectionism and indecision.

References have already been made in relation to the EDP style of personality to a sort of 'strategic' perfectionism aimed at minimizing the chances of negative evaluation. This kind of perfectionism shares certain features with both self-oriented perfectionism – the search for an ideal model – and socially-prescribed perfectionism – conformity to others' expectations.

In the case of obsessive personalities, by contrast, the search for perfection is related to an impersonal system to which the subject refers in order to attain stability. Perfectionism here represents an attempt to secure or re-establish certainty with regard to the meaning of the subject's experience; in its pathological form, it leads to the performance of a series of repetitive actions of control (which may involve other people, asked to reassure the subject by confirming his actions), to scrupulousness and accuracy in the performance of even insignificant actions, to an exaggerated attention toward detail that would strike an external observer as irrelevant. At the heart of perfectionism lies this need to conform to certain criteria which maintain or re-establish personal stability in feeling situated. From this principle derives the anxiety-reducing power of rituals, which consist in the performance of behavioural or mental acts according to an established sequence.

The search for perfection that is a constitutive trait of obsessive personality should not be confused with perfectionist behaviour. To quote Hewitt and Flett (1991), 'self-oriented perfectionism involves the self-directed perfectionistic behaviours'. On the basis of this distinction it is possible to trace a further one: between the perfectionism that affects the personality in question as a whole, and that which is connected to the obsessive disorder – although the line between the two is not always clear-cut. The perfectionism of this personality is a structural one, in the sense that it is implicit in the need to adhere to a meaning system in order to co-perceive oneself. Indecisiveness clearly exacerbates this tendency by engendering its pathological variants; yet, precisely because perfectionism is a constitutive element of the personality, it would be misleading to argue that it arises as a consequence of indecisiveness (as maintained by Guidano and Liotti, 1983). It is instead possible to argue that symptomatic perfectionism is instrumental, for it serves to reduce anxiety, as is clear in the case of compulsions.

Given these premises, it is possible to distinguish between structural disorders of this personality, such as scrupulousness, compulsive hoarding and logical complacency, which thematically concern the order on which the personality is founded, and obsessive-compulsive disorders, which more generally affect the individual's relation with himself, others and the world.

Besides perfectionism, the other essential trait that must taken into account when analysing obsessive personality is indecision: *la folie du doute*, as Ribot (1904) termed it, emphasizing the hesitation and impotence of the will that characterize the disorder.

Indecision and doubt concern the present, as they prevent actions and decisions from being taken; yet they are also connected to the foreseeing of the possible consequences of a more or less voluntary act, predicted on the basis of the present condition of indecisiveness – of a condition, that is, characterized by an inability to distinguish what is relevant from what is not. The subject's feeling of indecisiveness not only affects his perception of ongoing experience, but is also reflected in the anticipation of the consequences of action.

The person who must act or choose thus finds himself in a condition to analyse the possible consequences and counter-indications of a given action or choice, without having any point of reference or system on which to rely in order to make the right decision. What may be adopted as a criterion in such a context, then, is the damage a given choice might cause. The meticulousness and slowness of a decision-making process based on an assessment of the most catastrophic results that might occur constitutes an attempt to limit the risk of unexpected consequences, the paradoxical effect of which is to increase the subject's indecisiveness. For an exaggerated prediction of negative consequences makes the anticipated outcome of a given choice, or of its opposite, so uncertain as to affect the present by blocking any initiative on the part of the subject and stifling his will.

The issue of responsibility and of the pathological perception of responsibility is related to this anticipation of negative outcomes. The origin of dysfunctional responsibility, which according to Salkovskis (1985, 1989) consists in the distorted appraisal of the power of one's actions to produce or prevent harm, must be traced back to the feeling of indecisiveness behind anticipation. What makes the subject feel over-responsible is his assessment of possible harmful consequences in the light of an incapacity to distinguish what is relevant from what is not. Responsibility here concerns initiative and hence the consequences of having put a system in motion (Von Wright, 1971). This aspect, which is particularly evident among subjects characterized by pathological checking, is exacerbated by obsessions about safety or the possible harming of others (Rasmussen and Eisen, 1989, 1992; Summerfeldt and Endler, 1998).

Thematic personality disorders

Scrupulousness

This is a form of structural perfectionism characterized by a peculiar anchoring system – consisting of a series of moral or religious issues – through which the subject gives meaning to his experience. In the light of this reference system, the discrepancy between the subject's actual experience and the sense assigned to that experience (on the basis of given rules) is perceived as a form of religious or moral uncertainty. In this interpretative context, the body and its various conditions play a central role, as the sources of experiences that do not agree with the person's principles and are thus perceived as sinful or immoral. One of the most common themes is the sexual one, yet other, morally relevant emotional themes, such as anger, envy or joy, are also common. Various epidemiological studies show that religious, sexual and aggressive obsessions can occur simultaneously (Leckman *et al.*, 1997; Mataix-Cols, do Rosario-Campos and Leckman, 2005; McKay *et al.*, 2004).

In order to understand better the dynamics behind scrupulousness, it is worth considering the origins of the disorder. Let us imagine a subject experiencing the emergence of a state of sexual activation that is not in conformity to the set of meaning principles on the basis of which he measures the correctness of his own behaviour: for instance, a sexual fantasy involving a friend of his wife. The subject in this case would perceive the condition of arousal, yet not acknowledge it as his own; rather, he would consider it something alien, depending on the extent to which it fails to conform to the reference system on the basis of which he co-determines his experience. This inconsistency will engender a condition whereby the subject perceives a personal experience as something alien to himself. Herein lies the origin of *incompletude* (uncertainty).

The most obvious consequences of this duplicity are the blurring of meaning, confusion and the alteration of situatedness. This condition triggers a more or less stable and profound sense of anxiety (which is assigned a pivotal role in the Freudian model of the obsessive disorder). While many individuals regard the emergence of the disorder, with all the changes it entails, as a momentous turning point in their lives, others see it as almost a natural consequence of their way of being. What all these subjects share in common is a way of perceiving their present experience and future prospects in the light of the uncertainty surrounding their moral or religious righteousness.[3]

As a consequence of this condition, subjects are led to examine their present, past and future behaviour with even greater meticulousness, out of a concern for their own perceived immorality. This leads to increased vigilance with regard to their thoughts, words, feelings and actions in the attempt to detect any moral violation or sinful act in even the most ordinary circumstances, thus amplifying their significance in the attempt to control them. The need to bridge the distance between their experience and rules reinforces the need to conform to the rules themselves (thus increasing perfection). This in turn leads to even more critical situations, which generates a self-sustaining loop.

This process, often entailing feelings of guilt and/or shame, also gives rise to doubts and repetitive mental acts; it fosters a fixity of attention and meticulousness of analysis that changes the subject's everyday horizon, worsening his sense of uncertainty. Patients may spend whole nights trying to reconstruct a given episode, in the attempt to grasp all its consequences through a detailed analysis of irrelevant details (*under-inclusiveness*), in order to measure the nature and extent of their own sins, and of possible punishments.

Another rather frequent and often acute source of discomfort is the emergence of intrusive images or unwanted thoughts. The subject attempts to get rid of these, with the paradoxical result of actually increasing their frequency. The individual in this context will often turn to his confessor in an attempt to conform once more to religious principles. Confession, as a ritual, can thus become a feature of the disorder itself. At times, the images are so sacrilegious and the thoughts so abominable as to be unmentionable. In such conditions, the subject may be led compulsively to perform rituals and repeat prayers or sentences that temporarily serve to reduce his anxiety, but which in the long run may settle in fixed patterns that can consume time and effort (Abramowitz, 2008) or cause serious depression. At other times, the feeling of experiencing images one would rather not experience, of acting against one's will, or of having sinful thoughts, corresponds to a twofold perception of Self: as if one part of the Self (the sinful part) were opposing the other (the virtuous part) by raising doubts, formulating accusations and putting it to the test by tormenting it with blasphemies. Inner dialogues among these two parts of the subject's Self can go on for weeks, only to be replaced by other equally inconclusive dialogues. Similar conditions can also engender various kinds of compulsion aimed at alleviating the profound feeling of anxiety that affects the subject.

Hoarding

This is a form of structural perfectionism that is similar to the previous one, but which particularly affects the subject's relation to the world. Frost and Hartl (1996: 342) have suggested that clinical compulsive hoarding consists of three major elements: '1. *The acquisition of, and failure to discard, a large number of possessions that appear to be useless or of limited value* 2. *Cluttered living spaces preclude activities for which those spaces were designed* 3. *Significant distress or impairment in functioning caused by the hoarding* (excessive anxiety about others moving or touching possessions, conflict with one's spouse over clutter, illnesses of family members linked to the clutter [e.g. allergies], inability to complete necessary activities due to clutter [cooking, paying bills, etc.], withdrawal from social relationships due to the clutter, etc.).'

In what sense does this form of perfectionism particularly affect the subject's relation to the world? Whereas, in the case of scrupulousness, the individual's reflection is based on the relation between his own experiences and a system of rules, which allow him to acknowledge the experiences in question as meaningful (for it this correspondence that generates certainty of meaning), in the case of hoarding, the alterity through which the person assesses his own behaviour is found in the system of coordinates that guides his connection to the inanimate objects he owns and accumulates.

The issue at the heart of this disorder is clearly the meaning of accumulating worthless objects such as newspapers, old clothing, paper scraps and so on, to the extent of turning one's living space into a storage area for clutter. To what perception of situatedness does this condition correspond? What order can be found amid piles of newspapers and clothes, along the path leading to one's bedroom through ceiling-high heaps of trash, or in a dining room littered with old bills, bank statements, junk mail and plastic bags?

A crucial study by Furby (1978) on the nature of possessive behaviour in humans, which inspired the equally important research of Frost *et al.* (1995; Frost and Gross, 1993; Frost and Hartl, 1996; Frost, Steketee and Williams, 2000; Frost and Tolin, 2008), has provided a cross-cultural exploration of the motivations behind possession and its various meanings across the ages. The most significant finding of this study was that, in all ages, possession has an instrumental function, as it makes certain activities and enjoyments possible. The possession of objects, that is, allows individuals to make use of things to effect desired outcomes in their environments. The motivational force behind possession is closely connected to control over one's environment and, hence, to one's sense of security. Not surprisingly, the same study reported that security was one of the factors most frequently invoked by adult subjects.

The other major cause of possession that emerges from Furby's study is what he calls 'affect for the object'. 'This dimension,' Furby (1978: 60) writes, 'is clearly of a different nature than the instrumental control dimension – it focuses on an emotion or feeling the owner experiences with respect to the object.' The material object, that is, acquires a special meaning for the subject as it is part of a significant experience for him. The person thus develops material possession attachment.[4]

By adopting this perspective on the nature of possession, it has been possible to analyse compulsive hoarding by relating the disorder to the alteration of the subject's sense of possession. In line with Furby's study, it has been possible to distinguish between a population of hoarders characterized by instrumental saving and one that is instead characterized by sentimental saving.

The first group comprises individuals who accumulate useless possessions to which they attribute the most extraordinary chances of being used. What is meant by 'extraordinary chances' is an anticipation of the most unlikely scenarios in which a given object – any object accumulated – may prove crucially useful. Alternatively, these subjects choose not to get rid of anything because 'you never know' what might come in handy. According to this principle, hoarders carry more 'just in case items' with them (Frost and Gross, 1993). The saved possession thus acquires meaning in relation to the potential use imaginatively assigned to it by the hoarder. The person here feels responsible for preserving an object in order to be ready to face the exceptional circumstances in which it will prove useful (Frost *et al.*, 1995). Each hoarded object represents the solution to a possible need, which allows the hoarder to exert control over the future.

The question that needs to be addressed at this point is: if – as Frost and Gross (1993) have argued, in accordance with Furby (1978) – hoarders collect the clutter as a form of security, why is it that they derive comfort from what others regard as junk?

The second group of hoarders comprises those who accumulate junk for sentimental reasons. Possession attachments mark significant moments in each individual's life, yet they are also traces of the passing of time: footprints, as it were, of time gone by (Kleine and Baker, 2004). Every individual owns certain objects that are dear to him: objects that are part of his personal story and which possess more than a merely instrumental value. In intertwining with the personal experiences of an individual, an object is contaminated, so to speak (Belk, 1988; Watson, 1992): it becomes as unique and irreplaceable as the experiences to which it is connected. The watch a person uses every day, for instance, might remind him of a dear friend and of the particular circumstances in which it was received. Just as this object brings a certain event to the person's mind, so 'possessions are often intentionally acquired and retained in order to remember pleasant or momentous times in one's past' (Belk, 1990; 670).

This kind of belonging of an object to a past situation – as if the concrete evidence of a thing could capture the fleeting nature of an event by attesting to its existence – has been documented in empirical studies showing the irreplaceability of special possessions (Grayson and Shulman, 2000). When participants were asked what they would lose if one of their irreplaceable possessions were to be replaced with a replica, they answered that without that 'real' link their personal connection with past events would be diminished. Despite having the memory of the experience, they felt that without the original object they would lose their physical connection to the past event. In everyday experience, therefore, irreplaceable possessions can be seen as a means of reference and verification with respect to the experiences to which they are linked.

The case of sentimental hoarders thus raises a different question: why is it that these subjects treat things such as old newspapers or grocery receipts as special possessions, like I treat my watch?

The first aspect the two forms of hoarding share in common is the relation between objects and experiences. Both in the case of the anticipation of a future need and in the need for evidence of a past event, the person's experience of his relation to the world finds certain confirmation in the possession of an object. The relation between personal experience and the order of things is here assured, and reduced to the subject's relation to an object he possesses. So, for example, if an individual believes he will need fenders for his car in the future, and that the model he uses may one day cease to be manufactured and thus no longer be available on the market, by buying fenders and storing them he will be reassured of the fact that these objects will be available, should he ever need them.

This sort of reduction implies that all possible relations to the order of the world can be traced to the objects linked to those relations. For instance, all the newspapers a person has kept for the past five years will reassure him of the fact he possesses important information regarding each single day over the course of those five years. The possession, that is, of each single paper is an indication and guarantee of a unique relation to the world. What this also implies is that the person's various relations to the world are reduced to his possessive connection to the objects linked to those experiences. It is this connection that assures the opportunity of effecting desired outcomes in his environment. What this indirectly suggests is that the source of the subject's insecurity, and hence the origin of the disorder, lies in the alteration of the relation between anticipations and memories on the one hand, and possible changes in world circumstances on the other.

The second feature the two kinds of hoarder have in common is the fact that their uncertainty concerns both past experiences and experiences that might occur. In both cases, possession of the object is part of a relation with the past and the future, which anchors the subject's memory or anticipation to a set of concrete, stable and controllable elements. It is as if each hoarded object, like an archive of personal events without an index, acted as a reference to a given situation, keeping the person's certainty about it 'alive' and bestowing stable meaning on his experience, both past and future. In this respect, the accumulated clutter and its hoarder point to a means of facing the uncertainty of memory and insecurity of expectation. Through hoarding, the elusiveness of time is crystallized, rendered concrete and visible at a glance.

Given it is accumulated objects that provide hoarders with a feeling of situatedness, it is easy to see why these subject find it difficult to abandon their possessions, why they react in a strongly negative way to the unauthorized touching or moving of their junk, and why they consider a source of security and a special possession what others may regard as trash. These dynamics also account for the fMRI data showing an increased activity in the anterior cingulate cortex (an area of the brain associated with autonomic control) when subjects are faced with the possibility of discarding their objects.

The same perspective also informs cognitive disturbances. Both the decision not to discard possessions and that to hoard them are based on the subject's need to link the realm of hoarded objects to that of possibility (anticipations and memories). It is the need for this connection that also underlines *underinclusion*, as the person's certainty regarding any possible or past experience is here assured through a one-to-one correspondence between the experience itself and the object possessed. This process causes impairment in the organization of information.

The same need can also be invoked to explain decision-making deficits, which rather than a cause of the disorder would appear to be a consequence of the pervasive sense of insecurity that forces hoarders to crystallize time through things. What can also be made sense of within this framework is subjects' lack of confidence in their own memory and overestimation of recording information (Frost and Hartl, 1996).

Logical complacency

In order to complete the present analysis of structural disorders, it is necessary to examine a specific form of the OCP personality that borders on the EDP. So far, we have stressed the impersonal character of the system of coordinates that allows the OCP individual to co-perceive himself; in the case of the EDP style of personality, by contrast, we have emphasized how the pole through which the subject simultaneously defines and demarcates himself is the co-perception of the other's reciprocity with his own way of being. These two modes merge into a hybrid form that may take on various inflections or emphases: a kind of logical or moral complacency. The other in this case, albeit seen as a centre from which to demarcate oneself and correspond to, is also perceived as something that embodies the value system one must conform to. The significance of the other thus derives from the fact that it represents a stable embodiment of the value system through which the subject co-defines himself.

This unique mixture of elements raises the question of how the subject can distinguish himself from his source of sense. The features of such a problem significantly differ from those of the rather similar problem posed by the EDP personality: for the meaning of the other's significance for OCP subjects is radically different. If self-demarcation with respect to the invasiveness of the other is based on opposition, it engenders a sense of guilt or shame (related to moral self-evaluation), as the other also represents the system of meaning to which the subject must conform. The subject thus evaluates his opposition through a meaning system assured by the very other he opposes. Shame or guilt arise from the negative evaluation of himself, or of the act performed in the light of the standards of reference provided by his system of sense. An individual, for instance, who feels irritated at having failed to meet a parental request, may perceive his feeling as a sign of his own unworthiness and ingratitude. Likewise, in the context of pathology, binge eating and the practices through which the bulimic person attempts to cope with negative emotions may be perceived by the subject as a sign of his own monstrosity and despicableness.

While self-demarcation from the other corresponds to an 'excess' of autonomy, independent choice-making is accompanied by a perception of emptiness, a sort of moral embarrassment or sense of guilt that arises from the subject's lack of conformity to the value system embodied by the other. In both cases, evaluative emotions are accompanied by an inflated sense of responsibility with regard to the act that is perceived as deviant.

A sense of guilt, shame and uncertainty may thus become a fixed trait of a way of being that – as Kafka has shown – is incapable of freeing itself from the other. 'It is as if the person were a prisoner and wished not only to flee – which might be possible – but also to transform his prison into a magnificent castle. If he flees, he cannot build; if he builds, he cannot flee. If I wish to free myself from the miserable relationship that binds me to you, I must do something that is not connected to you in any way. Marriage would secure the greatest and most honourable form of independence, but it is most closely connected to you' (Kafka, 1966: 52).

This is the theme of an amazing story by Kafka (1995), in which the protagonist over the years constructs a labyrinth he inhabits and which separates him from others. This burrow – which gives the story its title – was first dug by the protagonist to keep him away from the world, but ends up becoming a prison to which he is confined.

On the other hand, the resentment, shame and sense of worthlessness connected to opposition, just like the embarrassment, emptiness and guilt connected to all independently made choices not in conformity with the subject's reference model, as well as, more generally, any condition that does not conform to his principles, engender a sense of uncertainty which may take the form of doubt or self-blame. The immobility deriving from this may cause the subject to refocus on his body, thus leading to eating disorders, but also hypochondria, dysmorphia, trichotillomania and other self-injurious habits (e.g. skin-picking, skin-scratching, nail-biting, self-harm, etc.).

One of the most debated issues currently, no doubt also in relation to the drafting of the DSM-V, is the relation between obsessive-compulsive disorders and eating disorders, particularly anorexia nervosa. Janet (1904) famously analysed anorexia in terms of obsession. In discussing '*obsessions de la honte du corps*',[5] he mentions the case of Nadia, a 27-year-old anorexic patient with obsessive symptoms. The same perspective is favoured today by authors who wish to include eating disorders in the obsessive-compulsive spectrum of disorders (McCabe and Boivin, 2008).

Eating disorders that affect obsessive personalities, however, can actually be understood in the light of the subject's conformity to a meaning system through which he defines himself, rather than merely as one means by which he regulates his relation to the other, as is the case with EDP personalities suffering from the disorder. The subject, that is, may give up food out of fear of contamination, to avoid the pleasure of eating, because of scrupulosity (Sharma, Kumar and Sharma, 2006) or out of disgust for food – as in the case of Kafka's (1995) 'A Fasting Artist'. All this differs from the use of food as a way to perceive one's body and thus regulate the dialectic between self-demarcation and the contemporaneous determination of Self through others. The various eating disorders can here be seen to acquire meaning in relation to a system of evaluation that is perceived as impersonal.

According to the perspective adopted so far, it is necessary therefore to distinguish between the two categories of disorders, even if the kind of symptomatology that characterizes eating disorders may also be framed within the obsessive-compulsive spectrum.

Obsessive-compulsive disorders

In outlining disorders affecting the OCP personality, three syndromes have been discussed. These are not exhaustive of the themes around which this psychopathological form is structured; rather, they are indicative of the three dimensions a subject's feeling of uncertainty can take in relation to issues that persist over time. For the scrupulous subject, personal experience acquires meaning in the light of a series of impersonal laws; hoarders find stability by relating to inanimate objects; logically or morally complacent subjects evaluate their own conduct by conforming to the value system embodied by others. One could replace the religion or morals of scrupulous subjects with logic, mathematics or music; similarly, we could replace hoarders with avaricious subjects, and their objects with money; in the case of complacent subjects, the moral system embodied by others could be replaced by a series of formal or aesthetic principles, or with social conventions shared by others. The replacement of themes, that is, would not alter the structural configuration of this disorder, which arranges the person's feeling of uncertainty according to its three fundamental components: relation to oneself, to the world and to others. It is precisely on the basis of this feeling of uncertainty that, in addition to structural disorders, the various symptoms characterizing the obsessive-compulsive disorder (OCD) can be defined.

The essential characteristic of OCD, which underlines its distinct symptomatological heterogeneity (Skoog and Skoog, 1999; Lochner and DaStein, 2003; McKay *et al.* 2004; Mataix-Cols, do Rosario-Campos and Leckman, 2005), consists of two components that may or may not occur in conjunction: obsessions and compulsions. The basic structure of this multiform symptomatology is one of the reasons why certain experts speak of a 'spectrum' of OCDs encompassing various conditions.

Obsessions, as Janet (1904) explains, are an intellectual phenomenon, for they concern ideas, thoughts and images that cause much discomfort (anxiety, anguish, fear, shame, sadness), both because of their content and because of the fact they emerge in a continuous and painful way even against the subject's will.[6] Hence, while the individual will perceive his obsessions as belonging to himself, he will not acknowledge them as his own. This contemporaneous sense of belonging and alienness raises the question of the origin of obsessions.

Compulsions, which are instead characterized by a need to perform behavioural or mental acts in a repetitive way and in accordance with pre-established rules, arise either spontaneously or as a consequence of obsessions. In subjective experience, the performance of mental or behavioural rituals reduces obsessive emotional discomfort. The question arises here as to the genesis of this mode of controlling emotional activation.

The interpretation we have provided of OCD (in its various forms) allows us to answer the question regarding the origin of the two distinctive components of this disorder. According to the perspective adopted so far, obsessions arise from the lack of correspondence between ongoing experience and the reference system through which the experience itself is assigned meaning. This lack of concordance engenders the peculiar feeling of simultaneous belonging to and alienation from the experience that lies at the root of the subject's emotional discomfort. The contents of the obsessions that thus arise will – so to speak – reflect the origins of the subject's uncertainty, in the sense that their themes will revolve around the subject's relation to himself (e.g. religious, moral and sexual obsessions, obsessions about crime and remorse, love, one's own madness, time and one's own death, or certain hypochondriac obsessions), the world (contamination, harming, hoarding, obsession with precision and symmetry) and others (dysmorphia, trichotillomania, hypochondriac obsessions, obsessions with envy and bodily odour). These various forms of obsession can mingle and change over time.

The origin of compulsions and their capacity to relieve present emotional discomfort is again related to the *sentiment d'incompletude*. Thanks to their structure, compulsions allow the subject to re-establish the connection between a given anticipated sequence and the (behavioural or mental) acts performed in relation to that sequence. This allows the subject temporarily to restore a sense of certainty.

In the case of compulsions, too, it is possible to draw a distinction with regard to the obsessive themes to which they are connected: for these must modulate the emotional discomfort arising from obsessions and the content of obsessions. The relation between obsessions and compulsions, therefore, extends to the very source of uncertainty, allowing us to distinguish between compulsions centred on the relation to oneself, to the world and to others. With regard to the relation to oneself, for instance, it is possible to link religious, moral or sexual obsessions to compulsions toward purification (prayers, rituals, washing) and obsessions about crime or remorse to compulsions toward control. With regard to one's relation to the world, contamination may be followed by washing; harming by checking or magical rituals; obsession with precision by ordering, verification and the search for both symmetries and opposite or contrary symmetries. As for one's relation to others, imagined ugliness, for instance, may be followed by a compulsion to gaze in the mirror or wear makeup; a feeling of emptiness or indecision may lead to a search for the perfect hair to pull out; the emotional discomfort engendered by a person's relation to his partner may be followed by hypochondriac compulsion, obsession about anger or envy through compulsive caring for others.

Compulsions can change over time for a number of reasons, ranging from a diminishment in their efficacy (if, for instance, they became automatic) to their becoming an actual cause of uncertainty, thus leading to endless rituals (as when a person perceives he has failed to perform required acts in the right order and is forced to repeat them). Recent studies nevertheless suggest that the symptoms of adult patients with OCD may remain stable in time (Mataix-Cols *et al.*, 2002; Rufer *et al.*, 2005).

In order to illustrate more precisely the three dimensions in which OCD can develop, we shall consider three clinical vignettes that show how the onset of obsessive-compulsive symptomatology is related to the emergence of a condition of uncertainty. As we shall see, *le sentiment d'incompletude* is triggered by those elements that cannot be understood in the light of the reference system through which a subject gives meaning to his ongoing experience.

6.4 Case vignettes

Uncertainty about one's own thoughts

Thomas is a 31-year-old married man and father of one child; he works as a truck driver for his father's company. The obsession he has repeatedly suffered from is characterized by his impression of being an unreal, imaginary person. This doubt has often triggered a second one, particularly when Thomas is on the road. Precisely because Thomas was no longer sure of being himself, when driving his truck he would often question his own spatial localization: Thomas, that is, felt he did not know where he was. Afraid of growing mad and of losing himself forever, on the occasions when the obsession manifested itself more acutely, Thomas was forced to quit his job.

The first time Thomas fell prey to these thoughts was 10 years earlier. When watching a film on television, he started wondering whether he himself was living in a movie: whether his life was real after all. A few months later, this symptomatology had gone, only to reappear, as if out of nowhere, some two years later, when it manifested itself in an even more marked way. While having a beer with some friends, Thomas suddenly began doubting the reality of what he was experiencing. Again, this symptomatology disappeared within a couple of months.

The same obsession, with the same characteristics, returned five years after the second episode; here too, it lasted no longer than three months. At present, it has been about seven months since Thomas started having doubts again about whether he is real or not. This doubt forced him to avoid all travel for a couple of months; and while he has now gone back to work, he is still tormented by the thought that he might lose his mind.

When we re-examine this recurrent symptomatology in the framework of Thomas' story, the clinical picture acquires a different meaning. The onset of the illness, which Thomas describes as sudden, was in fact triggered by his separation from his first girlfriend. Thomas' sense of unreality, that is, can be seen to arise from the feelings connected to this loss, which he perceived but failed to acknowledge as his own. Thomas' doubt as to the reality of his own existence originates from this incongruity between ongoing experience and the meaning system through which he can interpret it. Hence, Thomas perceives himself as double: as simultaneously real and unreal. The disappearance of the symptomatology after a few months corresponds to Thomas' new interest in another girl, later to become his wife. This new condition mitigated and then stilled those emotions connected to separation, which had given rise to Thomas' sense of uncertainty with regard to his own experience.

Although, according to Thomas' narrative, the episodes that followed the first ended as suddenly as they had begun and for no apparent reason, they can actually be seen to present the same recurring pattern over the course of a decade. Just as the episodes were initially triggered by an emotional state that could not be understood in the light of the subject's reference parameters, their remission occurred through the realignment of his experience according to a system of coordinates to which to conform.

In the second episode, Thomas' obsession can be seen as concomitant to the emotions stirred by the news of his wife's pregnancy; the episode ended when, a few months later, Thomas was awarded a financially favourable job promotion. The third episode was triggered by a series of disputes and conflicts (accompanied by intense anger) between Thomas and his father about the sharing of rights, duties and profits within the company between Thomas and his brothers. The obsession vanished when Thomas bought a new truck and started his own business. The latest episode, which is still in course, was triggered by the emotions stirred by Thomas' separation from his wife.

The crucial point with regard to this disorder is the fact that the subject's obsession about the reality of his own experience can be seen to arise from the uncertainty surrounding his own inner conditions. When the meaning of those conditions is realigned with the subject's reference system, both his uncertainty and his obsessive doubt disappear.

Uncertainty about one's actions and their consequences

Lucy is a 24-year-old woman, a university student and the eldest of two daughters. Lucy is currently single and works three evening a week as a bartender. For the past five months, she has been obsessed by the thought of causing fatal car accidents by getting the dosage of her cocktails wrong. In order to avert this danger, Lucy performs a series of rituals involving the repetition of magical formulas.

The context of Lucy's emergent disorder revolves around two significant events.

The first was when Lucy moved in with her sister, who was having a long convalescence following a car accident she had had with her husband. The couple, who had fractured their arms and legs, asked Lucy to help them look after their three-year-old son. Lucy perceived this request as a duty that any good sister would fulfil. The second event – which signalled the onset of the symptomatology – was the ending, on the initiative of Lucy's boyfriend, of a sentimental relationship that had started a few months earlier.

Like Thomas, Lucy describes the onset of the symptomatology as a sudden event. Although, during her adolescence, she experienced some recurrent thoughts about the possibility of damaging others as a result of her actions, only in the past couple of months have these become obsessive thoughts, which cause feelings of anxiety and fear she seeks temporarily to alleviate through compulsions with a magical content. A closer look at the two events that changed Lucy's life in the past few months reveals two elements which, combined, acted as a trigger for her obsession.

The first element is the development of a strong aggressiveness against her sister and brother-in-law, which did not agree with Lucy's set of principles and which she thus perceived as something alien. The fact that Lucy was forced to take care of the couple's house and child as if she were their maidservant caused her an intense anger, and one she could not understand on the basis of her own meaning system – for it is not possible to look after one's sister, when she asks for help, while at the same time bearing a grudge against her because of her request! Hence Lucy's uncertainty with regard to her own goodness and honesty.

What Lucy perceived as even more alien was the range of emotions associated with her breakup from her boyfriend. Lucy had started that relationship after much hesitation and doubt, as the young man in question had just ended a long sentimental relationship he had yet to fully distance himself from. Yielding to some insistent courtship, Lucy had gradually overcome her initial doubts. A love affair thus began, which ended only a few months later, when the man returned to his previous lover.

Concomitant to this event, Lucy became obsessed with the dangerous consequences of her actions. After work, she meticulously attempted to recall all the cocktails she had served in the course of the evening, in order to judge how precisely they had been prepared, whether they might have contained too much alcohol, and hence whether they were likely to cause any damage. Once the offending cocktails had been located, what followed was a compulsion to neutralize their effects.

Whereas, in the case of Thomas, the problem lies in the relation between the subject's conditions and the reference system on the basis of which he assigned meaning to those conditions, Lucy's uncertainty would appear to be due to the discrepancy between the principles that guided her action and her actual experience of the results.

Both in helping her sister and in yielding to courtship, Lucy anticipated a series of consequences in keeping with the principles that had guided her decisions: joy and satisfaction for the help furnished to her sister when she needed it, peace and well-being for a relationship that made her feel loved and wanted. The actual (and in Lucy's eyes discordant) experience that followed those choices was instead one of anger and resentment against her sister, and of desire toward the young man who had seduced and then abandoned her. Lucy's actual experience of the results thus proved utterly inconsistent with the principles that had informed her choices. The uncertainty that arose in this case can be seen to concern the feeling of being able to effect desired outcomes in one's environment, hence the possible consequences of a given act. It is from this insecurity that obsession originates; in turn, obsession contributes to exacerbate the uncertainty that lies at its root.

Uncertainty about one's sense of self

Marta is 18; she is in the final year of high school and is an only daughter. Her father works as a mathematics teacher, her mother as a land registry clerk. For the past two years, Marta has been suffering from a form of trichotillomania that has caused her much hair loss, to the point of exposing her scalp. The girl claims that her hair-pulling behaviour occurs when the action she is performing does not turn out in the best possible way, as this does not allow her to be how she would like to be in a situation. For instance, if Marta is translating a passage from Latin and fails to do so smoothly, her lack of correspondence to the expectation she had of easily translating the text acts as a trigger for her hair-pulling behaviour. Clearly, this form of trichotillomania is different from that which emerges during periods of relaxation – the so-called *non-focused* or *automatic pulling* – which is characterized by little awareness of one's behaviour (Christenson and Mansueto, 1999; du Toit *et al.*, 2001). Marta, by contrast, carefully chooses which specific hair to pull out on the basis of precise criteria that distinguish that hair from other hairs: only if the hair she has chosen meets those norms does Marta pull it out. The unfolding of this sequence brings a sense of relief; hence, Marta now repeats the sequence throughout the day. 'I estrange myself from reality by focusing on a series of acts that have nothing to do with reality. The more their concatenation becomes an accomplished, exact thing, the more I must devote my attention to it.' Every hair Marta pulls out also entails a perception of pain.

As already mentioned, the disorder first manifested itself two years ago. For the whole of her career as a student, Marta had been top of the class. Marta's excellence in school, acknowledged by both her classmates and her teachers, was the guiding principle on the basis of which she judged her own behaviour and regulated her social relations. Marta's experience, that is, acquired meaning through the reference system she also shared with others.

When Marta passed from the 10th to the 11th grade, the group she belonged to was suddenly disbanded: her old class was merged with a new one, and only eight of her classmates remained. In the course of the first three months of this new school year, Marta realized that she no longer personally corresponded to those principles of excellence that in past years had provided her sense of situatedness: for the first time, there were some students who were better than her. Marta, however, did not perceive this as a matter of comparison or competition; rather, she regarded it as a sign of her own inefficiency and imprecision. Marta reacted to this situation, not only by increasing her study hours, but by controlling the way in which she studied. She became so obsessed with the perfect revision of what she had studied that, even after several revisions of the same subject, she was no longer sure as to whether she was at all prepared. Her perfectionism with regard to preparation led her to slow down her study pace substantially, to the point where she fell behind in all subjects. 'It was not my wish to do so much revision, but still I did it, painfully, as if a person superior to me had commanded it – a judge I could not ignore.' At this point, the chosen speed at which a given task (e.g. a Latin translation) had to be performed became the principle on the basis of which Marta assigned meaning to her experience. If in this process something hampered that speed and did not allow Marta to meet her expectations, she was overcome by a paralyzing sense of confusion, uncertainty and emptiness. It was this emotional condition that in those early months triggered Marta's search for a perfect hair to pull out. In order to face her mounting discomfort, Marta refocused her ongoing experience on the exactness of the sequence and its repetition, which allowed her to 'forget' about the problem. 'Awareness of the fact that I am pulling my hair out, far from helping me solve matters, complicates them further: it doesn't help me avoid this behaviour at all.'

The disorder can here be seen to spring from the subject's lack of sense of her own situatedness; it becomes a way for the subject to face the loss of her sense of Self (resulting from her lack of adherence to the set of principles embodied by others), in a process that causes a recurrent sensation of pain. Trichotillomania shares this feature with other obsessive-compulsive disorders characterized by the need to find a way of perceiving one's body.

Endnotes

[1] Kleist's theme is made even more poignant by the fact that it was further developed by Kafka in 'In the Penal Colony'. By touching upon the same theme as Kleist, Kafka, who described *Michael Kohlhaas* as a heavenly piece of work, illustrated the shocking lack of humanity that human beings are capable of. His work, like that of Kleist, sheds much light on paranoia, here seen as 'the chronic development of an enduring system of delusion alongside a complete preservation of mental clarity' (Kraepelin, 1893: 384–434).

[2] 'Could it not be that he (i.e. the patient) has indiscriminately generalized a feeling caused by a genuine psychological imperfection and applied it to an insignificant act? . . . I would be inclined to think so: I believe the problem in the case of scrupulous patients is that of finding what this psychological imperfection might be.'

[3] From this perspective, it is evident that the distortion of beliefs which cognitivists talk about arises from a modification of one's experience of Self: a change in one's religious or moral certainty.

[4] In the field of marketing – from a Jamesian perspective – this dimension will be seen as a type of extension of the self (Belk, 1988).

[5] 'Obsessive shame of one's body.'

[6] Intrusive and unwanted impulses (e.g. compulsive play or sex) are triggered by thoughts, images or ideas.

7 Personalities Prone to Hypochondria-Hysteria

The fundamental feature of Outward styles of personality is that alterity is the orienting polarity with regard to how one perceives ipseity to be situated. As we have seen, both EDP and OCP subjects perceive alterity as a reference system through which to assign meaning to their own experience.

The personality style prone to hypochondria-hysteria, by contrast, is characterized by a way of perceiving the Self and of feeling situated that relies on a frame of reference that simultaneously employs a body-centred (Inward) coordinate system and an externally-anchored (Outward) one. 'Simultaneously' here means that the two polarities – Inward and Outward – are combined, to the point of jointly orientating the subject's search for personal stability. Although it is clearly the case that all styles of personality employ both polarities, what distinguishes this specific personality style from the rest is the fact that it is both inclinations, intertwined with one another, which provide the stable traits at the basis of personal identity. What this implies is that situatedness is constructed through the coordination of the two polarities. In such a way, the hypercognition of basic emotions that characterizes the Inward polarity is integrated with the fundamental characteristic that marks the Outward polarity: co-perception of one's own emotional experience by way of an engagement with others. This integration leads to unique emotional combinations, for the more specific elements of one polarity can amplify or trigger the components of the other. For instance, lack of validation at the hands of others, by engendering a feeling of emptiness, can act as a trigger for fear. Similarly, a manifest condition – such as anger, fear or sadness – can trigger an increase in one's sensitivity with regard to the judgment of others, while anticipation of, and complacent conformity to, the intentions of others can serve as a means to avoid situations where one may lose control over one's emotional sphere. Different combinations of these polarities thus cause a range of experiences, which, albeit mutually integrated, will tend more toward one polarity or the other, depending on the subject's personal story, the specific context and the period of his life.

The difference and mutual integration between a visceral, physical way of perceiving emotional experiences and one that is more perceptive and focused on the other is a defining trait of this style of personality, and one that more clearly emerges in the

Selfhood, identity and personality styles Giampiero Arciero and Guido Bondolfi

psychopathological conditions this style engenders. The configuration of any disorder is characterized by repetitive patterns that tend to fix the meaning of the subject's experience by accentuating the inclinations of his personality, which in this case we have described as prone to hypochondria-hysteria. In psychopathology, a clear example of this variety of polarization is found in the contrasting ways in which the 'sick body' is perceived by subjects suffering from hypochondria and hysteria, two conditions that focus on the Inward and Outward polarities in different ways.

One recurrent feature shared by all disorders connected to this style of personality, and which represents an experiential factor common to all of them, is the subject's way of perceiving the visceral, somatic and musculoskeletal dimension of his emotivity. Particularly when emotional intensity increases, but even in chronic forms of the disorder, the bodily dimension of emotional activation is perceived as an affliction that absorbs one's attention in a very distinctive way. For instance, in the case of the two pathological forms that may be seen to lie at the opposite ends of the spectrum (and to define its limits) – hypochondria and hysteria – subjects perceive their own bodily emotive experience as something central, while at the same time perceiving it as though from the outside. In the case of both conditions, that is, not only is this experience pervasive, but it is also perceived as something external, as if it only concerned the body. What form does the dialectic between ipseity and alterity take in the case of these two disorders, and what role does the body play?

In accordance with what has been argued so far, it is interesting to note that this shared sense of externality of emotional experience is perceived in diametrically opposite ways in hypochondria and in hysteria. In the case of hypochondria, where the combination of the two polarities inclines toward the Inward side, the subject can be seen to fall back on to his bodily experience, as if this were something other than an emotional experience. The person here sees his visceral, somatic and/or musculoskeletal emotional activation, not as the embodied meaning of a given situation, but as a sign of the sickness of his body or one of its organs; hence, emotional activation will here be perceived as a threat 'to the very basis of one's existence' (Ladee, 1966), both present and future. What accounts for the dramatic character of hypochondria is the fact that in subjective experience this condition corresponds to the actual alteration of one's perception of personal stability. As here the sense of permanence of Self is mainly centred on a reference frame that employs a body-centred system of coordinates, any (unexplainable) disturbing change affecting the body threatens to undermine the subject's perception of his own stability. The distinctive egocentrism of hypochondriacs must be viewed in relation to this intense visceral involvement, which 'forces' the subject to adopt a mode of 'internal' polarization and to monitor each change of intensity, here perceived as a threat to personal integrity. These alterations of personal stability are regulated through the search for a cure or, rather, for someone who can provide a cure: an internist, specialist, psychologist, psychiatrist or even exorcist, who is asked to explain the meaning of the affliction. The more intense the emotional condition perceived as an illness, the more acute the search.

What is no doubt revealing of the significance of this disorder is the considerable number of functional symptoms found among primary care patients: somatic symptoms that cannot be explained on the basis of general medical conditions account for between a quarter and a half of presentations in both primary and secondary care (Mayou *et al.*, 2005).

In the case of hysteria, by contrast, the same sense of externality which accompanies the subject's emotional experience – and can manifest itself through a variety of disorders, ranging from hysterical paralysis to non-epileptic seizures – is perceived as either a condition to be displayed or as something of little concern, to the point it may even disappear, depending on circumstances. The same bodily condition, that is, will have different effects in different contexts. Dependence on ongoing circumstances of ostentation or detachment with respect, for instance, to a form of paralysis, implies a dialectic with alterity and a perception of Self that is very different from that experienced by hypochondriacs. In discussing the external polarization that characterizes hysteria, Jaspers (1964: 434) writes: 'Suggestionability manifests itself in the entire nature of hysterical subjects, as they are capable of adapting themselves to every environment. They are so easily influenced that they appear to lack a nature of their own. These subjects are like the environment they happen to find themselves in: criminal, religious, industrious, enthusiastic about the ideas by which they have been suggestively inspired, and which they so promptly uphold, with greater intensity than their original author, only to abandon them again in favour of new influences'. As in the case of Outward personalities, the reference frame through which ipseity finds its own stability is externally anchored; yet, at the same time, a body-centred reference frame is also adopted. Hence, the paralysis of a limb may be openly displayed, ignored, or may even vanish: an external focus allows the person to regulate his distance from his 'own emotional body', to the point of pretending nothing is happening.

Hypochondria and hysteria thus reveal how focus on each of the two emotional polarities corresponds to different ways of perceiving the physical dimension of one's emotivity. In both cases, emotivity is perceived as an affliction. We shall consider the genesis of this common experience when discussing the disorders.

In order to define the forms of ipseity that originate within this style of personality, it is important to understand how viscerally-perceived emotional experience is combined with an attunement to external sources of reference. To illustrate how in the course of one life the integration of these dimensions can manifest itself according to preferential inclinations, we shall turn once more to literature.

7.1 *The Loser*

In what follows, we examine T. Bernhard's *The Loser* (*Der Untergeher*) (Bernhard, 1992). This is the story of two friends, the narrator and Wertheimer, whose lives undergo violent change following an encounter with an extraordinary man: Glenn Gould. The novel follows the interweaving destinies of these characters as though it were the sonata of a trio, where the figure of Glenn Gould is the basso continuo modulating the varying life rhythms of his two friends. After meeting a man of such great talent, one of the two virtuous aspirants becomes a loser, the other an ineffectual person. It is precisely the different development of the two characters' life variations that reveals two differently inclined forms of ipseity within the same style of personality.

The story starts from the epigraph that introduces the theme of the book: Wertheimer's suicide, something 'calculated well in advance ... no spontaneous act of desperation' (Bernhard, 1992: 3). What follows is a digression in which the narrator constructs and reconstructs a series of events, searching for the meaning of the suicide.

The narrator begins his investigation from the time when, 28 years earlier, he, Wertheimer and Glenn Gould were sharing an apartment in Salzburg, while attending Horowitz's specialization piano course. It was then, after hearing Glenn Gould play, that the narrator and Wertheimer stopped playing. 'I myself played, I believe, better than Wertheimer, but I would never have been able to play as well as Glenn and for this reason (hence the same reason as Wertheimer!) I gave up the piano from one moment to the next' (Bernhard, 1992: 8). Such was the explosive impact a comparison with Glenn Gould's greatness had upon the two friends: it brought an end to the careers of the two piano virtuosi and ruined their life plans.

A few pages later, the narrator, in one of his digressions, turns to his original reasons for becoming a pianist. He had devoted himself to music on account of his family, which hated all art and artistic talent. His choice had thus been a way of fighting his family, of punishing and opposing it. The same was also true of Wertheimer and Gould: they too had devoted themselves to artistic pursuits in order to oppose their parents, whom they sought to persuade of their own artistic genius. Gould alone, however, had succeeded in this task. The narrator had failed just like Wertheimer; yet unlike Wertheimer, he had not been excessively distraught by this, for he had never seriously believed he could be a piano virtuoso. Hence, he had not been utterly annihilated by Gould's greatness.

Comparison with Gould had instead shattered Wertheimer. For over 20 years he had then found comfort in his sister, to whom he had bound himself so closely as to prevent her from having any contact with other men. Wertheimer justified his new lifestyle by arguing that he has stopped playing because he had to take care of his sister: it was for her, he claimed, that he had given up his career as a virtuoso.

One day, Wertheimer's sister met a Swiss industrialist at the doctor's. When she secretly left the house to marry this man, Wertheimer was overwhelmed. He locked himself in the dark for 15 days, and when he finally went out in the street again, in need of food and human contact, he collapsed. Thanks to a relative who happened to be passing by, Wertheimer was brought back home rather than sent to a mental asylum. After some time, he left Vienna and withdrew to Traich, where he stayed in a hunting chalet that belonged to his father.

Wertheimer, who was charmed by his own unhappiness and failings, had later often talked about his sister's behaviour with an air of self-commiseration.

It is in Traich that we meet the first-person narrator again: in the local tavern, he is waiting to visit Wertheimer's chalet in the hope of finding traces of his writing. Here a new digression unfolds, which first touches again on Wertheimer's unhappiness and the flight of his sister, and then discusses Gould's death and the sister's flight together: these circumstances would now appear to be the crucial elements behind Wertheimer's suicide. After his sister's wedding, Wertheimer had spent months walking around in Vienna; he had done so, the narrator explains, to save himself. Wertheimer had then attempted to write a book, but had made so many changes to the manuscript that all that remained was its title: *The Loser*. This is the epithet he had been given by Glenn Gould on account of his moaning. Wertheimer loved unhappiness: he yearned for unhappiness and fed on it. He would read books on illnesses and death, visit hospitals, cemeteries and old people's homes. Then one day he had left for Chur and hanged himself one hundred metres from his sister's house.

Suddenly, the first-person narrator intervenes again to ask why it is he finds himself in this tavern rather than in his house at Desselbrunn, which is only ten kilometres away. This offers him the chance to tell of his departure from that place after the meeting with Gould had brought his studies as a pianist to an end. A stay in Vienna is then followed by one in Sintra (Portugal), where, after nine months of inactivity, it occurs to the narrator that he might write something on Glenn. He spends weeks assembling several unsatisfactory drafts, and only in Madrid does he finish the manuscript, at its eighth draft. The narrator, however, has now started having new doubts as to the value of his project, and thinks he may want to destroy the manuscript upon his return. 'How good it is that none of these imperfect, incomplete works has ever appeared, I thought, had I published them, which would have posed no difficulty whatsoever, today I would be the unhappiest person imaginable, confronted daily with disastrous works crying out with errors, imprecision, carelessness, amateurishness' (Bernhard, 1992: 75). From his piece on Glenn, the narrator moves on to consider the central influence this man had on both his life and that of Wertheimer: the destructive power Glenn Gould had exercised on their existence and the terrible direction he had imparted to their story since the days when they were sharing a house in Salzburg. 'For there's nothing more terrible than to see a person so magnificent that his magnificence destroys us' (Bernhard, 1992: 83).

This is a central moment in the narrative, for the various threads that link the destinies of the three men are finally brought together. The transformations in the lives of the two friends and their different developments are grafted upon the exceptional character of Gould. The narrator discloses the crucial difference between Wertheimer and himself: both were shattered by Gould and both are losers, but while he himself is alive, his friend has killed himself. Wertheimer, who wished to become a piano virtuoso, had failed as soon as he had come face to face with reality. This failure he had then turned into a constant excuse for unhappiness. The narrator, by contrast, had only used his no-doubt considerable talent for the piano as a means of postponement.

While Gould's music had killed Wertheimer, it could not kill the narrator. The narrator explains that while Wertheimer had felt trapped when listening to Gould play, through Gould's notes he himself had only discovered that he could not be the best: hence, that it would be better for him to be nobody. Wertheimer had always been an emulator and would always have wished to be someone – a new Gould, Mahler or Mozart; as it had not been possible for him to excel, he had been forced to end his own life. The narrator, by contrast, had always avoided all confrontation, leaving the game out of laziness, boredom, indolence and arrogance. 'He has taken his own life, while I have not' (Bernhard, 1992: 135).

While the first-person narrator is deeply absorbed in these thoughts, his attention is suddenly drawn to the tavern again: to the conversation he had with the innkeeper's wife, and to a lonely, cold and mouldy room. Here he had gazed in the mirror and noticed some herpes on his forehead, perhaps the sign of some nasty illness his doctor was concealing from him. For the first time, an explicit reference is made here to the narrator's concern with illness, a concern soon forgotten as he turns to a new digression.

After speaking with the innkeeper's wife, who gives him some information about Wertheimer's last days, the narrator finally sets off for the shooting lodge in Traich. It is on the road to Traich that a final variation is made on the theme of Wertheimer's death, which is now linked to that of Gould: for Wertheimer had not been able to cope with Gould's death. As he had given up the piano after hearing the latter play the Goldberg Variations and the Well-tempered Clavier, as he had fed his own unhappiness and come to terms with his own failure through a comparison with Gould, Wertheimer had felt he could not survive the man's death. This is the narrator's final thesis.

Upon reaching Traich, the narrator traces the last weeks in his friend's life thanks to Franz, Wertheimer's faithful servant. In his final two weeks, Wertheimer, who had always been a shy man, had inexplicably invited a cheerful group of acquaintances to his chalet. These people had spent the whole time in merriment. The strangest thing of all, however, was the fact that Wertheimer had received a completely out-of-tune piano from Salzburg the day before the arrival of his acquaintances, on which he had played Bach and Handel for two weeks straight. Franz still remembered how, when calling to order the piano, his master had repeatedly insisted that he wanted 'a completely worthless, a horribly untuned grand piano' (Bernhard, 1992: 170). Wertheimer had used this instrument to play Bach and Handel without interruption. He had then sent everyone away, and had spent two days in bed.

The narrative at this point shifts back to Wertheimer's house. The narrator has Franz take him upstairs to his friend's room.

> *I asked Franz to leave me alone in Wertheimer's room for a while and put on Glenn's Goldberg Variations, which I had seen lying on Wertheimer's record player, which was still open (Bernhard, 1992: 170).*

Here *The Loser* ends: a monolithic novel that describes two characters who take Glenn Gould, the exceptional man, as a reference point to give ultimate meaning to their own lives – one by stabilizing his life through a focus on unhappiness, the other through a focus on his own incapacity to dare.

The two tendencies of these characters become polarized through an encounter with a genius. Thus Wertheimer turns every event into an excuse for dejection, exploiting 'the mechanism of the losing man' to the maximum. The self-commiseration, moaning and unhappiness that await around every corner are combined with a need for another to emulate or crush, fear or oppress. The second character, by contrast, that of the first-person narrator, always takes part in the events in retrospective, as if he were never fully involved in them, but were only pretending – as if each circumstance provided a new excuse to continue hiding. His is a strange commixture of listlessness and conceit, fear and complacency, egocentrism and regard for others.

For both characters, Glenn Gould serves as a term of comparison: he is the source of their self-definition, and hence the origin of their failure. Wertheimer, however, makes Gould the very crux of his own unhappiness and even death. The narrator, instead, sees Gould as a mere pretext to abandon a game he had never placed all his bets on; once his career as a pianist is over, he becomes an unlikely essay-writer who works again and again on Glenn, indefinitely postponing the publication of the book. What makes all the difference is precisely the different emphases the two characters place on the alterity through which they define themselves, and hence the unique weight of that emphasis on the meaning of their individual experiences.

It is alterity that gives meaning to Wertheimer's discomfort and unhappiness: to his feeling of being trapped and sense of being a loser. Comparison with the other forces

Wertheimer to evaluate his own unhappiness by reference to Glenn Gould, as if Glenn Gould were its cause. For this reason, the notes of the Goldberg Variations Wertheimer had heard when Gould was studying with Horowitz had paralysed him forever.

The narrator, by contrast, experiences alterity through a form of detachment that allows him to enter the game while feeling that it is not a decisive one; thus, he is in a position to manipulate the outcome. The narrator does not destroy his own life by meeting Glenn Gould; rather, he gives up the piano and a career he had never truly believed in, and somewhat reluctantly tries to write a book. The power unleashed by the meeting with Glenn Gould is here reabsorbed into a kind of stability that revolves around the possibility of fleeing, avoiding comparison and postponing evaluation, by embracing the role of the underachiever as if it were his choice in life.

The different inclinations shaping the destinies of these two subjects provide an interesting example of the way in which this style of personality may incline toward one pole or another. Wertheimer's sense of his own experience depends on the measure he derives from a comparison with the other; the narrator – who structures the stability of his own experience according to a precise and intentional detachment from things and people – instead sees the other merely as an indirect point of reference.

7.2 Disorders

The personality style prone to hypochondria-hysteria lies at the crossroads between the Inward and Outward polarities, which it integrates and combines in a large variety of ways. The specific and more-or-less bodily- or externally-centred inclination this style can engender and stabilize, in relation to given circumstances, represents the underlying factor behind the disorders. The symptomatology of the disorders, that is, will be oriented according to the specific polarity on which the personality of the subject has become stabilized in different periods of his life, although the opposite polarity will also be integrated in a peculiar way when a disorder manifests itself.

It is possible, for instance, to come across a symptomatology that is characterized by panic attacks triggered by a particularly devastating comparison; on the other hand, the same condition may trigger a form of anorexia marked by a manipulative and controlling attitude. Although the objective symptomatology is indistinguishable from that of panic attacks in the first case, and anorexia nervosa in the second, a closer inspection – one that takes account of subjective experience – suggests that the symptomatic picture here is altogether different. The symptomatology of the two cases in questions will reflect the emotional structure on which it is grafted: in the case of panic, it will also be associated with an attention toward others; in the case of anorexia, to a manipulative attitude that is not found in the case of anorexia nervosa – which, as previously emphasized, is rather marked by a tendency toward the radicalizing of one's personal independence. If the first case may be regarded as a panic attack connected to a social situation (social phobia) (Stein, Shea and Uhde, 1989), in the second case it might be worth speaking of a secondary anorexia that differs from anorexia nervosa. The symptomatology of anorexia would here appear to be integrated with hypochondriac attitudes or with a self-assertive, controlling or theatrical attitude.[1] This brings to mind the distinction drawn by Sollier (1891) between 'primitive anorexia', which revolves around a fixed idea, and 'secondary anorexia', an often temporary disorder that occurs in relation to hysteria. A rather common form of this disorder encountered in clinical practice is secondary anorexia marked by difficulty swallowing (globus pharyngis).

The same diversity in polarization also explains two of the possible dimensions of social phobia, which were explored by Hofmann *et al.* (Hofmann and Barlow, 2002; Hofmann, Heinrichs and Moscovitch, 2004): fearfulness and anxiousness. Fearful social phobics attribute their fear of performing to panic attacks or bodily symptoms (such as blushing or sweating) that may occur in the course of their performance. The fearful type 'would show stronger physiological than cognitive or behavioural reactions to a challenging social task' (Hofmann, Heinrichs and Moscovitch, 2004: 777). Anxious social phobics, by contrast, report greater distress and worrisome thoughts about evaluation by others while performing a specific task.[2]

Another interesting aspect of this style is the way in which its polarization can vary through different periods of the subject's life, to the point of engendering disorders with apparently irreconcilable characteristics. The same subject, for instance, may show an anorexic symptomatology at the age of 20 and a hypochondriac one associated with panic attacks at the age of 30. Depending, that is, on the form taken by the subject's situatedness in different moments of his life, a series of disorders may arise that are grafted on to his emotional background, thus fixing its characteristics. This point will be illustrated in the case vignette that follows.

Claudia is a 42-year-old clerk; she is divorced and has a daughter aged 16. For the past three years or so she has been suffering from a very peculiar form of anxiety that arises from a 'fixed idea' (to quote Janet, 1898). For this reason, her case has been – mistakenly, in our view – diagnosed as one of obsessive-compulsive disorder. Claudia spends most of her day imagining that her present partner – whom she actually considers to be only a temporary one, and for whom she does not feel a strong attraction – is secretly meeting other women. So not only are Claudia's days marked by a series of episodes she evokes in her imagination, but it is on the basis of these episodes that Claudia organizes her time: she acts as a detective, rushing out in the middle of the night to check if her partner's car is parked by the house, checking the phone, changing her working hours in order to walk in on her partner when he least expects it. Claudia's entire life, in other words, is organized according to the plot of the 'detective movie' she constructs every day. It is worth examining the history of her disorder, which first emerged 13 years ago in the form of serious hypochondria. After two years of happy marriage, Claudia had a baby daughter, whom she looked after full time until the girl started going to the nursery. This change stripped Claudia's life of its meaning, for at the time she didn't have a job. Claudia's days thus grew long and boring, the time she spent alone a heavy burden. Claudia felt that her husband was not caring or present enough: the complicity that marked their relationship before the birth of their daughter seemed to have been irredeemably lost. Claudia thus began to ruminate on an extramarital affair; at the same time, however, she grew concerned about the possibility of contracting sexually transmitted illnesses (AIDS, hepatitis C, etc.). As Claudia focused her attention on changes in her body – imaginary changes arising from her fear of those illnesses – the dread of getting cancer gradually took hold of her. For two years she organized her life on the basis of new symptoms, medical results, examinations at specialist clinics and hospital stays for checkups. Then Claudia started working. Suddenly, her days became busy again, and her clinical picture changed: the hypochondriac symptoms subsided, but Claudia started having a recurrent fear that her husband might be cheating on her. Claudia's marital situation progressively worsened, and a few years later she decided to leave her husband. What is interesting is the fact that, even three years after separation, at a time when she had already embarked on the relationship with her current partner, Claudia continued to worry that her ex-husband might be having affairs she knew nothing about. Only recently has Claudia gradually started to look at her new partner with this same concern.

Among the vast range of disorders connected to this personality style, two in particular can be seen to lie at the opposite ends of the spectrum: hysteria and hypochondria. Both these disorders are characterized by the pervasive experience of the externality of the body, perceived – in different ways – as an autonomous and unreliable entity beyond one's control.

Hysteria

Because of its history, which intertwines with those of psychology, neurology, psychiatry, literature and psychoanalysis, right up to contemporary neuroscience, hysteria is certainly one of the best known and most controversial disorders of the modern age. Precisely perhaps because of its excessive use, this term – which has a distinctive decadent ring to it[3] – has gradually lost the original meaning it possessed through a slow process of consumption. From a clinical context it seeped into the culture of *fin-de-siècle* Paris; filtered through Freudian psychoanalysis, the term came into use again a few decades later in clinical psychiatry, where it was used with strong psychoanalytical connotations. Evident traces of this can be found in the current terminology of DSM-IV, which has replaced the expression 'hysterical neurosis', adopted in the previous manual, with that of 'conversion disorder'.

Since the days of Charcot, the problem posed by this disorder has been that of explaining symptoms and deficits that mirror a neurological symptomatology chiefly connected to voluntary or sensitive motor functions: from paralysis to aphonia, deglutition and micturition disorders, through tactile or pain anesthesia, diplopia, blindness and deafness, down to epileptic seizures. This formulation of the problem, which has sought the origin of the phenomenon in psychological mechanisms, has progressively reduced clinical experience to an explanation that no longer takes account of subjective experience. The neuroscientific research that over the past 10 years has sparked new interest toward hysteria appears to suffer from the same problem, for it is focused on the experimental study of the nervous circuits connected to the disorder, rather than on the integration of those alterations of cerebral functioning with the patient's experience. Why is it that hysterical subjects become paralysed or lose consciousness?

This question cannot be ignored if, along with the changes in natural dynamics that the neurosciences have drawn new light upon, we also wish to understand the alterations of personal experience that characterize the hysterical disorder. As we have consistently done throughout this second part of the book, we shall take the patient's experience as a starting point to examine both the origin of the disorder and its relation to the activation of those cerebral structures that constitute its neural substratum. In the following sections, we shall consider a case of psychogenic non-epileptic seizures and then one of bilateral hand paralysis.

Case vignette

Dora is a 33-year-old housewife, married to a 37-year-old metalworker, and the mother of a girl aged five. Dora is visiting our studio because of a symptomatology prevalently consisting of headaches, migrant pains and sudden fainting. Dora is also complaining about recurrent thoughts about the death of her husband and mother.

Dora's symptomatology, which began after the birth of her daughter, had initially manifested itself in the form of a frequent concern with illness. This had first been triggered by a recurrent abdominal pain, frequently accompanied by vomiting, caused by gallstones. The clinical picture that had emerged following the birth of the baby was gradually worsened by a pervasive feeling of fear and sadness, which significantly affected Dora's relationship with her daughter, thus making her feel profoundly guilty and inadequate. About one year after the onset of these symptoms, Dora had her gallstones removed. While her abdominal pain ceased, the hypochondriac symptoms inexplicably became stronger, and were worsened by strong headaches and a fear on Dora's part of losing her mother or husband. As Dora's daughter grew older, Dora felt increasingly incapable of discharging the responsibilities the rearing of a child entailed: she felt more and more inadequate as a mother. 'I haven't even been capable of breastfeeding her, as my own milk was no good.' At times, Dora would grow so dejected at these thoughts that she would blame the baby for having been born: she would see her daughter as the actual cause of her disorders. This situation further worsened in the course of the past year because of sudden bouts of fainting – apparently unrelated to any stressful event – that awakened in Dora a fear of having a brain tumour.

On the sole basis of Dora's account, it is not only difficult to make sense of her symptoms, but impossible to explain her hysterical symptomatology. The easiest way to account for Dora's clinical picture would then be to search for a mechanism capable of engendering it.

A clinical methodology that also takes the patient's story into account, however, will seek to uncover the coherence of the events described – and this by associating it with the underlying mechanisms. In such a way, all symptoms will be envisaged within the context of the configurative unity represented by the patient's construction of her own story, thus acquiring new determinations. In order to understand Dora's symptoms, they must be inserted in a web of circumstances that predate their emergence (Arciero, 2006). For if we examine the context of the baby's birth (which Dora regards as the root of her problems), we unexpectedly discover that when Dora was pregnant the factory where she had worked until then closed. This event elicited no immediate reaction on Dora's part because she perceived her pregnancy almost as a vacation. When the baby was born, however, Dora suddenly found herself in a condition where not only was she invested with new responsibilities, but where looking after her daughter made her feel lonely and scared. It was in these early months that Dora realized she would no longer have a job and that maternity was a blind alley. Dora's viscerally perceived fear and sadness – as will become evident in the section on hypochondria – account for the exacerbation of her abdominal pain, which forced her to undergo surgery. Yet the removal of the gallstones did not alter the hypochondriac picture: now deprived of any organic anchoring, it actually became more diverse, as Dora came to perceive all bodily change in the light of illness. Whenever Dora feels alone, the fear that accompanies her self-perception is immediately amplified by an anticipation of the even more severe conditions of loneliness that would be brought about by the death of her husband or mother.

At other times, Dora instead grows angry at her daughter, whom she blames for her own discomfort.

The more Dora's daughter grows independent and develops her language skills, the more Dora's sense of inadequacy increases. When the girl, like all children from about the age of three, started challenging the limits forced upon her, Dora perceived her behaviour as a sign of her own incapability and inadequacy as a mother: 'I never know when to say no and have my words obeyed'. In such a context, it is the child who has the upper hand: Dora's parental role is inverted.

The situation, which had grown increasingly worse when the child was still of pre-school age, suddenly worsened one day when she came home from the nursery. Dora's daughter decided she wanted to go and play with her friend, who lived in the house opposite theirs. Dora objected to this request. The child started arguing with her mother and then shouting at her. Dora not only felt that she was at her daughter's mercy, she also feared that the child's shouting might attract the attention of their neighbours and thus make them realize she was not up to her role as a mother. This anticipation caused Dora a feeling of instability: her head began to spin, her legs became wobbly and she started fearing she might faint. With little conviction, Dora attempted to silence the child, who just kept on shouting. Dora grew increasingly troubled by the fearful prospect of losing consciousness, something she sensed could happen any minute. Dizzier and dizzier by the minute, Dora could hardly feel her legs anymore; her daughter's shouts faded into the distance and her own vision blurred; in the grip of terror, Dora fainted. This sequence of events was destined to repeat itself several times in the course of the year. Now, each time the intensity of the conflict with her daughter crosses a certain level, Dora feels a kind of aura and has a non-epileptic seizure.[4]

The central theme of Dora's disorder, which makes her lose consciousness, would seem to be connected to an amplification of fear through a mechanism similar to that of panic, the main difference being that the immediate source of danger for Dora is the body in its motor and/or sensorial function. The fear engendered by an intervening situation, somatically perceived, leads to an anticipation of the inability of the body to function: a process not unlike the immobilization reaction triggered by a threat. This condition, in turn, leads to an increase in fear and – in a vicious circle – to a modification of the subject's perception of the body, which may even lead to various forms of epileptic seizure. The same process, as we shall see, can also lie at the basis of hysterical paralysis, and emerges with particular evidence in the case of lesser disorders such as the difficulty to initiate swallowing (globus pharyngis). From this perspective, the abrupt and discontinuous transition emphasized by those who follow the dissociation theory would appear to be the result of a process of self-amplification (which may become automatic over the course of time), a process first triggered by an emotionally significant situation.[5] The data gathered in some recent pioneering studies of functional neuroimaging would appear to support this perspective, although the particularly large variability of hysterical symptomatology (Janet, 1907; Ron, 1996) suggests that any results must be evaluated with extreme caution.

The neuroscientific perspective

Tiihonen *et al.* (1995) used electrical stimulation of the left median nerve in a single-case SPECT study both during an acute episode of psychogenic left-sided paralysis and paresthesia and after the recovery of the patient. Prior to recovery, there was increased perfusion in the right frontal lobe (+ 7.2% compared with the left side) and hypoperfusion in the right parietal region (–7.5% compared with the left side). After recovery, change in right parietal lobe perfusion was greater on the left side, as expected, during stimulation of the left median nerve. The interpretation of the results suggested that the paresthesia was associated with the inhibition of somatosensory cortex by frontal areas. These conclusions would suggest that specific psychological conditions can trigger changes in brain physiology, to the point of engendering specific symptoms.

Similar conclusions are suggested by an fMRI study, conducted by Mailis-Gagnon *et al.* (2003), of four chronic pain patients with 'hysterical' anaesthesia. Through the brush and noxious stimulation-evoked brain responses of the affected (unperceived stimuli) and normal limbs (perceived stimuli), this study found that unperceived stimuli were associated with deactivations in the primary and secondary somatosensory cortex (S1, S2), posterior parietal cortex and prefrontal cortex. The authors of the study suggest that the inhibition of somatosensory areas following deactivation may be connected to the recruitment of limbic areas concerned with emotion and attention, thus emphasizing the role of emotion in the development of the disorder.

Vuilleumier *et al.* (2001) carried out an fMRI study of seven patients with psychogenic unilateral loss of motor function, with or without concomitant sensory disturbances in the same limb, by employing a controlled stimulation involving the bilateral vibration of both affected and unaffected limbs. They further compared brain activation during the acute stage of the illness and again two to four months later. The regions in motor and sensory systems that showed hypoactivation in response to vibratory stimulation (associated with the hysterical symptoms and regressing with recovery) were the controlateral thalamus and basal ganglia circuits. These areas are part of the fronto-cortical circuits that subserve both motor and cognitive functions. The thalamus, in particular, is a main relay of afferents to the cortex and may control cortical areas involved in motor, sensory and cognitive functions. Stimulation of the central nuclei of the thalamus can trigger movements that are intentionally carried out, or inhibit voluntary actions. Vuilleumier *et al.* further point out that the damaging of those nuclei (e.g. through strokes) can cause 'intentional' motor neglect despite normal motor and sensory function – a clinical conditional similar to hysteric paralysis.

The basal ganglia, on the other hand, are neural structures within the motor and cognitive circuits (Graybiel *et al.*, 1994). The globus pallidus – but also the thalamus – receives signals from the amygdala and the orbitofrontal cortex. These circuits provide potential pathways through which limbic signals might affect sensory processing, or result in a selective inhibition of action. Hence, an intense and sustained emotional activation may impair motor readiness and initiation through the modulation of specific basal ganglia and thalamocortical systems.

Case vignette

Both the triggering and the automation process of the disorder can further be elucidated by examining the case of Carla. A 34-year-old woman who works at home as a hairdresser, Carla is the wife of a 43-year-old electrician and the mother of two children; she suffers from hysterical paralysis of the hands. Like Dora, Carla describes the onset and development of her symptoms as if they were completely unrelated to the everyday context in which they manifest themselves. According to Carla, her disorder first started abruptly, about two months after the birth of her second son. One afternoon, after dozing more than she ought to have, Carla suddenly woke up and realized she could not move her hands. Panic-stricken, she asked her eldest son to call for help. The child got in touch with his paternal grandmother, who lives in the apartment below, and Carla was taken to hospital, where she was administered intravenous diazepam, after which the symptomatology subsided. The same condition of bilateral paralysis had unexpectedly emerged several times over the course of the previous six months, with no apparent connection to existing circumstances. As in the case of Dora, if we accept Carla's story we can only explain her disorder in terms of an unconscious mechanism.

This kind of explanation becomes even more appealing if we examine the context in which the first episode manifested itself. Only one week had passed since Carla had started working again: the disorder emerged on her first day off. That morning Carla's mother-in-law – with whom she had a conflictual relationship – had asked for an afternoon appointment to get her hair done. Carla felt she could not turn down this request. The symptomatology that manifested itself that day may therefore easily be interpreted as a 'secondary gain'. Carla's paralysis, that is, may be explained as a means of saving face when an expression of distress would have been counterproductive, as an explicit refusal would further have worsened the conflict between the two women.

Upon closer inspection, however – one that seeks to understand the experience from the point of view of the subject experiencing it (and thus avoids applying any preconceived notions to the story of an individual life) – a different perspective on this first episode can be seen to emerge.

Carla had already started feeling that she could not take it any longer one week earlier, when she had been forced to get back to work in order to avoid losing any clients. Suddenly, after a rather long break, which lasted a couple of months, she had found herself having to work at three jobs at the same time: as the mother of a newborn baby who needed to be breastfed every three or four hours; as the mother of an older child who needed help with his homework and daily activities; as a hairdresser who had to meet her clients' needs during the little time she had left. Carla was given a hand in all this by her mother-in-law, who would take care of the baby when she was working, and by her husband, who would look after her eldest son after work.

On the Monday when the first episode occurred, Carla had fallen asleep for about half an hour after having breastfed the baby. Upon waking up, she anticipated the whole afternoon in one moment: she needed to fix her mother-in-law's hair, clean the house, pick up her son from school – all this without the help of her husband, who had started a new job on that very day and would not be home till late. The feeling of constriction that had accompanied Carla's days ever since she had started working again suddenly became so pervasive that she felt utterly trapped: Carla froze. She then focused her attention on her hands, and started feeling a tingling sensation in her fingers, which increased to the point where she could no longer move them... Carla could no longer open her hands.

In the months that followed this first episode, each time emotional pressure increased, Carla would anticipate this sequence, which always led to the same outcome: the paralysis of her hands. The same effect, however, could also occur 'with no reason': it was enough for Carla mentally to anticipate her incapacity to move her hands in order to trigger the process leading to their actual paralysis.

Carla's case poses an interesting problem, as impairment of movement here is not only caused by a given emotional activation, but also by a conscious anticipation of the incapacity to initiate action. The hysterical paralysis that emerges through a reaction somewhat similar to freezing would thus appear to be supported by a conscious mechanism – rather than by unconscious conflicts – capable of making the normal processes of the motor intentional system dysfunctional (Athwal *et al.*, 2001). Indeed, the very movements that cannot be made voluntarily will be made unconsciously: for instance, when the patient must balance herself, when she is distracted or sedated.

The neural substratum

A series of cerebral imaging studies can be seen to support this hypothesis.

Marshall *et al.* (1997) conducted the first PET study recording the brain activity of a patient with left-sided paralysis of 2.5 years' duration as she prepared to move and attempted to move her paralysed (left) leg; they compared this to a recording of when she prepared to move and did move her good (right) limb. As expected, voluntary movement of the unaffected right leg was found to activate the controlateral primary sensorimotor and premotor cortex and, bilaterally, the dorsolateral prerfrontal cortex (DLPFC), secondary somatosensory areas (inferior parietal cortex) and cerebellar hemispheres. Also as predicted, preparation to move the unaffected right leg activated the same network but not the left primary sensorimotor cortex. In contrast, readiness to move and attempt to move the affected limb failed to activate the controlateral primary sensorimotor and premotor cortex. Furthermore, when the patient tried to move the affected leg, controlateral anterior cingulate and orbitofrontal cortices were significantly activated. The authors interpreted this activation as an inhibiting of the movement of the affected leg through the disconnection of the cortical areas (DLPFC) subserving motor planning. In other words, it was the intention to move that triggered the incapacity to move through the activation of the anterior cingulate and orbitofrontal cortex.

This perspective, which emphasizes the role of the prefrontal inhibition of the motor and sensory cortex, is further supported by a single-case PET study conducted by Halligan *et al.* (2000). This research shows how hypnotically-induced paralysis in a healthy 25-year-old man activates the anterior cingulate and controlateral orbitofrontal cortex in the attempted movement of his paralysed leg without similar activity in the motor cortex. The activation of these areas, which – in agreement with the previous study – was seen to overlap with the regions recruited in the course of hysterical paralysis, led the authors to interpret hypnotic paralysis as a model for hysterical paralysis. The two studies further suggest that inhibition of the sensory-motor regions can be produced not only by limbic regions, but also by maintaining a certain level of attention: through the involvement, that is, of prefrontal regions. The symptomatology was thus seen to subside with the distraction or sedation of the subject.

The importance of prefrontal areas in the genesis of the disorder was the focus of a PET study conducted by Spence *et al.* (2000). This study recorded the brain activity of two men with hysterical left-arm motor symptoms and one with hysterical right-arm monoparesis in order to examine the difference between hysterical symptoms and those feigned during the attempted movement of a limb. All three patients exhibited relative hypoactivity of the left dorsolateral prefrontal cortex (DLPFC) when compared to both controls and feigners (healthy individuals who were required to pretend they had difficulty moving a limb). The left prefrontal hypofunction was common to all patients irrespective of symptom lateralization. Feigners instead exhibited relative hypofunction of the right anterior prefrontal cortex. Since DLPFC is activated by the generation and selection of action, its dysfunction in hysterical paralysis was interpreted as a volitional disturbance.

Spence (1999: 209) notes that: 'The problem in hysterical motor disorders is not in the voluntary motor system per se; it is in the way that the motor system is utilized in the performance (or nonperformance) of certain willed, chosen actions'. According to this perspective, the fact that hysterical patients are unperturbed by their dysfunction does not mean that they are not concerned about their paralysis; rather, it suggests the opposite. *La belle indifference* is a way of pretending nothing is happening: it represents a way of showing one's paralysis to others by manipulating their judgment through an attitude of indifference.

This attuning oneself to the other reveals a fundamental characteristic of the disorder, one that tends more toward the Outward side of the spectrum: the need for validation at the hands of others. This aspect of the disorder is connected to a series of traits that have induced people to speak of hysterical personality in the past and of histrionic personality disorder today: a need for attention, sexual provocativeness, seductiveness, emotional discontinuity, instability, an overemphasizing of one's affective state, as well as the kind of suggestibility Janet (1907) famously listed among the most important stigmas associated with hysteria. Although this aspect also characterizes EDP personalities (as we have seen in Chapter 5), the manifestation of traits typical of the Outward tendency is more marked, more amplified and more openly displayed in the case of hysteria. The much vituperated expressive theatricality of these subjects is perhaps due to the unique combination of a particularly intense way of emotioning and an equally strong need for another through which to feel situated. The utterly unique element of the disorder is precisely this integration of acute emotivity with an equally compelling need to co-perceive oneself by means of others. Hence, the intensity of the subject's emotions is here combined with his situational discontinuity,[6] as if a series of circumstances 'naturally' elicited over-the-top reactions. The violent changes these subjects experience in relation to their own sense of Self may lead to dissociative identity disorders or to mood swings.[7] From a clinical perspective, it is worth emphasizing one final and highly revealing finding we have made in the course of our clinical practice: the uncommonness of the association of these traits with conversion symptoms (Kretschmer, 1926; Bowlby, 1940; Chodoff and Lyons, 1958). It is as if these two conditions corresponded to two different modes of articulating the same combination of elements.

Hypochondria

In what follows, we shall refer not only to hypochondria in the strict sense of the word, but to a hypochondriac spectrum that also includes the somatization disorder and the undifferentiated somatoform disorder. These two disorders share a common characteristic: the presence of visceral, somatic or somatoskeletal symptoms that cannot be explained by organic findings (De Gucht and Fischler, 2002), although they may be associated with other medical illnesses. Unlike hysteria, hypochondria is more oriented toward the Inward polarity, which predominantly stabilizes self-perception on one's bodily state, here immediately perceived – if beyond a certain range – in the form of worrying symptoms. Thus transient pains such as intercostal pangs, or more marked physiological conditions such as exertion tachycardia and visceromotor or musculoskeletal conditions associated to basic emotions, may trigger a 'self-reflexive' process in the body that amplifies the subject's discomfort and engenders one or more symptoms. As Lipowski (1988: 1358) notes, this distinction had already been recorded with surprising clarity by Sims in 1799:

> *'He offered a modern definition of hypochondriasis, characterizing it as a disorder whose main feature was that the patients had "the mind almost entirely taken up with the state of their health, which they imagine to be infinitely worse than it is" (13, pag.392) and believed themselves "afflicted with almost every disorder they have ever seen, read, or even heard of" (13, p.398). Hypochondriasis could affect either sex, resembled melancholia, and featured diverse symptoms. It differed from hysteria by being always associated with a low rather than a changeable mood'.*

The crucial distinguishing element of hypochondria is precisely its constant preferential anchoring to the body – perceived as ill or about to fall ill – rather than a form of variability dependent on context and thus associated with a changeable mood, as in the case of hysteria.

It is evident, in the case of disorders that fall within the hypochondriac spectrum, that subjects perceive significant changes of circumstances on the basis of a system of coordinates that has the (sickly) body as its fixed point of reference. The sick body is here the condition through which subjects feel emotionally situated. It is on the basis of this condition that significant variations of situatedness may be perceived as symptoms: as the signs of a body that, on account of its illness, is governed by a dangerous degree of autonomy, and is thus perceived as something external to oneself – as a sick body. In the case of hypochondria proper, the subject's unpleasant experiencing of a given symptom is associated with his certainty of suffering from an organic disease, and with 'rumination' about illness.

While focus on the sickly or diseased body accounts for a variety of symptoms – ranging from palpitations to breathlessness, from headache to tinnitus, diarrhoea, thoracic constriction, muscle and abdominal pains – it also raises a crucial question: how do these symptoms arise? One of the most misleading concepts invoked to answer this question has been that of somatization, which is still in use in DSM-IV and continues to be a source of controversy (Fava and Wise, 2007; Kroenke, Sharpe and Sykes, 2007; Mayou *et al.*, 2005; Sharpe and Mayou, 2004; Wise and Birket-Smith, 2002). The term 'somatization' was first introduced as a neologism to render the word *Organsprache* ('organ-speech'), originally used by Stekel and Adler to describe 'the hereditary susceptibility of an organ to be diseased' (Marin and Carron, 2002: 250). With the introduction of the neologism 'somatization', the concept of *Organsprache* was translated and reinterpreted in Freudian language to describe the conversion of emotional conditions into physical symptoms. Traces of this meaning can still be found in the use made of the term in DSM-IV.

According to our own perspective, it is clear that the issue of how the symptoms in question arise cannot be solved by envisaging them as a translation of the emotional sphere on to a physical level, for those subjects who experience and convey their emotional distress in the form of physical symptoms (Lipowski, 1988) prevalently perceive emotivity as a body-centred phenomenon. Those who construct their own stability in time, chiefly through basic emotions, clearly show a hypercognition of the visceromotor and musculoskeletal manifestations usually associated with each of those emotions (Rainville *et al.*, 2006). An evident example of this is fear and anxiety, which are associated with an increased heart rate, hyperventilation and muscle tension, as well as in many cases temporary dizziness or confusion, nausea, increasing perspiration and dryness of the mouth. The emotional dimension of these subjects, rather than being converted into physical symptoms, is thus prevalently connected to the perception of bodily signals; as we have seen, the dimension in question represents a peculiar form of embodiment. In this respect, the original notion behind the term *Organsprache* can be seen to acquire new meaning: the inclination to perceive one's own stability chiefly through a focus on Inward conditions makes the subject more perceptive toward his own inner organs.

The question that needs to be addressed, therefore, is how hypochondriac subjects manage to transform their perception of bodily signals into one of signals from a diseased body. The simplest answer would be that the erroneous interpretation of the subjects is due to distorted beliefs about care habits, or about perceived personal weakness and vulnerability, or a narrow concept of good health (Abramowitz, Whiteside and Schwartz, 2002). A similar perspective (uncritically) assumes that the meaning of the subject's experience arises from a reflection, from 'the ego bending around backward and staring at itself' (Heidegger, 1988) to grasp itself (see Chapter 1). It should be noted that, while cognitivist explanations indeed illustrate the mistaken interpretation of someone at risk of developing hypochondriasis, they do not solve the chief problem posed by this disorder, for they fail to explain the origin of the experience at the basis of the distorted beliefs. If the hypochondriac subject did not feel prey to his body, he would feel prey to his illness. It is interesting to note, in this respect, that often hypochondriac individuals who suffer from a real physical illness are not concerned with it, choosing rather to focus their attention on – and hence organize their existence around – the symptoms of a nonexistent illness.

Another important aspect of this disorder is the fact that it is precisely the hypochondriac subject's perception of his body as stricken by an illness, which does not actually exist, that leads him to mistrust doctors, to constantly search for new cures, to press for new diagnostic tests, to search for information concerning the possible forms a given illness might take and the complications it might bring, to concern himself with the illness to the point of fixation, or to complain in a more or less open way about his own health and the general dreariness of life. The incongruity, that is, between the opinion of doctors – who will generally tend to play down the significance of any functional symptoms – and what hypochondriac subjects personally feel, is strongly perceived by the latter and lies at the root of their constant dissatisfaction with both diagnostics and therapeutics, making them seek ever new consultations.

The experience hypochondriac subjects have of their own body is of an object whose actual or potential alteration regulates their everyday life. A patient of ours, Andrea, who is now 34 years old, changed all his habits and started living like a 70-year-old man; since that one restless night when he was 22, he has been shaken by several attacks of tachycardia. Now every evening before going to sleep, Andrea prepares his clothes, in case he is forced to leave for the hospital in the middle of the night. Ever since that first episode occurred, Andrea has perceived his body as a capricious tyrant.

This perception of a sovereign alterity – that of one's own body – attracts the subject's attention, determines his priorities and, most importantly, dictates his sense. The 'intimation' inexplicably and unpredictably given by the body is perceived as an ever-impending danger, which can manifest itself with different degrees of intensity, to the point of causing terror. This intimation from the body is of an emotional nature and speaks the language of organs: *die Organsprache*. Andrea, for instance, the day before the eventful night that 12 years ago made an old man of him, had unexpectedly been left by the only girl he had ever loved. It is on that very night that Andrea was terrorized by tachycardia: for one whole night he was hostage to his heart!

Andrea could not see that his anguish was caused by the fact that he found himself alone after a relationship that had lasted for five years: the intensity of the anguish was such that his whole attention was hostage to the perception of the uncontrollable autonomy of his own body. Tachycardia thus ceased to be a sign of anguish for Andrea by becoming a symptom that could be triggered by the most disparate circumstances: a sign of the dangerous autonomy of his cardiocirculatory system.

The severity of hypochondria depends on this sense of uncontrollability of the body, whose disorders become a point of reference for the structuring of one's life. It is hardly surprising, therefore, to find the relation between negative affectivity (anxiety, guilt, hostility and depression) and physical symptoms emphasized in certain studies (Costa and McCrae, 1980, 1985).

When the feeling of being emotionally situated through a set of references prevalently anchored on the body crosses a certain level of intensity (which varies from person to person), it leads hypochondriac subjects to increase their focus on the body and – more generally – on a wide range of bodily states and/or conditions. This would appear to be confirmed by study data suggesting a correlation between somatic symptoms and hyperarousal (Lipowski, 1988; Hammad, Barsky and Regestein, 2001).

It is possible to suggest, therefore, that in cases of hypochondria marked by somatic symptoms, the over-polarization of attention on 'inner' states removes the subject's feeling from its reference to the world, thus transforming it into a worrying bodily sign that is perceived as something almost external and governed by a logic of its own: that of illness. The amplification of the symptom is thus due to the focusing of the subject's attention on the very heart of the experience: it is the intensity of experience – and hence its quasi-extraneousness – that leads to increased attention being directed toward the subject's body, thus affecting its sensitivity.

The physiological mechanisms at the basis of this phenomenon are far from clear. One of the most interesting hypotheses, which could account for the processes underlying visceral hypersensitivity in particular, but also muscle tension, takes account of the role played by afferent neurons (peripheral sensitization), spinal cord dorsal horn neurons (central sensitization) and descending stimulating or inhibitory influences on spinal cord nociceptive neurons (Anand *et al.*, 2007; Hobson and Aziz, 2003).[8]

The heightened perception of visceral or somatic sensations may be due to the sensitization of primary afferent nerves by the kind of inflammatory mediators (such as K, ATP, bradykinin, prostaglandins, cytokines) that are released in emotionally significant or particularly stressful circumstances (Black, 2002; Janssen, 2002). Through the 'neuroinflammation' of tissues (leading to the activation of nociceptors), the peripheral sensitization triggered by the inception of stability-threatening events of an acute or enduring nature produces changes in the activity of dorsal horn neurons. This activation causes the development of a hypersensibility field that extends far beyond the initial area of inflammation, and which is due to an amplification of the reaction to noxious stimuli and a perception of pain following innocuous stimuli.

Such a phenomenon, known as central sensitization (Woolf, 1983, 1991, 1995; Woolf and Salter, 2000), leads to an increase of sensitivity to pain in the organ in question that may persist over time (without any evidence of ongoing inflammation), causing long-term sensorimotor disturbances that can worsen in relation to triggering conditions. Several studies would seem to suggest that central sensitization plays a crucial role in a series of disorders and functional illnesses, such as irritable bowel syndrome, functional dyspepsia, non-cardiac chest pain, cutaneous hyperalgesia and fibromyalgia (Dickhaus *et al.*, 2003; Schaible, Ebersberger and Von Banchet, 2002; Staud *et al.* 2003; Treede *et al.* 1992; Sarkar *et al.*, 2000; Van Oudenhove *et al.*, 2004, 2005). It would thus seem that this mechanism lies at the basis of the transformation of bodily signals into symptoms. The sense of extraneousness of one's feelings with regard to the perception of a given symptom – and, more generally, of a given emotion of particular intensity – leads to a state of hypervigilance. Although hypervigilance is a normal condition of the nervous system in response to perceived threats, hypochondriacs – with or without somatic symptoms – develop a chronic condition of hypervigilance with regard to visceral and/or somatic stimuli that will vary in accordance to the perceived significance of given events.[9] Because of this condition, certain hypochondriac subjects are likely to suffer from panic attacks caused by a vicious circle of somatic symptoms and catastrophizing anticipatory thoughts followed by an increase in the intensity of the symptoms, which in turn triggers more fear (Fava *et al.*, 1990).

According to our perspective, the essential element that explains the various disorders within the hypochondriac spectrum is the 'self-reflexive' mechanism affecting the body. This mechanism, which arises among certain patients in response to sustained and acute stability-threatening events, engenders a certain sensibility and fosters a tendency in the subject to experience some bodily sensations as intense, noxious and disturbing. It is this experience that underlies the 'distorted beliefs' about care habits, or about perceived personal weakness and vulnerability, that congnitivists talk about. Through the heightened perception of visceral and somatic sensation, individuals with hypochondriasis develop a concern for their health and convince themselves that they are suffering from a serious disease, thus creating a vicious circle that amplifies the intensity of the experience by increasing the subject's attention toward perceived or possible symptoms.[10] As shown, for instance, by Berman *et al.* (2008), anticipatory down-regulation of the activity within the CNS network, activated by potentially aversive interoceptive stimuli, is inhibited by negative emotions (stress, anxiety, anger) in irritable bowel syndrome patients during the expectation of pelvic visceral pain.

Barsky (1992; Barsky *et al.*, 1988) is quite right in defining somatosensory amplification both as a trait that may be learned during one's upbringing and as a transient state that may emerge in response to various sensations across different periods of one's life (Barsky *et al.*, 1993). The mere presence of this trait, however, does not imply any concurrent medical disease or psychopathology (Barsky and Klerman, 1983).

The greater sensitivity toward bodily sensations certain individuals appear to develop in the course of their lives, and which at particular times is amplified to the point of causing a series of secondary effects (concern with, and fear of, an illness, the seeking of medical advice, etc.), should not be mistaken for obsessive-compulsive disorder (OCD). Although seeking reassurance from physicians and adopting anxiety-reducing behaviours, such as feeling one's lymph nodes to check their size, are practices aimed at reducing the anxiety deriving from one's concern about illness (and indeed these may be read as signs of OCD), their significance is markedly different from that of OCD symptoms. As we saw in the last chapter, obsession emerges from the lack of correspondence between ongoing experience and the reference system that gives meaning to that experience; this statement also holds true in the case of hypochondriac obsession. A person's lack of desire toward his wife, for instance, may lead him to believe he is suffering from a disease of the prostate, a belief that in turn will lead to the frantic search for an unequivocal diagnosis and to a range of behaviours aimed at verifying it. The disorder, that is, originates from a sense of insecurity and is based on an obsessive idea about illness that engenders forms of behaviour aimed at acquiring new certainty (doctor-shopping, diagnostic tests, the testing of one's sexual potency), which in turn amplify the obsessive idea, thus contributing to the anxiety and distress of the subject.

Things are very different when it comes to hypochondria, be it with or without somatic symptoms. Although patients with high levels of disease conviction tend to have increasingly severe somatic symptoms, whereas patients with high levels of disease fear tend to be more anxious or phobic (Kellner *et al.*, 1985), in both cases the disturbing and noxious perception of one's own body or organs is crucial. It is precisely the body-centred perception of oneself that engenders and fosters one's behaviours, fantasies and thoughts about illness. By contrast, the attention of OCD patients is only drawn toward the sick body on account of an 'intellectual phenomenon': obsession (Greeven *et al.*, 2006).

As previously noted, emotional discomfort may be associated with one or more physical symptoms, even if the clinical picture is not characterized by the fear and belief of suffering from an organic disease. This is, for instance, the case with the somatoform disorder, the onset of which we shall illustrate through a case vignette.

Case vignette

Peter is a 30-year-old computer engineer, an only son who still lives with his parents. From the age of 19, when he first started university, Peter has been suffering from muscular pain, concentration difficulty, headaches, fatigue, nausea and intestinal bloating. These various symptoms, which were a constant feature in Peter's life as a student, worsening at exam times, turned into a full-blown disabling disease in 2004. When Peter came back from his summer holidays that year, he found himself in such pain that he could no longer study. Piercing pain in his back and joints prevented him from getting any sleep, while an annoying intestinal irritability forced him to go on a strict diet. Peter's condition worsened over the course of the following months: the pain grew more intense and Peter could no longer concentrate, to the point that he was thinking of abandoning his studies. At this prospect, he grew even more dejected, and his health further worsened: he began running a constant temperature. In March 2005, Peter decided to ask to be admitted to hospital for a general checkup.

It is interesting to re-examine Peter's symptomatology within the framework of his life. Before leaving for his holidays, in 2004, Peter had sat and failed the most difficult exam in his course. Upon returning from his holidays, faced once again by this insurmountable obstacle, Peter started fearing he might never pass. As his anxiety grew, he was no longer able to concentrate. Peter spent his days tormented by what he perceived to be a pain sine causa, wavering between a feeling of failure and the impossibility of abandoning his studies. In February, stricken by excruciating pains,

Peter chose to leave university. This move on his part coincided with his admission to hospital for some checkups. The various diagnostic enquiries yielded no results: Peter was discharged and prescribed 20 mg of paroxetine. Within a few weeks all pain disappeared, and in a few months Peter managed to complete his exams. On the day after gaining his degree he stopped taking the paroxetine. A few months later, Peter started working for a software company, and for a couple of years all seemed to go well. A few months before his wedding, however, Peter started suffering again from fatigue, headache, irritation, muscular pain, dyspepsia and abdominal colic, and turned to us for help.

One of the most interesting questions raised by Peter's case, and one which can be extended to the somatoform disorder and to functional disorders more generally, concerns the relation between a certain way of perceiving oneself and the onset of organic diseases (Geeraerts *et al.*, 2005; Kubzansky *et al.*, 1997). The issue of the extent to which these disorders may predispose subjects to certain illnesses suggests that dialogue and joint research with the study of clinical pathology ought to be renewed. The neurosciences may thus provide a new way of linking psychology and medicine.

Endnotes

[1] One need only to think, for instance, of anorexic subjects who cook a large meal they force their families to eat while they themselves fast.

[2] This difference in style also applies to sexual performance. Sexual dysfunction in fearful subjects will be characterized by difficulty in achieving an erection, in anxious subjects by premature ejaculation.

[3] See, for instance, the use of the term in Rachilde's (2004) *Monsieur Venus*.

[4] It is necessary to point out that there are no episodes of childhood abuse in Dora's story.

[5] The manifestation of the disorder is thus related to the modification of a wider context, which ought to be the focus of therapeutic attention.

[6] This discontinuity is reflected in the symptomatological variability which led Janet (1907: 271) to observe: 'And you know that to express the changeableness of hysteria, Sydenham called it "That Proteus that cannot be laid hold of"'.

[7] Janet also emphasizes this point: 'dual personality is the hysterical form of periodic depression' (Janet, 1907: 283, quoted in Merskey, 1995). Indeed, many alleged cases of double personality were perhaps manifestations of a cyclotimic disorder (Merskey, 1995).

[8] The biological substratum of this reciprocal connection is the so-called brain–gut axis (Van Oudenhove *et al.*, 2004).

[9] Sustained and acute stability-threatening events can be seen to play an important role in the onset and modulation of non-ulcer dyspepsia and irritable bowel syndrome among hypochondriac patients when compared to healthy controls (Locke *et al.*, 2004).

[10] In a study examining how the extent of an injury (as measured by number of teeth extracted) and the attention paid to the injury (as measured by frequency of pain ratings) affected the pain level of patients, it was found that the more frequently postoperative patients were asked to rate their pain, the more intense they rated it to be (Levine *et al.*, 1982).

8 The Phobia-prone Style of Personality

The fundamental characteristic of this style of personality is the subject's stable anchoring to a reference frame that predominantly uses a body-centred coordinate system in order to face situational variability. As was repeatedly stressed when discussing the Inward tendency, the fact that an individual's sense of permanence of Self is predominantly centred on his perception of bodily signals is something related to the hypercognition of basic emotions. The subject's particular mode of feeling, that is, can here be seen to draw his sense of personal stability over time toward a context of reference that is focused on 'inner' conditions, and which affects the very quality of his experience. Over time, this tendency will settle, leading the individual who possesses this personality style to focus – in his relation with others and the world – on the visceral aspect of his emotions, thereby allowing his personal stability to coincide with the stability of his own bodily condition.

A crucial role in the above process is clearly played by interoceptive awareness,[1] for this way of feeling represents the most significant means for the subject to feel situated when it comes to the variability of events and his relations to others. Interoceptive awareness provides personal situatedness with a sort of defined gravitational field, a baseline level whose fluctuations will engender a state of alarm when they extend beyond a given limit.

This form of inclination of personal stability emerges even more clearly in the unique dialectic between ipseity and alterity that characterizes this style of personality. The distinctive trait of this dialectic is represented by the fact that alterity is reduced to ipseity, so to speak, or rather to the 'internal psychological economy of the organism': to bodily variations and the way these are perceived by the subject. This dialectic is perhaps best described in the words of William James: 'My thesis is that *the bodily changes follow directly the* PERCEPTION *of the exciting fact, and that our feeling of the* p.190 *same changes as they occur* IS *the emotion.* Common sense says, we lose our fortune, are sorry and weep; we meet a bear, are frightened and run; we are insulted by a rival, are angry and strike. The hypothesis here to be defended says that this order of sequence is incorrect, that the one mental state is not immediately induced by the other, that the bodily

Selfhood, identity and personality styles Giampiero Arciero and Guido Bondolfi

manifestations must first be interposed between, and that the more rational statement is that we feel sorry because we cry, angry because we strike, afraid because we tremble, and not that we cry, strike, or tremble, because we are sorry, angry, or fearful, as the case may be' (James, 1884: 189–190).

James argues that the perception of a given thing may trigger a bodily change, and that it is precisely the feeling of this change that makes us experience an emotion. The bodily signal represents the information the body generates to face environmental perturbations, whereas the awareness of that signal *is* the emotion.

In the case of the phobia-prone style of personality, strong interoceptive polarization corresponds to an equally strong attention toward a range of situational aspects that may lead to an alteration of the baseline interoceptive-emotional level of the subject. While the person's feeling of interoceptive stability here acts as the reference system regulating his position with respect to the world and others, it also opens possibilities for action aimed at maintaining the stability itself: for instance, the pulling or pushing away from certain people, situations or contexts, always for the sake of stability. In this respect, alterity (both that of the world and that of others) is reduced to the maintenance of that permanence of Self the organizing of which, at every moment, defines the range of actions possible by 'submitting the world to one's own conditions'. It is precisely this central role played by bodily conditions, and hence the preservation of a given bodily milieu over time, that allows us to state that the construction of identity in the case of Inward styles of personality is based on what are almost essential traits of the subject's character.

8.1 Interoceptive awareness and emotional experience

In the course of the past decade, particular efforts have been made in the field of the neurosciences to find neural structures that may account for this way of feeling: what a widely cited article describes in its title as 'Neural Systems Supporting Interoceptive Awareness' (Critchley *et al.*, 2004). The most recurrent question in studies of this matter concerns the role played by interoception in the perception of emotional experience. To what extent does greater interoceptive sensitivity affect the intensity of one's emotional experience? And besides, does a more marked tendency to experience certain emotions correlate with an ability to perceive visceral responses?

Heartbeat detection is the methodology of choice for the indexing of people's interoceptive ability.[2] In one study (Wiens, Mezzacappa and Katkin, 2000), where subjects were presented with sets of two film clips targeting different emotions (amusement, anger and fear), good heartbeat detectors reported experiencing more intense emotions than poor detectors – and this without the two groups displaying any substantial differences in terms of heart rate and electrodermal activity. In another study, people who were more sensitive to their heartbeats showed more arousal focus (Barrett *et al.*, 2004); additional data also suggest that different types of emotion are associated with different kinds of visceral activity (Rainville *et al.*, 2006; Critchley *et al.*, 2005). Several studies thus seem to suggest not only that a correlation exists between people's sensitivity to visceral signals and the intensity of their emotional experience, but also that this correlation accounts for the different way in which emotional states are perceived by certain subjects

The above interpretation appears to be confirmed by a series of studies reporting interoceptive sensitivity to be subtler among subjects with high basal anxiety level (Ehlers and Breuer, 1996; Zoellner and Craske, 1999; Stewart, Buffett-Jerrott and Kokaram, 2001) or suffering from anxiety disorders (Mumford *et al.*, 1991; Van Der Does *et al.*, 1997, 2000; Eley *et al.*, 2004). This would seem to indicate that individuals who are more prone to feeling emotions such as fear and anxiety, which are related to visceromotor activation, will also develop a greater sensitivity toward interoceptive signals. Further confirmation comes from a highly significant study showing how people who are more interoceptively aware can use visceral cues (gut feelings) to predict the consequences of subliminal stimuli (Katkin, Wiens and Öhman, 2001). The particular significance of this study derives from the fact that it illustrates how certain subjects (who are better able than others to detect their own heartbeats) are able to anticipate negative stimuli through their perception of interoceptive signals.

A direct consequence of the correlation between more precise interoception and more intense emotional experience is the fact that neural structures responsible for interoceptive regulation also seem to be engaged in the generation of emotional processes (Damasio *et al.* 2000). Clearly, this entails a partial overlap between the interoceptive neural system and the areas associated with emotional activation. One of the most significant studies exploring the neural substrate that underlies both interoceptive awareness and the conscious experience of feeling is that conducted by Critchley *et al.* (2004). This study employed fMRI to scan the brains of 17 subjects during a heartbeat detection task, in which the subjects judged the timing of their own heartbeats (an interoceptive event) relative to feedback notes, interleaved with trials in which the participants were asked whether one of the notes had a different pitch from the rest (exteroceptive control task).

The study found that when the subjects focused on their heartbeats (rather than the pitch of the notes), they activated the bilateral anterior insula and anterior cingulate cortex. The subjects' accuracy in heartbeat detection, moreover, correlated with the activity in the right anterior insula and with self-reported measures of negative emotional experiences. This suggests that interception plays an important role in emotional experience and that the anterior insula represents the common substrate of both interoceptive sensitivity and emotions. This shared element may explain why, in the case of many phobia-prone subjects, emotional activation coincides with a more acute perception of the physiological conditions of the body.[3] As we shall see, the perfect equivalence of emotion and interoception – as if the situation that elicits an emotion were separate from the emotion itself – is probably one of the most significant features in the inception of panic disorder.

Another equally significant trait of this style of personality – which tends to preserve the sense of permanence of Self through the stability of interoceptive activation – is the need it feels to face and anticipate conditions that may alter stability by generating fields of action to buffer environmental stimuli. Thus the subject's dialectic with alterity here centres on a range of interoceptive modulations that both secure a stable perception of Self – by bestowing meaning upon his strength or frailty – and allow the individual to manage and foresee contingent situations, to the point where he is able to avoid what he deems as excessively activating circumstances.

The above perspective provides a better understanding, both of those studies showing a correlation between avoidance-oriented coping strategies and increased levels of anxious responding to bodily sensations, and of the fact that a greater tendency to use avoidance strategies is found among people experiencing panic attacks than among those without histories of panic (Feldner, Zvolensky and Leen-Feldner Ellen, 2004). In this light, it also becomes clearer as to why in structured conditions of agoraphobia or claustrophobia subjects feel as if the source of their sense of danger were the situation itself.

8.2 'The stuffed bird'

A story by Pirandello (1994), 'The Stuffed Bird', can be seen to blur the lines between agoraphobia devoid of panic attacks and hypochondria. In just a few pages, Pirandello describes – to the bitter end – the life of a man who is living in constant fear of the danger – that of illness – posed by his dealings with the world.

The story opens with the picture of a defunct family, most of whose members – the mother, brothers, sisters, uncles and aunts – have died of phthisis, with the exception of the father, who died of pneumonia. This beginning establishes the context in which the lives of the remaining brothers, Marco and Annibale Picotti, unfold. As survivors, the two brothers have structured their lives in such a way as to triumph over disease, and live in constant fear for their own safety. Both men are particularly cautious when it comes to food, their daily rhythms, the weather and seasons: out of their fear of illness, they avoid all excesses. A first change occurs, however, when Annibale, the youngest of the two brothers, yet the most robust, having passed the age reached by his deceased family members, starts loosening his control, as if he has already passed the limits that nature wishes to impose upon him. When Annibale gives in to a few transgressions and excesses, Marco reacts, urging his younger brother to restrain himself. Yet, at the same time, in his heart Marco feels a sense of curiosity toward that which he glimpses lying beyond the limits of his strict conduct. One day, Annibale suddenly announces that he is about to get married. Marco grows furious at these words, for he can already foresee the death of his brother and that of his brother's future son. Marco insults Annibale and his bride, but to no effect: Annibale actually tells him that he would rather die than continue living as he is doing. Marco, worried at having become so worked up, tells his brother he does not wish to be disturbed, and that if Annibale has decided to get married, that is none of his business: Annibale is free to leave the house.

Marco then pays a five-minute visit to his future sister-in-law, but won't even speak to her; he does not attend his brother's wedding, and continues living as he has always done: in a room that stinks of medicines, where he spends his time worrying about draughts and foretelling misfortunes.

A few months later, on Christmas Eve, Annibale and his wife burst into Marco's house: merry, lively and full of joy. The two seem drunk to Marco, who has a hard time falling asleep that night: it is as if he has been stunned by his brother's happiness and freedom. Suddenly, Marco is overwhelmed by a desire to turn over a new leaf and to stop living like a stuffed animal. A few days later, he visits Annibale and stays at his place for dinner, intoxicated by a vortex of emotions. Marco then returns home and falls ill for several days. To no avail, Annibale attempts to persuade his brother that his illness is merely due to his excessive fears. But Marco only grows more frightened when on his brother's face he read the signs of impending death he knows only too well.

Sometime later, Annibale dies.

Marco does not attend his brother's funeral and avoids all contact with people because he wishes to avoid any excessive emotions. He now takes extra care of himself, seeking to banish all thoughts of his brother. One day, Annibale's widow, her eyes full of tears, pays Marco a visit. He views the visit as an outrage and sends the woman away. That night he bursts into tears, yet wakes up the following morning as if nothing has happened.

As the seasons go by, Marco continues behaving as cautiously as ever.

Finally, he turns 60 and feels he has reached his goal: he is past the limit. Marco abandons his rules, but is now tired and annoyed, and feels that life has had no meaning. Has he won? Something, he thinks, is missing. Marco stares at his stuffed bird, which was a family memento; perhaps he can see the whole course of his life unfold – as dry as the straw that fills the belly of that bird and the armchairs of his room. Marco walks over to his desk, takes a revolver out of the drawer and shoots himself in the head, bringing the final operation to an end.

Subjects can regulate their need to maintain a stable level of activation, not merely through self-management, anticipation and avoidance behaviour, but also by exercising direct control over their own interoceptive-emotional condition through various strategies (such as distraction, wishful thinking and the suppression of emotion) aimed at limiting emotional intensity to the point of suppressing it. An exclusive focus on these states, and a concomitant lack of attention toward the circumstances that brought them about, leads the subject to perceive his own body as the primary source of danger. This condition may then trigger panic disorder and panic attacks.

8.3 Zuccarello the distinguished melodist

Another short story by Pirandello (1994), 'Zuccarello the Distinguished Melodist', develops in an extremely refined way a theme often found in his writing: that of the danger posed by the world, and of the need to shield oneself from this danger by keeping away from intense emotions through the stable construction of a life centred on avoidance situations. The uniqueness of this short story lies in the fact that the avoidance behaviour around which the existence of its protagonist is structured simultaneously concerns the dangers of the world and over-intense emotional conditions. Sentimental involvement is the domain in which all situations are perceived to be potentially dangerous, precisely on account of the intense emotions they can elicit. As it is the sphere of love that represents a source of danger here, emotional stability is derived from the foregoing of sentimental involvement. It is on these notes that Pirandello begins his story, which is reminiscent of Maupassant in both style and structure.

Perazzetti, the protagonist of the story, married a woman 'so as to avoid the danger of getting a wife for real' (Pirandello, 1994: vol. 3, page 2132). In the meantime, 'he had long devoted himself – for what reason I do not know – to the study of philosophy' (Pirandello, 1994: vol. 3, page 2132).

The narrator's premise is followed by a section in which the protagonist, speaking to a group of friends, relates an episode in support of his thesis that every man, without knowing it, is in search of an 'absolute': of a centre that might bestow meaning upon his life; but that when he has found it, he then discovers how useless it is and how vain was his search. And yet, it is precisely from this centre that a small seed will sprout: a seed destined to grow and make each man 'the master of a world'.

After presenting his thesis, Perazzetti moves on to describe his encounter with Zuccarello.

One evening, as he was walking down a busy street, he was struck by a red poster beside a café. It read:

MR ZUCCARELLO

DISTINGUISHED MELODIST

Perazzetti was impressed by the description. A man, he thought, who labelled himself a *distinguished melodist* – not an excellent or renowned melodist, but a *distinguished* one – must surely have found that absolute centre within himself and feel no need to aspire to be anything other than himself: 'it is enough to call oneself a *distinguished melodist*. This much and nothing more. This is enough for him to be himself rather than someone else' (Pirandello, 1994: vol. 3, page 2134).

Driven by a desire to converse with Zuccarello, Perazzetti entered the cellar café and music bar. Several patrons were sitting at the counter. Perazzetti gave the waiter his ticket in order to be shown a seat; with a feeling of surprise and indignation, he found the hall to be half-empty. Annoyed, Perazzetti turned on the waiter, reproaching him for having said that Zuccarello's exhibition attracted no clients. He then asked to speak to the proprietor, whom he addressed with vehement words, emphasizing both the exceptional quality of 'distinguished melodist' as a label and the fact that it was quite unbecoming for a distinguished melodist to sing in front of an audience of empty chairs. Perazzetti's outburst caused such bewilderment, laughter and turmoil that it took little effort for him to persuade the proprietor to invite the patrons of the bar to sit in the hall for free. When Zuccarello appeared on stage, the place was full. Zuccarello was a perfectly ordinary man who, just as Perazzetti had expected, gave what he could without a trace of effort: 'This much and nothing more, in his voice as well as in his gestures and smiles' (Pirandello, 1994: vol. 3, page 2139). This was the sort of perfection Perazzetti was searching for.

After the show, an angry Zuccarello faced Perazzetti, reproaching him for his thoughtlessness at having exposed him to the risk of a fiasco and, hence, of losing his job. Perazzetti did his best to appease Zuccarello and invited him to a night café, in the hope of learning more about the life of a man who was the master of a world of his own. Zuccarello told Perazzetti the most obvious, trite and banal things, which all radiated from that 'absolute' centre in which had sprouted the seed of the world he had become a master of. This was a small world, comprising a cellar cafe with empty chairs and performances, and small country towns in which Zuccarello could boast that he had sung in a theatre-café in Rome. But the greatest proof of the fact that Zuccarello had attained perfect equilibrium came from one of the shadows that had followed them as they left the music bar and entered the night café. This was a badly dressed woman – wearing cheap men's shoes – at whom Zuccarello uneasily glanced from time to time.

No doubt, this woman was his wife. 'I was sure that he still kept her, not just so that she could be at his service, like a slave, but so that he might also measure the progress he had made through her. Likewise, I was also sure of the fact that without a word of complaint she was doing everything she could to keep him like a dandy'(Pirandello, 1994: vol. 3, page 2140).

Perazzetti's supposition was confirmed when, leaving the small hotel to which he had accompanied Zuccarello, he met the woman, who bowed deeply as if to pay homage to a man who had honoured her husband.

Perhaps, just like himself, Zuccarello too had been careful to avoid the danger of getting married for real!

Affective relationships play a particularly significant role for the phobia-prone style of personality, which favours the stability of interoceptive activation as a way of preserving the sense of Self. Feelings of love represent a highly variable sphere, and hence a possible cause of the alteration of the bodily interoceptive milieu. After all, both Zuccarello and Perazzetti, who 'marry [women] in order to avoid the danger of getting a wife for real' (Pirandello, 1994: vol. 3, page 2132), embark on an affective relationship in order to avoid the risk of becoming involved in any real love story. The two men can thus be seen to regulate their own emotional stability by choosing a condition of predictability and control of their partners, which – from the point of view of interoceptive awareness – corresponds to an avoidance of the peaks of activation that could alter the meaning of their situatedness. An alternative version of this form of intimacy is represented by dongiovannism. Here the goal of seduction eclipses all possibilities of affective involvement, as emotional tension is entirely aimed at conquest: directed, as it were, at the capturing of one's prey. Once the goal is reached, the emotional tension is lost.

Although these modes of managing one's intimacy represent borderline cases, they still reveal one general trait that phobia-prone subjects display in their sentimental attitude: the need for predictability on the part of their partners, coupled with a need to preserve their own freedom of action. The establishment of significant relationships is characterized in these cases by the attainment of a dynamic balance between the individual's perception of the reliability of his partner (a feature associated with the stability of one's personal interoceptive space) and his feeling of being able to face environmental perturbations without being restricted by, or being dependent upon, this reliability (something associated with one's control over ongoing situations).

This sentimental style can be understood more clearly in the light of the fact that, on the one hand, the subject's sense of permanence of Self here corresponds to his emotional-interoceptive stability, and, on the other, that this stability is always matched by the opening of new possibilities aimed at its preservation (through anticipation and the avoidance of critical situations). While the individual, therefore, will perceive any sign of unreliability on the part of his partner as a danger, for this leads to emotional-interoceptive instability, he will perceive any duties deriving from his relationship in the same way, as these limit the control he exercises over his own stability. Any bond may thus be perceived by the subject as a genuine threat to his own personal integrity.

According to this perspective, the development of any affective relationship would appear to be marked by a subtle ongoing balance that changes across the various phases of the relationship itself: from the initial meeting between the two partners, to the strengthening of their ties in the early months of the relationship, to their social debut as a couple, down to cohabitation, marriage, honeymoon, the birth of their children and so on. Each of these transitions may represent a critical moment, as it alters the relation between perceived stability and the feeling that limits have been imposed upon the subject's life. Clearly, these moments may coincide with the onset of symptomatic pictures, or even trigger significant changes in the trajectory of life.

In order to illustrate the significance that one of these critical moments may have for phobia-prone individuals, we shall outline the story of one of our patients, who sought help when, for the fourth time in fifteen years, she was about to leave her new fiancé a few months before their wedding.

8.4 Case vignette

Giovanna is a 41-year-old accountant, the only daughter of a divorced couple. The unexpected separation of Giovanna's parents, which occurred when she was 28, opened a new chapter in her life: she perceived this as a liberation from a range of limits and controls that, despite her age, were still imposed upon her by her parents. On the other hand, Giovanna, who was engaged to a colleague at the time, whom she planned to marry and start a family with, was overcome by a strong feeling of precariousness following the separation of her parents, and started putting pressure on her partner to speed things up. A few months later, the two set a date for their wedding the following year. Suddenly, Giovanna started experiencing a feeling of thoracic constriction and suffocation. While she still felt as if she were in a cage, she also realized that life outside the cage continued to be off limits for her: previously the cause of this had been her parents, who through countless expedients had sought to restrain her; now that she was free, she could feel the noose of marriage tighten around her neck. As the days went by, Giovanna's feeling of being trapped increased, as did her desire to flee. She thus systematically sought to argue with her husband-to-be, displaying an unprecedented degree of aggressiveness. Frequent clashes and violent rows took place between the two, and they broke up several times before leaving one another for good.

At the age of 30, Giovanna, finally a free woman, experienced the best period of her youth. 'I was missing a portion of my life, and I finally got it back.' It is with these words that Giovanna justifies her first flight.

At the age of 32, Giovanna embarked upon the most passionate of all her love stories: one that ended two years later, a month before the wedding. Giovanna describes this second flight of hers as if it had been caused by the religious disaccord between herself and her former fiancé, who was Jewish (although he did not actually practice the religion!). A closer inspection of this period in Giovanna's life, however, reveals a series of circumstances strikingly similar to those found in the previous situation. Following the promise of marriage, Giovanna had started to experience the same feeling of suffocation, the same anxiety and angry desire to break free that had brought her previous relationship to an end. The final episode, in the course of which the two partners had heatedly discussed their religious divergences, had served as a pretext for Giovanna, who claimed that a marriage between them would never work. The truth of the matter is that this was only the last in a series of clashes that had started with the couple's decision to get married.

Following the end of this second relationship, Giovanna devoted herself to her professional career. Only after five years did she start a new relationship, one that matched the previous two almost perfectly, the only difference being that it took far less time in this case for Giovanna to flee: she left her partner only one week after the promise of marriage. For the first time, however, Giovanna became aware of the course her relationship was taking, and started asking why the most important love stories of her life had always ended in the same way.

The same question is emerging in the context of Giovanna's present relationship. This too, like the previous ones, started with a struggle in which Giovanna aimed to assert control over the life of her partner, something clearly related to an attainment of interoceptive stability on her part. Once this was acquired, the next step lay in defining a shared plan: usually involving marriage and family. Transition from the definition of the plan to its implementation constituted a turning point: the strengthening of the bond came to be perceived as a trap, a feeling of restriction that caused anxiety and a desire to escape. It was at this point that Giovanna started looking for fights and exacerbating any contrasts, to the extent of severing her sentimental tie with the man she felt constrained by, on the alleged grounds that their relationship could not work.

In the case of the phobia-prone style of personality, the modes of self-regulation aimed at ensuring a sense of personal stability are not limited to avoidance behaviour, to the anticipation of dangerous situations or to direct control over emotional conditions. A rather unique mode of self-regulation is the establishment of critical situations in which one's stability is exposed to the constant risk of being disrupted by extreme emotional conditions. The need to maintain a manageable level of activation, that is, may lead to an active drive toward the experiencing of novelties, the facing of dangers, the overcoming of limits and the challenging of natural bonds, by engendering a feeling of mastery over both ongoing situations and the interoceptive-emotional variations to which they are connected through action. This mode of self-regulation often characterizes what we may describe as 'risk careers' (e.g. those of pilots, explorers, firemen, paramedics, lone sailors, policemen), as well as attraction to extreme sports. The person here constantly renews his feeling of invincibility by confronting the most dangerous situations, even to the point of facing death. An exceptionally relevant piece of evidence, which amplifies the distinctive characteristics of this way of being, to the extent of making them come across as self-evident, is the autobiographical conversation between Reinhold Messner – often cited as the greatest mountain climber of all time – and Thomas Hüetlin, a journalist from *Der Spiegel*.

The central theme of this interview is already outlined in the first chapter of Messner's book, which is significantly entitled *Childhood and Rocks*: on the one side stands the world, which for Messner as a child did not extend beyond the valley; on the other, the curiosity he felt for what lay ahead, beyond the limit. '*What lies beyond?* This has always been an underlying question in my life' (Messner, 2006: 20). When Messner began his extraordinary career, this curiosity turned into an incessant desire to cross the limit, and to overcome the fear that coincides with it. 'What I would dream of was to succeed in climbing a given gorge the following summer, to make my way up a given face or reach the level we had been too scared to cross the year before' (Messner, 2006: 22). Fear is here seen as a condition to be challenged; and Messner's is no ordinary fear, but the very fear of death itself. 'This is the key to mountaineering. This is the contradiction that no one will understand about my way of facing the mountains. No one who practices mountaineering would like to find himself in a similar situation (i.e. the loss of a fellow climber), where he must survive. As for me, I was torn between the desire to avoid going through that experience once more and the desire to feel new strong emotions. As men, we only get to know our humanity when we face death' (Messner, 2006: 91). What is at stake, therefore, is survival itself: one must escape danger and overcome fear, for to 'resist the challenges of death' (Messner, 2006: 57) is to push that limit a little further. Herein lies the source of that strength and feeling of security from which Messner has derived his awareness of belonging to an elite ever since he was an adolescent. 'Where it becomes difficult to go beyond on this earth, we shall be the ones to succeed: for the others have never learned to survive in a world full of obstacles' (Messner, 2006: 47).

When Messner turned into a young man, he extended his challenge to the highest mountains of the world. The first person ever to have ascended all the 8000 m peaks of the world, Messner lost his brother Günther in a tragic expedition on the Nanga Parbat. This terrible event, however, the memory of which haunted Messner for years, did not put an end to his Himalayan adventures. Rather, his lonely fight against the dread of death became even more extreme. 'I hope never to live through an experience like the one I had on the Nanga Parbat, I hope never to experience anything like that. Yet, I cannot live without extreme experiences. If I had to define my "disease", I would describe it as: the desire to live by constantly putting one's life at stake' (Messner, 2006: 92).

After facing the great challenges of high peaks in the attempt to experience 'the tension, fear and happiness of getting in touch with an utterly new world' (Messner, 2006: 78), Messner started taking expeditions on foot, driving himself to the farthest limits of civilization.

8.5 Disorders

The distinguishing trait of this style of personality is the fact that in each case it perceives alterity by focusing on bodily signals (ipseity). The configuration and intensity of these signals, that is, assigns meaning to both the subject's experience and to ongoing events. If interoceptive-emotional polarization here represents the sense matrix at the basis of the maintenance of personal stability over time, its alteration, perceived as a signal that lies outside the range of bodily experiences familiar to the subject, elicits a sense of either possible or imminent danger, which corresponds to an acute feeling of anxiety. For instance, the increase in cardiac frequency associated with profound joy, a feeling of great tiredness and the inebriation induced by an excessive intake of alcohol may all be perceived as instantly alarming conditions, as they lie beyond the interoceptive-emotional baseline.

The distortion of personal stability

In subjective experience, any move beyond the familiar range of emotions is indistinguishable from a state of anxiety. Be it in the case of joy, tiredness or inebriation – to refer to the previous examples – an increase in the intensity of the sensation or emotion beyond the baseline that regulates the personal stability of the subject is immediately perceived as a symptom, rather than as a variation of the feeling in question. Virtually every sensation and emotion, therefore, whose intensity goes beyond a given limit, may be perceived as noxious and engender a state of anxiety that changes the very way in which the person perceives himself within his own body, thus affecting his sense of situatedness.

For the person who experiences it, this state of altered stability corresponds to a broad perception of frailty (a sort of decrease in self-efficacy) that increases vigilance toward bodily sensations, amplifying the sensations themselves and contributing to an increase in the overall feeling of danger. Thus the increase in body vigilance and attentional focus – which enhances the probability of perceiving threatening interoceptive cues[4] – is a function of the subject's perception of instability. For, given that the sense of permanence of Self is predominantly body-centred in the case of this style of personality, the greater the instability perceived, the greater will be body vigilance and the likelihood of perceiving threatening sensations. The available data suggest that enhanced interoceptive ability may be considered a risk factor in the development of panic attacks. Abundant evidence suggests that people with panic disorder are able to record changes in heart rate with greater precision than nonclinical panickers (Ehlers and Breuer, 1992; 1996). Moreover, nonclinical panickers have better cardiac interoceptive accuracy than non-anxious controls (Ehlers and Breuer, 1992; Zoellner and Craske, 1999), and trait differences regarding interoceptive acuity are intensified by state anxiety (Zoellner and Craske, 1999).

On the other hand, the person who feels he is in this state of frailty progressively distances his experience from its intentional object: for, as we have seen, in order to maintain stability, the subject shifts his attentional focus from the ongoing situation to his bodily sensations. For instance, the increase in cardiac frequency that occurs when the subject climbs up a few flights of stairs will no longer be perceived by him as something related to physical exertion; rather, it will be seen as an exclusively somatic event, one that is amplified through attentional focus and removed from the condition that engendered it. By means of this operation (which separates one's body from the world), an ordinary case of tachycardia triggered by exertion comes to be perceived as a tachycardic heart that threatens the whole organism, thus further increasing the person's sense of frailty. The tachycardic heart that here causes alarm, however, is not quite the 'almost infarcted' heart that is perceived during panic attacks.

This 'absolutization' of interoception manifests itself in an even more surprising way in the case of emotions. This is, for instance, the case with the hyperventilation associated with a state of fear that follows the avoidance of accident. Once hyperventilation is removed from the situation that elicited it (through an increased attentional focus on the body), it is perceived as the symptom of an altered breathing. The emotional state triggered by a given situation, that is, loses its reference to the situation and is reduced to a bodily sign that goes beyond the baseline and hence becomes a danger for the stability of one's own organism. The hyperventilation deriving from the manifestation of fear becomes the symptom of an altered condition that puts the integrity of the subject at risk. Clearly, though, shortness of breath is not yet quite the sense of imminent suffocation that characterizes panic attacks.

The fear of fear

In both examples, increased attention to bodily perturbations (tachycardia and hyperventilation) also increases the subject's sense of frailty and hence his perception of instability. In order for a panic attack to occur, however, the state of anxiety associated with the sensations and emotions that are perceived as noxious must itself become a cause of fear. What this means is that the condition of instability that surfaces when the subject moves beyond the interoceptive-emotional baseline must be so intense as to trigger an alarm with respect to his whole organism. This well-known phenomenon is the fear of fear, which most theories suggest lies at the basis of spontaneous panic disorder and the symptoms related to it. This peculiar form of fear consists of the fright caused by an acute state of anxiety, which in subjective experience corresponds to an intense perception of personal instability, which is perceived by the person as an alteration of interoceptive stability. Not surprisingly, spontaneous panic is associated with an enhanced awareness of interoceptive cues (Richards, Cooper and Winkelman, 2003). It will be useful once more to recall the fact that, for this style of personality, interoceptive stability represents the reference point through which the subject in each case regulates his own position in the world.

According to the perspective we have adopted so far, the fear of fear cannot be the consequence of a panic attack, which is what Goldstein and Chambless (1978) have argued (although interoceptive conditioning may play a role in maintaining proneness to panic). The behaviourist approach suggests that the cause of the phenomenon lies in a process of Pavlovian conditioning, whereby panic attacks are considered to be conditioned responses to interoceptive cues that have preceded panic in the past.

Likewise, the fear of fear cannot be seen to derive from catastrophic misinterpretations of bodily sensations, as suggested by cognitive theories (Clark, 1986), although cognitive processes can certainly play a significant role in the genesis of panic attacks. From a cognitivist point of view, this type of fear would emerge as a consequence of inappropriate threat beliefs (catastrophic thoughts) about internal bodily perturbations. 'Once perceived, the bodily sensation is interpreted in a catastrophic fashion and then a panic attack results' (Clark, 1986: 463). The question this approach leaves unanswered, however, is why, once perceived, the bodily sensation should then be interpreted in a catastrophic fashion. In other words: why should a person who panics and can feel his heart pounding believe that he is about to die? What is the origin of this catastrophic thought?

The construct that most clearly expresses the peculiar phenomenon represented by the fear of one's own state of anxiety is known as *anxiety sensitivity* (AS) (Reiss and McNally, 1985). This refers to the fear of anxiety-related sensations. In a well-known paper originally published in 1991, Reiss stresses that AS is an individual dispositional variable, one that differs from both trait anxiety and anticipatory anxiety[5] (Reiss, 1991; McNally, 2002). Reiss further traces a basic distinction between fundamental fear and ordinary fear; he writes:

> *'Consider the rational relationships among three different fears: (a) the fear of snakes; (b) the fear of heights; and (c) the fear of anxiety. Fears of snakes and heights are rationally unrelated to one another, in the sense that having one of the fears is not a reason for having the other fear. It makes no sense for a person to say, "I am afraid of heights because I am afraid of snakes." On the other hand, the fear of anxiety is rationally related to the fear of snakes and heights. A rational person might say, "I am afraid of snakes and heights because I am afraid I would have a panic attack if I encountered those stimuli"' (Reiss, 1991: 147).*

According to Reiss, the fear of anxiety symptoms (anxiety sensitivity) is thus the most fundamental fear, for it gives reason to avoid all situations that may engender the stimuli a person fears. Regrettably, Reiss does not follow his arguments to their inevitable conclusion, which is the raising of an even more crucial question: why is it that there are many people who are afraid of heights and serpents but not of anxiety perturbations? Why is it that only individuals with high AS perceive such sensations as personally harmful? To express the matter even more succinctly, how does the fear of anxiety-related sensations emerge?

The above question appears all the more legitimate given that the level of AS not only varies among different individuals, but may also change in the same individual, in relation for instance to anxiety-relevant stressors (Schmidt, Lerew and Joiner, 2000) and specific events or circumstances, prior to the inception of panic attacks (Donnell and McNally, 1990) and in particular moments of life (Faravelli and Pallanti, 1989; Pollard, Pollard and Corn, 1989; Roy-Byrne, Geraci and Uhde, 1986).

The answer expectancy theory gives to our question is that the fear of anxiety-related sensations is caused by beliefs about the harmful consequences of experiencing certain bodily perturbations (McNally, 2002; Reiss, 1991; Reiss and McNally, 1985; Reiss *et al.*, 1986; Taylor, 1995).

As the fear of fear, therefore, is produced by the belief that certain sensations have harmful consequences, not only can individuals be seen to vary from one another according to whether or not they hold this belief, but the fact that the AS level of an individual may change over the course of his life suggests that specific circumstances or conditions contribute to modify the belief in question. What this means, in concrete terms, is that in different moments of his life an individual may perceive the same sensation in completely different ways. A few months before his wedding, for instance, a person may take heart palpitations to be the sign of a serious, life-threatening condition such as a heart attack, while he may regard similar palpitations as merely an annoying sensation just one year after his marriage.

The fact that the same individual may interpret the same bodily sensation in different ways – which in the above example would be due to the transition from a condition where a life change is imminent to one where the change has been stabilized – must be seen as something related to a change in the subject's beliefs about bodily perturbations.

Just how an impending marriage or more generally a life event may change a person's beliefs about bodily perturbation is unclear. It may be, however, that what AS theorists call 'belief', rather than representing the crux of the interpretation of anxiety-related sensations, may actually come about as a consequence of the subject's state of anxiety. This alternative view implies a radical shift in perspective, one that affects the very foundation of cognitivism: for belief would have to be regarded as merely a way of *grasping* one's own experience – which would already possess meaning pre-reflexively – rather than as the primary method of generating meaning. Only then could self-awareness clearly be seen to derive from one's relation to the world, rather than from any reflection upon one's own actions. This is indeed one of the underlying themes of the present book.

What is the origin of distorted beliefs?

It is on the basis of this reading that we regard the change of beliefs associated with certain life events as due to an anxiety triggered by an alteration of the emotional-interoceptive stability of the subject, in concomitance with the events in question. The meaning of this form of anxiety – which may or may not explicitly be grasped and fixed as a belief – is that of feeling one is in danger; and danger is here triggered by a situation that elicits an acute feeling of instability with regard to one's whole organism, and which coincides with a state of anxiety.

This condition of altered stability simultaneously engenders a range of anticipations concerning the possible consequences of the ongoing situation (of danger). As we have seen in Chapter 4, the perception of oneself as being in a given affective state always concerns the way in which one *finds oneself* in a given situation, and how one situates oneself in relation to the present circumstances. A condition of acute anxiety, therefore, perceived as a threat to the integrity of one's organism, simultaneously corresponds to the generation of thoughts and images aimed at anticipating the possible developments of the ongoing situation.[6] From the perspective, that is, of the person who is experiencing a profound alteration of his sense of permanence, the catastrophic misinterpretation described by Clark (1986) represents an attempt to foresee the possible developments of the situation. We may argue, therefore, that forecasting here serves as a means to face the ongoing situation by anticipating its possible outcomes. For instance, if exertion tachycardia is perceived as a symptom (as it lies beyond the interoceptive baseline), and if this sensation causes an acute feeling of danger with regard to one's whole organism, the anticipation of the outcomes of tachycardia cannot but be a heart attack (and what follows it: the arrival of the ambulance, hospitalization and, eventually, death). These anticipations, which represent attempts to face an acute condition of instability in order to regain control over an ongoing sequence of events, actually trigger fear; hence, they increase bodily symptoms, leading to a vicious circle that culminates in a panic attack.[7] Despite behaviourists' suggestions, therefore, the fear of anxiety symptoms may be seen to arise from sources other than the direct experiencing of panic, although once this fear is perceived it may function as a conditioned response to the bodily sensations that were already present before it.

The intensity of the anxiety-related feeling that can trigger a panic attack depends on the emotional-interoceptive level regulating the subject's sense of personal stability. Particularly challenging moments in the emotional life of a person will correspond to an increased focus, and hence an acute amplification of his bodily sensations, as well as to increased amygdala responsiveness, probably via a direct spino-thalamo-amygdalar pathway: for the way in which individuals regulate their own situatedness is within a framework of reference that predominantly uses a body-centred coordinate system. While this increase in attention toward bodily perturbations raises one's chances of perceiving threatening interoceptive cues, it also adds to the condition of perceived instability by making one more vulnerable, and thus more prone to regarding innocuous bodily events as dangerous (to one's own stability).

Interesting evidence, in this respect, emerges from studies on the neurological basis of the close association between balance disorders and anxiety. Anatomical and physiological data may shed light on the genesis of one symptom in particular, psychogenic dizziness, which has high incident rates among patients suffering from panic attacks and agoraphobic avoidance. As these subjects are particularly dependant on proprioceptive balance cues to maintain their balance, while they lend insufficient weight to vestibular and visual-balance information (Jacob *et al.*, 1997, 2001; Staab, 2006; Staab and Ruckenstein, 2007), they may experience inadequate stability in situations where the sense of the physiological condition of the entire body is altered (as is the case in a state of fear). A key role would here be played by the parabrachial nucleus, which represents an area of convergence of vestibular signals and somatic and visceral sensory-information processing in pathways that appear to be involved in avoidance conditioning, anxiety and conditioned fear (Balaban and Thayer, 2001; Balaban, 2002, 2004).

On the other hand, the fear of anxiety-related sensations may develop into a subacute or chronic form of hypochondria, accompanied by agoraphobia or panic attacks.[8]

Although both hypochondriacs and those who suffer from panic disorder may share the general tendency to become fearful in response to bodily perturbations, several studies suggest a role of the amygdala in the rapid, automatic and initial processing of fear-relevant stimuli, and also suggest that its activation is not sustained (LeDoux, 1998; Öhman and Mineka, 2001; Larson *et al.*, 2006). Other evidence reveals that, in some cases, anxious individuals sustain attention to threat-related stimuli longer than other people (e.g. Fox, Russo and Dutton, 2002). Several studies, moreover, have reported an absence of amygdala activation during sustained periods of symptom provocation, which suggests that the sustained processing of phobogenic stimuli and corresponding affective reactions may be based on the activation of regions other than the amygdala (e.g. Mountz *et al.*, 1989; Fredrikson *et al.*, 1993; Rauch *et al.*, 1995; Reiman, 1997; Paquette *et al.*, 2003; Straube *et al.*, 2006; Straube, Mentzel and Miltner, 2007). There are good reasons to believe, therefore, that not only the amygdala[9] (through various modes of activation), but also the recruitment of other areas of the brain, plays a key role in the symptomatology that characterizes both hypochondriasis and panic disorder.

In order to prevent, or limit, those situations which may alter his sense of permanence, the subject may adopt a number of avoidance behaviours that, while temporarily reducing the range of negative sensations, in the long term will heighten his physiological/emotional precariousness, leading to a stable condition of agoraphobia.

To sum up, different circumstances in life, and, more generally, different anxiety-relevant stressors, do not affect the degree of AS of the subject by altering his beliefs; rather, they do so by altering his level of interoceptive stability. Empirical data suggest that it is because of their more acute sensitivity to bodily variations that subjects with a higher level of AS respond with greater panic, fear and distress to biological challenge procedures, such as hyperventilation challenge (Sturges *et al.*, 1998), caffeine challenge (Sturges and Goetsch, 1996) and carbon dioxide challenge (Forsyth *et al.*, 1999; Schmidt and Trakowski, 1999; Zwolensky *et al.*, 2001). Similar conclusions were reached in the studies conducted in a naturalistic environment by Schmidt *et al.* (1997, 1999). By taking a large nonclinical sample, these studies found that subjects with a higher level of AS were more likely to develop spontaneous panic in particularly stressful conditions.

What makes some persons prone to perceiving bodily sensations as harmful is the way in which they construct and maintain their own sense of personal stability. It is these individuals who possess what we have termed a phobia-prone style of personality (Arciero, 2002, 2006; Arciero *et al.* 2004; Bertolino *et al.*, 2006). As an important role in the processing of fearful stimuli is played by individual differences in the amygdala response modulated by serotonin transporter (5-HTT) polymorphism (Hariri *et al.*, 2002), the allelic variation between individuals may contribute to the different reactivity of the amygdala among those possessing this style of personality (Bishop, Duncan and Lawrence, 2004; Mathews, Yiend and Lawrence, 2004; Cools *et al.*, 2005). Individual differences in the activity of the amygdala – expressed as increased sensitivity to fear-related stimuli – may arise as an emergent property from the association between genetic and psychological factors. In other words, the 5-HTT's allele predisposes a more reactive arousal system that, through experience as well as other genetic and environmental moderators, may manifest itself among certain subjects in the form of phobic-proneness (Bertolino *et al.*, 2006).

As we have seen, the condition of acute vigilance that follows the perception of harmful bodily perturbations may have a number of consequences, even leading to the emergence of spontaneous panic and the symptomatic pictures associated with it. The clinical phenomenology deriving from this may be characterized by a panic disorder, which may or may not be followed by a condition of agoraphobia; alternatively, albeit far more rarely, it may be characterized by an agoraphobic syndrome associated with no panic attacks, and which may later be followed by panic disorder (Bienvenu *et al.*, 2006). The reason why agoraphobia without a history of panic is so rare is both that individuals affected by this condition are less likely to seek psychiatric care (Wittchen, Nelson and Lachner, 1998; Andrews and Slade, 2002) and that the heterogeneous sources of the disorder make its manifestations and possible complications rather varied.

Agoraphobia

It is possible to distinguish at least three origins of agoraphobia. (1) A clinical picture of 'social agoraphobia' that may revolve around the fear of a negative evaluation by others – something that makes it close to social phobia and that may be worsened by panic attacks. (2) An agoraphobic picture similar to, yet clearly separate from, the previous one, and that cannot be worsened by panic attacks. For in this case, social avoidance, while equally marked by the systematic shunning of any confrontation with others, is motivated by the fear, not of harmful feelings, but of how negative evaluation at the hands of others may engender a feeling of nullification of Self. (3) Agoraphobic syndrome proper, which may be identified with that described by Pirandello in *The Stuffed Bird*, and which consists in the perception of the world as a place where danger lies around every corner; and danger here can only be faced by anticipating those situations that may alter one's sense of personal stability and trigger panic attacks. Thus, in the framework of this clinical picture, two more-or-less distinct symptomatological conditions may emerge that often alternate with one another, or merge one into the other. (a) A condition associated with the nonpredictability of possible situations, for instance when the subject finds himself in an unknown place, or in a space too wide to be under his control (as the very etymology of the term 'agoraphobia' suggests). The symptomatological profile associated with this condition is mostly of a psychasthenic type, marked by a feeling of weakness, vertigo, stuffed head, wooden legs and aches of various sorts and of different degrees of intensity. (b) A condition linked to the impossibility of anticipating the consequences of a given situation, as the person feels that his own sphere of action is being limited through external forms of coercion: burdened, for instance, by irremovable bonds (e.g. the birth of a child or marriage), controlled by other people (e.g. during an airplane journey or at the barber's) or tied to a given place (e.g. a concert hall, tunnel, highway or elevator).

This second condition, which corresponds to the perception of being trapped (as the very etymology of the term 'claustrophobia' suggests[10]), is associated with a symptomatological profile that is mostly of the constrictive type: intercostal pain, hunger for air, the feeling of having a lump in the throat and of suffocating, and, in some cases, even the imminent and impendent feeling that one is going mad, that one is about to act in a heedless manner and that one is losing one's bearings.

In both conditions, the systematic avoidance of what are regarded as excessively activating circumstances is a way for the subject to maintain a stable perception of Self. From this perspective, and in agreement with the empirical data (Bienvenu *et al.*, 2006), not only does panic disorder appear to be a potent risk factor for agoraphobia, but agoraphobia in turn appears to be a risk factor for panic disorder.

In the light of the above perspective, moreover, several phobias ought to be reassessed which have been characterized as specific phobias. Sensitivity to specific threat-related stimuli, even when subjects are distracted or unaware of these stimuli (Straube *et al.*, 2006; Straube, Mentzel and Miltner, 2007; Carlson, Moses and Claxton, 2004), should often be viewed in the framework of an agoraphobic perception of the world. The animal, natural event, situation or blood-injection-injury condition feared, that is, represents reference points to be avoided at all costs, and on the basis of which a viable course may be marked out in what is perceived as dangerous territory. This, of course, is not to rule out the possibility that the disorder in question may have come about through the classical conditioning pathway (as is the case, for instance, when a person comes to fear dogs after having been attacked by a dog), or indeed through indirect pathways (as is the case when the fear of dogs is vicariously passed on to his child from a parent who was once attacked by a dog); nor does the above view imply that the disorder in question must necessarily occur as part of a clinical picture. Although specific phobias form a heterogeneous class of disorders, characterized by various aetiologies and different degrees of intensity (for a review, see Merckelbach *et al.*, 1996), most of these phobias are only the most evident symptom of an underlying agoraphobic condition. As shown in the clinical vignette that follows, often what seems to be a specific phobia of the natural environmental type is actually one of the symptoms of 'social agoraphobia'. In order to complete our discussion of these disorders, we shall then follow this first vignette by examining the case of Judith, which emerges as one of 'spontaneous panic' later worsened by agoraphobia.

8.6 Case vignettes

Specific phobia?

Victor is a 20-year-old history student and the eldest of three brothers. His father works as an electronics shopkeeper and his mother as a speech therapist. The problem that has been tormenting Victor is a specific phobia: the fear of thunderstorms. Victor perceives thunderstorms as a physical malaise: 'a threat to my vitality'. The alleged cause of this terror is Victor's fear of being struck by lightning. Each time a storm breaks out, Victor locks himself in his room, where he remains waiting, in a condition of existential precariousness, for the rain to stop.

The first time Victor felt this fear was at the age of 10, when on the day of his grandmother's birthday, as he and his family were about to go to a restaurant; he was left in the car with a female cousin a few years older than he was, to wait for the end of a violent storm. Victor's cousin then told him a series of stories about the tragedies caused by storms, stories that produced a strong effect on him. Although Victor believes this episode to lie at the origin of his disorder, it was only after he had entered high school that the fear of storms became an increasingly serious concern in his life. By the time Victor was finishing school, both his daily routine and his mood varied according to the clouds.

Once again, as in all previous clinical cases we have considered, the symptomatology of the subject can here be seen to receive new determinations of meaning, determinations that cannot be grasped by means of empirical analysis alone, once it has been examined in the framework of his life.

When Victor was 10, his life was shaken by another, far more significant event, concomitant to the emergence of his fear of storms. As in the course of his school years Victor had proved to be a studious and responsible child, but also a shy and awkward one, his teacher decided she needed to 'help' him overcome his shyness. She thus forced Victor to read his essays in front of different classes, with the result that on the one hand Victor started suffering from a bad stutter, and on the other, his fear of others' judgment and self-exposure increased. Stuttering was Victor's most serious problem when he began junior high school, although things improved as his feeling of acceptance on the part his school mates increased. By the time Victor had entered senior high school, his stutter had almost disappeared; his fear of storms, on the other hand, had steadily grown worse.

Control over the weather became Victor's chief way of regulating his relation to others. Even his sentimental debut was postponed by blaming the weather: 'I could not invite a girl over, as I could not plan anything ahead: the weather might have changed and I might have embarrassed myself.' Phobia is thus what allows Victor to find a way through various ongoing situations by monitoring a danger – that of storms – which becomes his way of defining his own position in what he perceives to be a hostile environment. 'It is as if this fear I have were crucial to my own survival. I find the prospect of recovery far more terrifying: it is as if I were heading towards an unknown danger, as I would have to change my own self completely.'

Spontaneous panic?

Judith is a 35-year-old MD specializing in internal medicine. She is the mother of an eight-year-old boy, and the wife of a 45-year-old lawyer. Judith visits our centre because of a panic disorder she has been suffering from for more than a year, and which in the last months has worsened, owing to her avoidance of crowded places like supermarkets, cinemas, theatres and banks, as well as her difficulty in moving about freely, as she is overcome by the fear of having a crisis as soon as she follows routes other than those familiar to her. Despite her caution and avoidance behaviour, Judith still suffers from unexpected panic attacks, which occur on a weekly basis and are mostly characterized by vertigo, a feeling of fainting and tachycardia.

Judith traces her first panic episode back to the time when, one year ago, as she was working in the ward, a nurse asked her to cannulate the vein of a bedridden patient. In order to perform this operation, which was a rather difficult one given the condition of the patient, Judith was forced to kneel and stay in that position for some time. When she moved to stand up, she felt a grip in her stomach, accompanied by tachycardia, nausea, a weakness in her legs, sweating and a feeling as if she were about to faint. Judith immediately asked for an electrocardiogram, and was astonished to find that her cardiac frequency, which she thought might be around 120 beats per minute, measured less than 100.

As her fear that she might be suffering from a cardiac pathology vanished, Judith regained her self-control and interpreted the event that had just occurred as something that was no doubt caused by a vagal reaction. Everything got back to normal; but one week later, when Judith had almost forgotten about the event, a similar situation elicited symptoms identical to those of the first.

Judith then began having serious concerns that she might be suffering from an organic pathology.

She visited a number of specialists, but her medical examinations showed no significant results; her fear, on the other hand, increased, as did the frequency of the attacks. Judith started dreading the thought that the same condition might surprise her when she least expected it, and no longer felt safe when leaving the house. 'I feel I have completely lost my bearings.' At this stage, Judith took the step she had always hoped to avoid: 'I thought I could cope on my own, instead I chose to visit a shrink.' It was with a feeling of shame and profound unease that Judith turned to us for help.

The emphasis of Judith's story is clearly on the medical aspects of her disorder: particular attention is paid to the unpredictability of the attacks, and hence to her constant worry that she might be overwhelmed at any minute. But when Judith's disorder is examined in the wider context of her story, her symptomatology acquires a rather different significance: for in the background of these events lies the marital crisis that had begun four years earlier, at the time of her father's death.

Although Judith owned a house with her husband, even after her wedding she continued living in a different area of town, in an apartment adjacent to that of her parents, forcing her husband and later her son to conform to the structure and everyday rhythms of her family of origin. The cornerstone of the family was Judith's unique relationship with her father: 'Whenever I needed to take a decision, I would turn to my father. I knew that I could trust him.' The death of Judith's father thus altered the existential balance that also sustained Judith's relationship with her husband. Not long after Judith had lost her father, she and her husband moved into the house they owned. Judith suddenly found herself face to face with a man who was her husband, but whom she had never really got to know: a stranger with habits, behaviours and ways of being that she was then witnessing for the first time, and which she did not like. Surprised, but also saddened and disappointed, Judith was struck by her own blindness: 'Why is it only now, after all these years, that I realize whom I have married!' Judith started increasingly distancing herself from her husband. After leaving the hospital, she started working in a private clinic, spending more and more time away from home. Gradually, Judith's relationship with her husband was reduced to a minimum: the two would see each other in the evenings, but hardly speak a word. 'If I talk, I have the impression that he is not listening: he always seems to be elsewhere. He is detached and indifferent.' Judith felt increasingly alone and realized she had to make a choice. A few days before the first episode, she confronted her husband, sharing her concerns and discontentment with him; the man reacted 'as if he didn't give a damn'. Judith immediately realized that her husband might be seeing another woman. Two days later she had her first panic attack.

Endnotes

[1] We are following Craig here in using the term 'interoception' to describe 'the sense of the physiological condition of the entire body, not just the viscera' (Craig, 2002: 655).

[2] It is important to add, however, that the ability to detect heartbeats correlates with the ability to detect changes in other autonomically innervated organs (Whitehead and Drescher, 1980).

[3] It is worth noting the existing correlations between thyroid function and panic (Kikuchi *et al.*, 2005), hypertension and panic (Davies *et al.*, 2008), asthma and panic (Hasler *et al.*, 2005), respiratory disease and panic (Goodwin and Pine, 2002), and colon motility and panic (Hyman and Cocjin, 2005). New forms of collaboration must be sought between psychology, the neurosciences and the various branches of medicine.

[4] Pennebaker *et al.* (1985) have found that inward-focused attention increases the probability of perceiving physiological changes.

[5] Trait anxiety denotes the specific tendency to respond fearfully to stressors in general, whereas anticipatory anxiety denotes an increase in distress occasioned by prospects of imminent threat (McNally, 2002).

[6] A key role in this process is probably played by the connection between the ventromedial prefrontal cortex (vmPFC) (which is associated with the processing and comparing of different goal-directed behaviours aimed at the avoidance of threats or distress), the amygdala and the periaqueductal grey (PAG). An fMRI study investigating the spatial imminence of a threat found that as the threat grew closer, brain activity shifted from the vmPFC to the PAG. This shift showed maximal expression when a high degree of pain was anticipated (Mobbs *et al.*, 2007). For an analysis of the influence of the phobia-prone style of personality on the modulation of prefrontal cortex activity during the cognitive evaluation of emotional stimuli, see Rubino *et al.* (2007).

[7] Once this vicious circle has been established, an acute state of instability may also be triggered by anticipation alone: a word or image is enough, in this case, to elicit fear of anxiety in the subject.

[8] The similarities between the fear of anxiety symptoms in panic disorder and the fear of somatic sensations in hypochondriasis are well documented in a study by Otto *et al.* (1992). Significant correlations between AS (measured according to the Anxiety Sensitivity Index) and hypochondriacal concerns were obtained for five of the seven Illness Attitude Scales: worry about illness, concern about pain, thanatophobia, disease phobia and bodily preoccupations. Commenting upon this relation between hypochondria and panic disorder, the authors point out that 'these questionnaires assess different aspects of a more general tendency to become fearful and aroused in response to somatic sensations, and that this tendency is central to both hypochondriasis and panic disorder' (Otto *et al.*, 1992: 100).

[9] Several anxiety disorders are characterized by an increased activation of the amygdala before emotional human faces, namely social anxiety disorder (Whalen *et al.*, 1998; Birbaumer *et al.*, 1998; Stein *et al.*, 2002; Furmark *et al.*, 2004; Phan *et al.*, 2006), posttraumatic stress disorder (PTSD) (Rauch *et al.*, 2000; Shin *et al.*, 2005), panic disorder and generalized anxiety disorder (Thomas *et al.*, 2001; Stein *et al.*, 2007).

[10] Although studies have stressed the difference between animal phobia and claustrophobia (Craske *et al.*, 1995), the latter is still counted among specific phobias. Were we to act in agreement with this definition of claustrophobia as a situational type of specific phobia, we would be forced to adopt the same classification in the case of agoraphobia as well!

9 The Depression-prone Style of Personality

9.1 The margins of the problem

'Depression, Bereavement, and "Understandable" Intense Sadness: Should the DSM-IV Approach be Revised?' So reads the title of an editorial published in the *American Journal of Psychiatry* in November 2008, in which Mario Maj poses a problem that is also the focus of this chapter (Maj, 2008). What is questioned in what follows is the relation between some central elements in the contemporary debate on the subject: the continuity and boundary between deep sadness, bereavement and depression.

Maj's argument begins with a premise: according to DSM-IV, the intense sadness that follows an unpleasant life event qualifies for the diagnosis of major depression if severity, duration and impairment criteria are fulfilled. The diagnostic decision, that is, is based on exclusively clinical criteria and does not take any contextual elements into account. The only exception to this rule is bereavement: while the intense sadness that follows the death of a loved one possesses certain clinical characteristics that would make it qualify for a diagnosis of major depression, it is not regarded as a mental disorder. The asymmetry between the criteria adopted is quite clear. Hence the chief question raised by Maj (also on the basis of empirical data) is whether bereavement-triggered and other loss-triggered forms of uncomplicated intense sadness should be excluded from the DSM-V diagnosis of major depression. What is at stake here is actually the introduction of a criterion to categorize the contextual element. The above question immediately leads to two caveats: (1) if in one's personal experience a given life event other than bereavement is perceived through a form of loss-triggered intense sadness, this may be due to a pre-existing depressive state or to the worsening of an already depressed mood (as in the case, for instance, of depressive personality disorder (DPD)); (2) it is difficult to draw any clear-cut distinction between what is contextual and what pertains to the constitution of the subject.

Beside this explicit problem, Maj's editorial also raises a more profound issue, which concerns the very history of the conceptualization of the disorder. What is at stake in the question raised by Maj is the integration between the perspective of German psychiatry and that of psychoanalysis, which by introducing the relation between bereavement and melancholy after 2000 years made a momentous contribution to the understanding of the disorder. In the light of this requirement to mutually integrate the two perspectives, we need to redefine a series of elements that come into play in the contemporary debate on the matter.

On the one side we find the sadness, depressive temperament and depression that have entered the contemporary psychiatric discourse in the wake of the German tradition of Kraeplin and later Krestchmer.[1] The origins of the perspective of German psychiatry can actually be traced back to the well-known *Problem XXX* attributed to Aristotle (Barnes, 1984; see Arciero, 2002; Pies, 2007). This treatise, which may be regarded as the first ancient monograph on melancholy, is based on the Hippocratic system of four humours: phlegm, yellow bile, blood and black bile. The last of these humours is termed *melena* in ancient Greek – hence the word melancholy. The Hippocratic perspective does not conceive of humours in pathological terms, as symptoms; rather, it regards them as predispositions toward certain illnesses. The prevalence of one humour over the rest is here seen to foster a particular tendency in the normal constitution of an individual, and thus to reveal pathological conditions or constitutional attitudes.

The above notion of humours provides the starting point for Aristotle's treatise; it is immediately thematized when a question is raised regarding the multiple manifestations of the melancholic temperament. At one extreme stands Herakles, with his fits of anger, followed by Ajax and Bellerophon – the former a man who 'utterly lost his mind', the latter one who 'wandered alone across the plain of Alea, pining away and shunning all human traces' (Barnes, 1984) – and then Empedocles, Plato, Socrates, poets and other well-known men. Some of these men, Aristotle adds, also suffer from physical illnesses due to their temperament. How to explain this variance among melancholic constitutions? Aristotle draws an analogy with wine, which drunk in great quantities can make people similar to those who are melancholic:[2] for wine, like the melancholic humour, affects the spirit; depending on how much of it is consumed, it changes the character of those who drink it. A quiet person might turn talkative; by drinking a little more, he might become impudent; and if he drinks even more, he might become insolent and choleric, or dull and sorrowful.

Wine, however, makes man abnormal only temporarily, whereas nature – which shapes the character of a man – like wine, permanently marks him. A melancholy humour may thus come about by nature, although in the case of most people black bile has no significant influence on character.

Aristotle, then, draws a first distinction between people temporarily possessing a melancholic humour and having a character naturally inclined toward melancholy.

Once he has made it clear that an excess of black bile can affect the spirit, Aristotle gets back to his initial argument: the variety of ways in which this character may manifest itself. To explain this phenomenon, Aristotle invokes the notion that heat and cold are mixed in various proportions in bile: when black bile is cold, people are 'sluggish and dull'; when it is hot, people are 'prone to anger and desire', to the point of suffering from 'fits of fervour or overexcitement'. Where a mean level is reached between heat and cold, people 'are indeed melancholic, yet more reasonable and less eccentric, and in many ways most apt in the fields of culture, the arts and the running of the state' (Barnes, 1984). It is the balance, therefore, between heat and cold that determines the alternation in everyday life between bad mood (*emeran athymias*) and happiness. There is something melancholic in all of us, 'but the persons in whom this element is deeply active certainly possess a peculiar character' (Barnes, 1984). These persons differ from others because they are prone to suffer from illnesses 'connected to black bile' (Barnes, 1984); some melancholic individuals are suddenly overcome by sadness for no apparent reason, while others are always sad; still others kill themselves. According to Aristotle, it is the alteration of the melancholic humour that explains the pathology affecting melancholic characters.

Melancholic individuals, however, also differ from average people because given the right mixture of heat and cold, they make exceptional individuals. Where does the exceptionality of people like Empedocles, Socrates or Plato stem from? The last section of *Problem XXX* aims to provide an explanation for this extraordinariness, which situates the man of genius between two opposite excesses: excessive cold, which leads to 'irrational desperation' and even suicide, and excessive heat, which causes fits of rage. Exceptionality is found when the individual is capable of preserving his own melancholic character (a constitutive trait that sets him apart from the majority of people) in the different circumstances of his life, while 'temperately' oscillating between heat and cold without yielding to either rage or desperation.

Problem XXX distinguishes four configurations which are still relevant today:

1. A 'temperate' melancholic constitution, which we shall term the depression-prone style of personality.
2. A 'melancholic temperament', which may be identified with the condition known as DPD.
3. A melancholic reaction characterizing temperaments other than the melancholic, which may be identified as a major depressive episode.
4. A melancholic reaction that may be identified as a major depressive episode, but which emerges in a melancholic character and corresponds to a strong accentuation of its distinctive traits.

This statement of the problem underwent its most significant modification following the Scholastic appropriation of Aristotle. While the excellence of the melancholic character then came to be regarded as a favourable condition for the life of contemplation,[3] the excess of black bile, or *morbum melancholicum*, came to be seen as a genuine disease. The reasons for this change, which introduced a form of discontinuity – disease – into the spectrum of manifestations of melancholic humour outlined by Aristotle, are to be sought in the need to account for the manifest madness to which some monks were subject. One great Scholastic, William of Auvergne, thus explained that melancholy individuals may be struck by the disease because they are particularly prone to leading a meditative existence, removed from mundane turmoil. Madness, while seen to signal a break in the life of these individuals, could not be considered a threat to their salvation: for if a person had been pious prior to falling ill, 'he could not lose his merit'; if he had been a sinner, 'he could not increase his guilt' (quoted in Klibansky, Panofsky and Saxl, 1964). Through the lenses of moral psychology, depression was destined to be regarded as something quite distinct from the melancholy character.

This statement of the problem, which may be defined as the Greco-Christian one, foreshadows the classic prospective held by Kraepelin (1921) and later Kretschmer (1936), both of whom – albeit with different emphases – posited a 'depressive temperament' as the basis of the manic-depressive illness. People with this temperament were characterized as being predominantly gloomy, sad, despondent, dejected, shy, inadequate, quiet, conscientious, serious, fatigued, lacking initiative and vitality, and so on. Kretschmer, however, whose views were closer to those of Aristotle, maintained that Kraepelin's 'fundamental states' were not enough to incline a certain personality toward melancholy: while they might predispose the individual toward the illness, what proves co-decisive is actual experience. Besides, Kretschmer's description of constitutionally depressive people is rather indicative of a perspective that has been seen to anticipate present dimensional models of personality and affect (Ryder, Bagby and Schuller, 2002). Kretschmer writes: 'If we ask directly about his [i.e. a subject with strong tendency to periodic depression] temperament, then we get something like this: "In normal times he is friendly; people like him; he never grumbles; he has a sense of humour; he joins in a laugh, and even makes a bit of a joke himself at times. Only tears come easily to his eyes, he can't get over even quite little things, and he grieves longer and deeper than other people over sad situations." That is to say: in the case of such individuals, it is not that the temperament itself is sad, but only that it is more easily roused by a sad condition' (Kretschmer, 1936: 129–130). We shall return often to this sharp intuition of Kretschmer's in the course of this chapter.

The concept of depressive personality first suggested by Kraepelin and later revised by Schneider (1959) was incorporated in the classification of depressive disorders with DSM-III (Akiskal, 2001). Particularly in the wake of the influential studies conducted by Akiskal (1983; Akiskal *et al.*, 1978, 1980; Yerevanian and Akiskal, 1979), in the early 1980s the category of dysthymia was introduced to describe any form of affectively-based chronic depression. 'Subaffective dystimia' (Akiskal, 1983) was distinguished from other characterologically-based depressions (which did not respond to antidepressant medications) chiefly on the basis of its response to treatment. As Huprich (1998) has emphasized, as dysthymia responded to antidepressants 'they reasoned that it was appropriate to think of all depressions as having a biological basis, which inherently reflects the idea that depression is a pathological, disease state' (Huprich, 1998: 489). Through Kraepelin, Schneider and Akiskal, then, the scholastic view of William of Auvergne, according to which depression is a discontinuity of character, entered the multiaxial classification system of contemporary psychiatry: 'dysthymia' was placed on Axis I along with the 'major depressive episode'.

While DSM-IV later continued to keep dysthymia on Axis I, in its Appendix B it included research criteria for DPD, thus reintroducing the Aristotelian and Kretschmerian problem of the relation of this construct to both mood disorders and normal character. This fostered much debate, particularly concerning the conceptual overlap between dysthymia and DPD (Huprich, 1998; Klein, 1990; Klein and Miller, 1993; Phillips *et al.*, 1993, 1998; Ryder and Bagby, 1999; Ryder, Bagby and Schuller, 2002, 2005; McDermut, Zimmerman and Chelminski, 2003). Even without discussing any of these debates in detail, if the problem is traced back to its original foundation, a series of questions can be seen to emerge that have already been addressed in *Problem XXX*. The most important of these questions concerns the relation between a particular non-pathological character type – which Aristotle described as the temperate melancholic constitution – and DPD, understood as a pathological condition of one's character. How to account for these two ways of being?

What is essential, given the above definition of the problem, is to understand: (1) how a particular way of feeling over time may become sedimented as a tendency to react emotionally that corresponds to the temperate melancholic constitution (the depression-prone style of personality); (2) what relation exists between this style of personality and the melancholic temperament (DPD). Only once we have clarified what continuity exists between normality and the psychopathology of the depressive character will it be possible to address an equally relevant question: that of the relation between personality and depression.

9.2 Enduring dispositions

An extraordinary contribution to research into what conditions may favour the development of a depressive personality has been made by psychoanalysis, which from its origins has been more interested in explaining the phenomena that underlie symptom formation than in developing diagnostic categories. In a well-known essay published in 1917 and entitled 'Mourning and Melancholia', Freud (1917) touches upon two themes that are crucial for any understanding of depressive reactions. The first is the strong similarity between bereavement and melancholy; the second is the hypothesis that this similarity may be due to a loss suffered in childhood, which would thus lie at the basis of the subject's predisposition toward melancholy.

The relation suggested by Freud between early loss and vulnerability to the depressive disorder was made the object of various longitudinal studies about half a century later. In 1978, a seminal study was conducted in Camberwell, London, by Brown and Harris, who analysed the role of psychosocial factors contributing to depression in a group of depressed female patients. This study identified triggering elements – significant recent losses – and factors of vulnerability – the failure of a trusted relationship with a partner, the loss of a mother before the age of 11, having three or more children under the age of 15, joblessness – the mutual interaction of which was found to be statistically significant for the onset of depression. In a subsequent study, which provided a more detailed examination of the data emerging from the first, Harris, Brown and Bifulco (1986) suggested that the lack of adequate parental care (negligence or indifference) that precedes or follows loss represents an important determinant of morbidity, to the point of making the individual twice as likely to develop depression in the course of adult life.

The potential impact of loss or separation in childhood on the risk, both present and future, of suffering from depression thus depends both on the child's attachment relations – and hence on the sense of Self that he constructed and developed up to the event – and on the degree of regulation that alternative attachment figures have been capable of providing after the occurrence of the loss. The above studies would seem to indicate that a dysfunctional parental style – ranging from extreme forms of rejection, as in the case of maltreatment, to indifference toward care requests – contributes more toward the development of depressive disorder than loss or separation (Parker *et al.*, 1995).[4]

The most interesting element that these studies – which were developed in the context of attachment theory (Bowlby, 1980) – bring to light is the fact that a chronic condition of lack of care (ranging from indifference to detachment, contempt, hostility and maltreatment) may affect the development of one's personality, to the point of making it more vulnerable to depression (for a review, see Alloy *et al.*, 2006). Unlike loss – which still elicits analogous emotional tonalities – parental rejection possesses a structural character; as such, it leads to a chronic eliciting of those emotions which are relevant to both depression and bereavement: sadness and anger.

The sedimentation of these tonalities over time as character traits may thus predispose individuals to develop a depression-prone style of personality or to suffer from DPD (Guidano, 1987, 1991; Arciero and Guidano, 2000). This process may account for the development of those enduring dispositions that both Kraepelin and Kretschmer believed to lie at the basis of the depressive temperament. These tendencies, however, far from being genetically determined,[5] would be seen to arise from recurrent experiences that present emotional characteristics similar to those of bereavement – as Freud had already sensed – but which can more clearly be traced back to chronic conditions of rejection and poor social support of various levels of intensity.

The above perspective appears to find confirmation in those studies that point to a link between the serotonin transporter (5-HTTLPR) (short allele) and the onset of depression following adverse life experiences, but only in individuals with histories of child maltreatment (Caspi *et al.*, 2003; Eley *et al.* 2004; Kaufman *et al.*, 2004, 2006; Kendler, 2005). Not only was the short allele not associated with an increased risk of depression in the absence of similar experiences, but available positive social support was found to moderate the risk of depression associated with a history of maltreatment and the presence of the short allele of the serotonin transporter (Kaufman *et al.*, 2004). As Kretschmer had already observed, actual experience is co-decisive for the development of a tendency toward depression. These traits may be inherited by the next generation if a given niche is again formed that favours the reproduction of this configuration (Griffiths and Gray, 2001).

In a replication of the study conducted by Harris, Brown and Bifulco (1986), by examining the history of the female patients under observation, Bifulco, Brown and Harris (1987) noted that, among the significant characteristics related to lack of care and subsequent depression, an unwanted pregnancy was listed, which was associated with emotional relationships devoid of intimacy and with unreliable partners. In the stories analysed, lack of adequate parental care was seen to increase the risk of young women embarking on premature marriages devoid of any mutual support. One of the most common factors leading to marriage was unwanted pregnancy, a frequent cause of problems in the relationships examined: extramarital affairs, financial hardship and the structuring of a context characterized by lack of caring. It is evident that similar conditions of parental care, strongly marked by the absence of any form of support, fostered a tendency in the offspring to repeat the cycle. The individual disposition toward depression was thus passed on from one generation to the next through the inheritance (i.e. reproduction) of specific conditions necessary for the development of the tendency.[6]

9.3 The depression-prone style of personality

The new contribution made by psychoanalysis and attachment theories to the problem of the genesis of the depression-prone style of personality is to be found in the study of those conditions (loss, separation, rejection, etc.) that in the course of one's development engender recurrent ways of feeling. These experiences, which become sedimented over time, incline the subject's sense of personal stability toward a context of reference that is prevalently focused on states of sadness, anger and anxiety. Hence, the individual's sense of permanence of Self is prevalently centred on the hypercognition of these basic emotions, which structure his situatedness according to the variability of circumstances and his relations to others. The endurance of this tendency is further reflected in the ways in which the person shapes his personal identity.

On the other hand, the differences between the depression-prone style of personality, DPD and affectively-based chronic depression would appear to hinge on the degree to which this mode of maintaining one's personal stability is absolute and rigid, and hence on the degree of intensity and mobility of the emotional states that characterize it. The analysis of these emotions – and sadness in particular – thus represents the thread to be followed in order to reconstruct the continuity between normality and psychopathology. Why do people become sad?

Sadness

Sadness may be elicited by a number of phenomena, ranging from disappointment to rejection, from separation (even temporary) to the loss of a loved one, or even – to quote Bowlby (1980) – 'any trouble or misfortune'. Sadness may thus be regarded as a normal and healthy way of feeling that emerges in response to an adverse and unalterable event. These two characteristics of the event correspond to two distinctive elements in the experiencing of sadness: on the one hand, goal blockage and/or goal loss, which may manifest itself according to various degrees of inactivity; on the other, unpleasantness, which in the case of intense sadness may even take the form of bodily pain. What is the relation between these two aspects of sadness?

No doubt it is one thing for a person to feel sad because he is forced to leave his family on account of his job, for instance; it is quite another for him to be pervaded by sadness following the death of a dear friend or the end of an important relationship, and another still to feel sad every day because his parents have no interest in him and take no care of him. Yet these three different experiences have something in common. What makes them similar to one another is the impossibility of changing the present state of affairs; only in the first case, however, is sadness a transitory occurrence, as the event that elicited it is a temporary one: sadness here indicates a transient impossibility. In the other two cases sadness endures, and its permanence is connected to the immutability of the events that triggered it.

The above conclusions would seem to run against the view on affectivity we have promoted so far. If e-motioning corresponds to the process of *motioning from* a given context by generating a renewed range of possible skilful engagements, then sadness would seem to prove that this way of understanding emotions is wrong. This problem has been addressed by several authors, who by adopting other approaches have come to regard 'propensities for action' as defining features of emotion. Lazarus, for instance, in his weighty study of emotions, writes that 'If we treat sadness as a mood, then we are relieved of having to resolve certain difficult issues such as specifying an action tendency'; he concludes, 'In sadness there seems to be no clear action tendency – except *inaction*, or withdrawal into oneself – that seems consistent with the concept of a mood...'[7] Lazarus thus maintains that sustained states of sadness are moods, and that it 'may be inappropriate to attribute an action tendency to a mood' (Lazarus, 1991: 251).

By criticizing Lazarus' approach, which we may term eliminationist (for it does not consider sustained sadness as an emotion), Power and Dalgleish assimilated the 'action tendency' to the relational aspect of sadness: 'Sadness prompts the individual to make demands for help from members of the social network especially in cultures in which help-seeking is a cultural norm' (Power and Dalgleish, 2007: 225). Yet even this approach, while taking emotion as a communicative gesture produced as a negotiating signal on the part of the emoter, fails to grasp an essential aspect related to emotion: *inaction*.

If e-moting constitutes an attempt on the part of one's organism to find a new orientation when faced with changing contexts through the generation of new meaning possibilities (action tendencies), sustained sadness may be seen to signal the impossibility of grasping the ongoing condition in any other way: this condition therefore remains the chief situation on the basis of which the person feels situated. Two characteristics of sustained sadness may be seen to clearly emerge in the light of the fact that this condition is elicited by various other kinds of loss besides bereavement, for instance: marital dissolution or conjugal infidelity, parental rejection, unexpected loss of social status, failure to attain important goals, unexpected job loss and chronic conditions of rejection. The first characteristic is the fact that the condition lost was fundamental to one's situatedness; the second, that it is precisely the unalterable nature of the condition (of loss or rejection) in which one *finds oneself* that makes motioning from it through the engendering of a renewed range of propensities for action and perception impossible. Inaction thus proves to be an essential component of sadness, for it emerges as a way of feeling situated that is characterized precisely by a sense that the adverse circumstances in which one *finds oneself* cannot be changed. Besides, if we regard the manifestation of sadness not merely as an emotional experience, but also as a negotiating signal, it is clear that sadness corresponds to a communicative gesture related to the impossibility of changing present circumstances: a cue that one needs help.[8] The displaying of sad expressions has long been known to inhibit aggression and elicit prosocial behaviour (Miller and Eisenberg, 1988; Eisenberg *et al.*, 1989).

The anger that often accompanies sadness – to the extent that the two may even merge with one another, as in the case of bereavement – represents an attempt to engender a field of action – and hence to open new possibilities of meaning – aimed at modifying the restraints posed by the immutability of the situation. The sadness–anger linkage is thus one of the most common forms of interaction among the emotions of human experience (Izard, 1991). Although each of these emotions is accompanied by the activation of specific neural patterns, in a study investigating neural responses to facial expressions of sadness and anger, Blair *et al.* (1999) found that the anterior cingulate cortex and right temporal pole were jointly activated by both sad and angry expressions. The researchers suggested that this conjoint activation of neural structures implies a degree of communality in the processes engaged by both expressions.

From this perspective, it is possible to understand the feelings of anger toward the deceased person that may emerge in the early phases of bereavement, as well as the anger directed at other persons who, in the circumstances at hand, may be considered responsible for the loss. Even unwanted separation is frequently characterized by persistent bursts of rage. In an ongoing separation, a common cause of anger is the fact that being misled, betrayed or disappointed by one's partner is something which disrupts personal desires, projects or goals (Izard, 1991). These conditions may become stabilized to the point of fostering hostile feelings, even leading the person to seek vengeance. Rejection often triggers anger and various forms of aggressive behaviour.[9]

It is no coincidence that early-onset depression is associated in adulthood with elevated rates of suicidal behaviours, criminal offences and significant social dysfunction (Fombonne *et al.*, 2001; Knapp *et al.*, 2002; Weissman *et al.*, 1999).

The experience of Suffering

Intricately connected to inaction is the tendency to focus attention inwardly. Hence the paradoxical nature of sadness: an emotion that binds us to the world while at the same time distancing us from it. Several theories and a variety of studies have been developed to account for this inward focus of sadness. According to some researchers, it is related to a unique *depressive attributional style* for one's loss of control over outcomes (Abramson, Seligman and Teasdale 1978); others have suggested that it is linked to a *depressive self-focusing style* characterized by the fact that self-focus sets off a self-evaluative process in which one's current and desired states are compared[10] (Pyszczynski and Greenberg, 1987; Pyszczynski *et al.*, 1989). Others still maintain that low moods are a determinant of attentional focus (Cunningham, 1988; Sedikides, 1992). None of these theories, however, has ever dwelled upon another fundamental aspect of sadness: the experience of suffering. According to our perspective, it is precisely this experience that polarizes the subject's attention, anchoring the depression-prone style of personality to a body-centred coordinate system.

As previously noted, the experience of pain consists of two components: pain sensation, whose neural substrate is found in the somatosensory cortex and the posterior insula, and pain affect, which is associated with the dorsal area of the anterior cingulate cortex (dACC). The sensory processing of pain provides information about ongoing tissue damage, whereas the feeling of unpleasantness signals the perceived aversive state and 'motivates behaviour to terminate, reduce, or escape exposure to the source of the noxious stimulation' (MacDonald and Leary, 2005: 204). As suggested in our own study, the affective component of pain is modulated by the emotional proneness of one's style of personality (Mazzola, 2009).

Not only do different languages employ the same expressions used for physical pain (hurt, injured, harmed, broken bones, etc.) to describe painful experiences such as rejection or the loss of a loved one (social pain), but patients with depression often present unexplained physical pain (Simon *et al.*, 1999; Bair *et al.*, 2003; Trivedi, 2004; Tylee *et al.*, 2005). The hypothesis that the brain areas recruited for physical pain may be similar to those recruited for social pain was tested in an fMRI study that investigated the neural substratum of social exclusion (Eisenberger, Lieberman and Williams, 2003). Subjects scanned in a situation in which they were prevented from participating in a game by other players showed increased activity in the dACC (areas 24′ and 32′). The degree of activation of the dACC strongly correlated with self-reports of social distress felt during the exclusion episode. This study provided evidence that the experiences of social and physical pain share a common neural substratum: the dACC.

Interestingly, frequencies of reported activation of brain areas during induced sadness across 22 relevant studies show that the ACC (areas 24′, 25′, 32′) is the second most prominent region recruited (after the basal ganglia) (Freed and Mann, 2007). This brain region, along with others, is also activated in cases of grief (Gündel *et al.*, 2003), separation from loved ones (Najib *et al.*, 2004), depression (Davidson *et al.*, 2002), distress vocalizations emitted by young mammals when separated from caregivers

(Lorberbaum *et al.*, 1999, 2002) and the maternal response of rodents to the vocalizations of their pups (Murphy *et al.*, 1981; Eisenberger and Lieberman, 2004). Hence, a range of evidence suggests that physical-pain distress and social-pain distress share overlapping substrates (Eisenberger *et al.*, 2006). The dACC also plays a part in functions unrelated to pain, such as goal conflict or expectation violations (Vogt, 2005). Eisenberger and Lieberman (2004) regard this discrepancy detection function as complementary to that which underlies pain distress; in the footsteps of Panksepp (1998), they envisage the general activity of the dACC as a kind of 'alarm system' of the brain. The function of this system would be linked, therefore, to two mutually related components – a discrepancy detection system and a distress system – just as a smoke detector is connected to the ringing of an alarm bell.

In the case of mammals, the surfacing of this 'alarm system' from ancient regions of the brain (Panksepp, 1998, 2005) has served to promote social integrity by allowing individuals to signal their exclusion from their groups of belonging through pain, thus making relationships with conspecifics crucial for survival throughout the course of one's life. It is probably on the basis of this process that awareness of the death of others, and the expressions of bereavement connected to it, developed in *Homo sapiens sapiens*. Rejection and loss may then be seen as two aspects of a single phenomenon that concerns exclusion or the end of one's relation with others.

From an evolutionary perspective, the dACC, which made its first phylogenetic appearance with mammals, would have provided the neural substratum for painful feelings triggered by threats of exclusion from one's group or by loss. The function of social pain would thus appear to be similar to that of physical pain. In particular, just as physical pain sensations focus the subject's attention on physical injury, motivating him to perform a series of actions aimed at mitigating his pain, the feelings of unpleasantness directly or indirectly associated with the breaking down of social relations (exclusion, grief, unwanted separation, rejection, unexpected loss of job or of social status, failure to reach important goals, lack of a viable life plan, etc.) attract the attention of others and direct the individual inwards, away from the current unalterable situation.

Inaction and inward attentional focus, then, are two aspects that are closely and mutually integrated in the experiencing of sadness, particularly in the case of conditions such as bereavement or chronic rejection, which are characterized by sustained sadness. For in these cases it is even more evident that the subject's impossibility of changing – by generating actions – the painful situation in which he finds himself (and which is of central importance to his situatedness) forces him to disengage from the situation by producing a change of experiential focus: almost a need to take care of himself and his own pain. This may be an acute need, as in the case of bereavement or unwanted separation (when it extends in various ways over time), or a need related to structural conditions such as the lack of adequate parental care. In both cases – albeit in different ways – situatedness is perceived by focusing on inner states connected to the unalterable situations, which are thus reduced to the effect they produce: a perspective that takes account of the analogy between bereavement and the melancholic character first sensed by Freud. Only in the case of sustained rejection, however, does the person's way of feeling incline his sense of personal stability over time toward a reference context focused on inner states, orientating his situatedness in this direction: for as the studies conducted by Harris, Brown and Bifulco (1986) have shown, an early loss is not enough to predispose individuals toward melancholy.

The fundamental characteristic of this style of personality (and of DPD) is the subject's anchoring to a body-centred reference system that allows him to focus on inward signals in order to face the multiplicity of situations and his relation with others. Ipseity here shapes the person's dialectic with alterity on the basis of visceral states. MacDonald and Leary have aptly observed in relation to the aversiveness of pain: 'We propose that painful feelings triggered by social exclusion also provide a mechanism useful for learning effective approach/avoidance regulation to avoid exclusion' (MacDonald and Leary, 2005: 204). The subject, that is, maintains his own sense of permanence of Self by avoiding situations and actions that may engender painful feelings, and by paying stable attention to his own inward states, the management of which monopolizes his cognitive resources.

Since Abramson (Abramson, Seligman and Teasdale, 1978), numerous studies have emphasized the above process, while stressing only its cognitive aspects (treated apart from the emotional states that determine them): aspects that have been explained as a dispositional tendency to make internal attributions. The strong reflexive engagement of the subject may actually be said to be completely subordinated to emotional activation, as the cognitive domain is here made to do what sadness does not, namely: engender a renewed range of possible skilful engagements in order to create new meaning possibilities in the ongoing situation. Sadness, by contrast, binds the person to the situation, deactivation of the motor system being but one clear sign of this. Cognitive engagement (supported by painful feelings) constitutes the chief means for this style of personality to change the aversive emotional states through which it feels situated by generating new meaning possibilities. Thus, Cioran noted in his *Cahiers*: 'It is incredible how everything in me, truly everything, starting from my ideas, derives from physiology. My body is my mind; or, rather: my mind is my body' (Cioran, 1997: 36).

It is precisely this crucial point that allows us to distinguish the depression-prone style of personality from DPD: the possibility and capacity on the part of the subject of disengaging from the situation that triggers sadness by grasping these affective states, not as destructive emotions but as a source of meaning – like a sense matrix that, while anchoring the person's understanding of himself, generates new possibilities of engagement in his relation to the world and others. Hence, Cioran can write: 'Thank God for my failures! I owe them everything I know' (Cioran, 1997: 469), and again: 'He who wallows in sadness is no longer the man of yore, but a poet' (Cioran, 1990: 72). This would also appear to be the suggestion Aristotle makes in *Problem XXX*, when he notes that what makes people possessing this character – poets, philosophers, doctors and well-known men – stand out is precisely their ability not to fall prey to sadness and anger.[11]

The ontological solitude

This origin of this personality is thematically reflected in the cognitive style that characterizes it, whose keystone is represented not only by a strong inward anchoring, but also by a feeling that reality is temporary and illusionary. The feeling that reality is precarious – corresponding to a form of sensitivity ready to grasp the most evasive and defective aspects of the human condition – focuses the subject's cognitive resources on the search for consistent and solid inner realities: for enduring characteristics which may allow him to face the perceived evanescence and fatuousness, or absurdity and pointlessness, of existence. The work of Rilke can be seen to illustrate this search.

In a short piece of writing entitled 'On Transience', Freud (1915) describes a summer walk he made in the Dolomites with a young yet already well-known poet – whom some have identified as Rilke – and a friend of his. Despite the beauty of the natural surroundings and the charm of the landscape, the poet was far from rejoicing; rather, he sensed the transience of all things. By the use of various arguments, Freud did his best to show the 'pessimist poet' that the value of that beauty was not diminished by its temporal limitedness, yet he failed in his task. Later, when Freud paused to reflect upon the matter, he realized that a strong affective element was troubling the visions of this poet: 'The idea that all this beauty was transient was giving these two sensitive minds a foretaste of mourning over its death. . .' Freud, who too readily associated that form of sensitivity with bereavement, failed to grasp that what the poet was sensing was the ultimate vacuity of all things – this being an element that leads to creative developments and new itineraries of meaning in a way that is different from that of bereavement. Another passage from Cioran's *Cahiers* sheds light on the meaning of this search: 'To perceive the element of unreality of all things, an irrefutable sign that one is progressing towards truth. . .' (Cioran, 1997: 18). Indeed, the flimsiness of human life represents the underlying theme in the journey that brought Rilke from his *Duino Elegies* to his *Sonnets to Orpheus*: a path leading to song as a stable place of existence in which frailty becomes a trace and testimony.

The other element which inevitably accompanies one's feeling that reality is precarious is 'ontological solitude'. For if the world is reduced to the meaning a person derives from the effect produced by his living experience of it, solitude can be seen to emerge from the perception of the profound originality of this meaning. It is this 'excess of inwardness' that makes solitude and uniqueness coincide: being unique makes one feel one is alone. Also deriving from this excess of inwardness is a difficulty in communicating: almost a feeling of shame to present one's being to others, which makes one feel alien, like an exile in the world. It is 'this very uniqueness' that induces the great Portuguese poet Pessoa to write (Pessoa, 1989: 68):

I abhor love: it is abandonment,
intimacy, the showing-off [. . .] of one's own being.

. . .

It would mean violating my deepest self,
and getting too close to men.

Pessoa leads this journey of restless solitude to its extreme consequence, so much so that in the third act of his *Faust* he speaks of 'metaphysical abhorrence of the other': another that always remains beyond his reach (Pessoa, 1989: 55):

. . . and I
remain within what I say, concealed
like the skeleton beneath this flesh,
an invisible support for what is visible,
different and essential. . .

These great themes, which represent creative sources of meaning for the depression-prone style of personality, acquire a rather different significance when it comes to DPD. Here the very sadness that represents a source of poetry in the first case is perceived through the other as a consequence of one's personal unacceptability: something due to one's intrinsically negative nature. The subject attributes any rejection or hostility on the part of others, which he perceives through negative feelings, to the defectiveness of his own being. It is this 'ontological unacceptability' that justifies others' perceived attitudes of rejection or indifference toward oneself, and which provides the foundation of one's own feeling of helplessness – a feeling several studies have pointed to. Yet, for some people, 'ontological unacceptability' is also a punishment to strive against. Hope and despair both depend on the outcome of this struggle: for the intensity of hopelessness will vary in the course of time (Young *et al.*, 1996; Hankin and Abramson, 2001), as the different events of one's life can have a profound impact on the outcome of the struggle. Indeed, the most apt observation made by Aaron Beck (Beck, Kovacs and Weissman, 1975; Beck *et al.*, 1985, 1990, 1993) with regard to the depressive disorder concerns the special clinical importance of hopelessness as a key factor in suicidal ideation, serious suicidal attempts and completed suicide.

It is the need to rely exclusively on oneself, combined with the fact that self-perception is characterized by a feeling of intrinsic unacceptability, that here guides the reflection of the subject and engenders convictions such as feelings of deficiency and inadequacy, or lack of self-esteem, and attitudes such as an inclination toward guilt, self-blame, pessimism, ill disposition and the criticism of others. While by seeing himself as the cause of his own unamiability the individual can stabilize his own sense of inadequacy within an acceptable range of intensity, this makes him all the more vulnerable to situations that lend themselves to being perceived through the lenses of rejection, loss, exclusion or indifference, thus leaving him more vulnerable to the onset of major depressive episodes.

The mode of feeling situated corresponds to an attitude of mistrust toward the world and particularly toward others, perceived as possible sources of intolerable emotions. Several studies point to the relational difficulties of subjects affected by DPD, ranging from distrustfulness toward one's best friend (Fraley and Davis, 1997) to the increasing of affective distance when one's partner is most in need of solace and support (Fraley, Davis and Shaver, 1998). On the one hand, therefore, the more intense and inarticulate the subject's feeling of solitude, the more vulnerable he will be and the more problematic his affectivity; on the other, it is the sentimental relationships themselves that, once structured, must secure a 'regulated' and accessible form of solitude and emotional distance from the subject's partner. This explains the difficulty individuals with DPD have in becoming affectively involved, a difficulty they frequently perceive as unbearable. This is also one of the themes of 'A Painful Case', a splendid tale featured in Joyce's *Dubliners* (Joyce, 1993).

A painful Case

The protagonist of the story, Mr James Duffy, lives alone in a gloomy house quite far from the crowds of Dublin. The story begins with a description of Mr Duffy's bare room: his bed, washstand, desk, writing materials and books, arranged on shelves of white wood.

In a few brief sentences, Joyce outlines Mr Duffy's face along with his character: his head was long, his face unpleasant and his cheekbones harsh, yet his eyes were benevolent and almost ingenuous.

Mr Duffy worked as a cashier in a bank, which he would go to every morning. He would have breakfast nearby and in the evening dine in an unpretentious eating-house where he felt sheltered from the crowd. He had neither companions nor friends, and only went to see his family for Christmas or when someone had died. Mr Duffy's only distraction was the occasional opera or concert. It was at one such event that he happened to take a seat next to two ladies. One of the two, a woman of about his age, made a passing remark which he took as an invitation to converse. The two then introduced themselves and Mr Duffy learned that the younger woman was the lady's daughter. The two met again: Mr Duffy sought greater intimacy with the woman, who quietly informed him that she was married to the captain of a merchant ship who was often at sea. That one daughter was her only child. After some time, Mr Duffy and the lady met again, and began seeing each other on a regular basis: Mr Duffy was introduced to the woman's husband and started visiting her home.

An intimate, but nonphysical relationship was established between the two: they exchanged their thoughts and ideas, and later a few secrets as well. Mr Duffy would frequently visit the woman and spend the evenings chatting with her. Wrapped in this sweet warmth, Mr Duffy sometimes caught himself listening to 'the strange impersonal voice which he recognized as his own, insisting on the soul's incurable loneliness. We cannot give ourselves, it said: we are our own' (Joyce, 1993: 98).

One evening like many others, as they were deep in conversation, Mrs Sinico, as the woman was called, took Mr Duffy's hand and pressed it to her cheek. Mr Duffy was baffled and avoided the woman for a week. He then chose to meet her in a small cake shop. The two went for a three-hour walk in the adjacent park, where they agreed to break off their intercourse: 'every bond, he said, is a bond to sorrow' (Joyce, 1993: 98–100).

Four years went by. Mr Duffy's father died and a partner of the bank where he was working retired, yet Mr Duffy continued to lead his usual life. He only stopped going to any concerts, so as to avoid meeting Mrs Sinico.

One evening, as Mr Duffy was dining in his usual eating-house, his eye fell on a paragraph in the newspaper. He read it several times and stopped eating. He took the paper, paid the bill and headed home. He entered his room and, muttering to himself, went through the paragraph again. The writing in bold read: 'Death of a lady at Sydney Parade'. The short article was about the death of Mrs Sinico, who had been killed by a train while crossing the railroad. From the investigations it seemed that Mrs Sinico had lately turned to alcohol. She had taken the habit of leaving her house at night to buy liquor.

Mr Duffy was appalled at this death: nauseated by the woman to whom he had opened his soul, and who had given herself to a contemptible vice like the lowest of drunks, only to end her life in such a heedless manner. He hated her.

Mr Duffy put on his coat and left the house. He headed for the eating-house, where he sat drinking until late. As the memories of the time he had spent with Mrs Sinico came to mind, he realized that she was truly dead. In an instant, Mr Duffy sensed how lonely she must have felt. Leaving the place, he crossed the park on foot. As he gazed toward the slope, he was gripped by despair at seeing two figures embracing in the dark.

Mr Duffy wanted no one: he had been excluded from the banquet of life.

9.4 Disorders

The most evident difference between a depression-prone style of personality and DPD is found in the role played by cognition. In the first case, cognition serves as an instrument that allows the subject to disengage from situations that trigger destructive emotions; in the second case, it represents a way of stabilizing and – in pathological forms – amplifying a negative perception of one's being in the world. As we have already emphasized, these different roles played by cognition are not primary ones; rather, they depend on the emotional structure of cognition. That is, the inability to disengage is connected to the pervasiveness (across situations) and recurrence (across time) of the painful feelings elicited in delicate moments in one's life, and hence to the difficulty of articulating these feelings. The particular emotive structure that underlies the construct we have termed DPD – and the cognitive configuration related to it – must thus be traced back to a repeated exposure to negative events (i.e. chronic conditions of emotional, but also physical and sexual, maltreatment) (Harkness and Lumley, 2008).

The kind of stability deriving from the above structure is centred not only on negative emotions, but also on a way of bearing these emotions that is determined by the emotions themselves, and is characterized by the development of personal themes of derogation, unacceptableness, unworthiness, defectiveness, unamiability and so on. The factors of vulnerability to depression, therefore, must be sought not only – and not chiefly – in the characteristics of cognition (Abramson, Seligman and Teasdale, 1978; Abramson, Metalsky and Alloy, 1989; Beck, 1967; Bondolfi, 2004; Bondolfi *et al.*, 2006; Abela and Hankin, 2008), but in the ways those cognitive forms stabilize a mode of feeling that by its very characteristics is susceptible to being disrupted by negative life events, and negative emotional stimuli in general. The fact that a given event may cause sadness and that this sadness – by taking hold of cognition – may come to be cognitively articulated in terms of one's own defectiveness is due to the characteristics of sadness itself, which – as we have seen – forces the individual to take care of himself in order to disengage from the situation that caused it. Unlike in the case of those who are not vulnerable to depression, this concern with oneself – with one's perceived unworthiness, for instance – rather than enabling a disengagement from the event, amplifies the sadness from which it originates, thus initiating a downward spiral that may lead to depression. Depending on the range of stability attained, which may vary in the course of one's life, every event capable of triggering negative emotions (such as sadness, anger or anxiety) exposes those who are vulnerable to an increase of negative affects and an inevitable amplification that may lead to a depressive episode.[12] From this perspective, it is possible to make sense of those studies that point to a greater change in dysfunctional beliefs following negative mood induction in formally depressed individuals compared to those who have never been depressed (Scher, Ingram and Segal, 2005). Vulnerability to the disorder would thus appear to be linked to a personality structure that, by its very way of maintaining stability, predisposes the individual to the development of depression following the occurrence of negative events. This personality may be identified with the depressive temperament, which, as Kretschmer has pointedly observed, 'is more easily roused by sad conditions' (Kretschmer, 1936: 129–130). What may possibly account for the subjects' susceptibility to depression is an abnormally elevated reactivity of different areas of the brain. Although there are no data directly supporting this hypothesis, some studies indicate that elevated amygdala activity, for instance, predisposes toward the recurrence of depressive episodes (Drevets *et al.*, 1992b; Post, 1992). Along much the same lines, Liotti *et al.* (2002) have shown that in patients with remitted unipolar depression there is a persistence of focal metabolism abnormalities (cerebral blood flow (rCBF) decrease in the pregenual anterior cingulate 24a) after transient sad mood challenge – changes which were not found in the healthy group under observation. The fact that certain regions of the brain may show signs of peculiar metabolic activity even after the complete remission of depression is also suggested by a PET study of tryptophan depletion (Neumeister *et al.*, 2004), which reveals an increased metabolism in several regions, including the anterior cingulate, orbitofrontal cortex and medial thalamus.

Although depressive disorders can be viewed as varying along a 'temperamental continuum', not all depressions can be traced back to a poorly functioning depressive personality. As already emphasized by Akiskal (Yerevanian and Akiskal, 1979; Akiskal *et al.*, 1980; Akiskal, 1983), 'characterologic depressions' may be divided into a predominantly subaffective form, which is characteristic of the depressive temperament, and a predominantly characterologic form, which emerges in temperaments other than the melancholic. Before ending this chapter, we shall briefly turn to consider the latter form of depression and its development by examining the case of Clara, which will allow us to shed light on the transition from DPD to major depressive episode.

9.5 Case vignette

Clara is a 42-year-old lawyer. She is single. She is visiting our centre, to which she was referred by her GP, because for the past three months she has been feeling depressed, apathetic and asthenic; her interest in all activities has markedly diminished, as have her powers of concentration. Clara spends her free time in bed. Her symptoms first emerged a few days before Christmas, with no apparent cause. Clara, who lives alone, spent her holidays in bed without seeing anyone. Each time we search for situations likely to have triggered Clara's present depression, we fail to find any significant event. Clara's depressive episode would seem to have come out of nowhere!

As is always the case, in order to understand the emergence of the symptomatology, our analysis must aim at a more detailed engagement with the life context that preceded the onset of the illness. It has been about 10 years since Clara last had a sentimental relationship. This exit from the banquet of life – as Joyce would put it – was made following the sudden termination of a relationship after five years of cohabitation. Clara was shocked by this event. Suicidal thoughts crossed her mind for a couple of years: thoughts aroused not so much by desperation at the unwanted separation, as by anger toward her own incapacity and inadequacy in life. Clara saw herself as an idiot who had yet again been fooled by her trust in another human being.

'Yet again': for Clara had already been deceived and abandoned twice in her life. Occasionally interrupted by bouts of tears, Clara began telling the story of how she had been cheated, as evidence of her inability to be part of human society.

The first person to deceive Clara had been her father, at the age of six, when she was playing at Happy Family with her sister. On one side stood Mother Bear, on another the Cubs, and on another still Father Bear. Clara's sister, who was one year older, was about to hand her Father Bear when Clara snatched the toy and threw it at her sister, telling her that their own father had promised them he would come back, but had never returned. The girls' mother happened to hear this exchange and uttered words like a sudden gunshot: 'Dad is dead'. For Clara's father had died of cancer in the hospital three years earlier.

Clara was later deceived by her mother. When Clara was 18, her mother found she herself had cancer, but only told her daughters that she had to undergo an operation: she went to a clinic without allowing them to visit her or enquire about her health. Clara only discovered her mother had cancer a few months after she had returned home from the clinic. As her health was getting worse, Clara's mother visited a doctor, who informed her that this was due to metastasis. One morning, when Clara was at school, her mother hanged herself in the garage.

Clara finally embarked on her love story, in the hope of having children and starting a family, but was again met by deceit, infidelities, lies and abandonment. Two hellish years followed. Gradually, a feeling of not being made to live among men became her way of structuring her life. Incapacity turned into resignation. On that Christmas day, the thought that she was destined never to have children or a family, that she was to remain alone for ever, suddenly flashed through Clara's mind. Renunciation turned into the impossibility caused by her intrinsic deficiency.

9.6 Is depression an adaptation?

Clara's story illustrates quite clearly how the fall into a depressive state is mediated by an emotional structure prone to sadness. If this sadness, once elicited, goes beyond a certain threshold, it becomes strongly pervasive, as it is amplified by forms of cognition that are meant to provide a meaning for it, resulting in the creation of a vicious circle. It is this circle that lies at the origin of depressive episodes.

If depression, therefore, is a state based on sadness, then in this pathological condition certain characteristics at the level of the neural substrate should be found that can be traced back to sadness: for instance, various degrees of alteration in the activity connected to goal blockage and/or goal loss, and different degrees of unpleasantness. Symptoms such as asthenia, apathy, anhedonia, loss of interest and profound suffering would appear to account for this continuity. Yet we also find new phenomena that come about when these states become chronic: for instance, the inability to take the initiative, difficulty in making decisions, recurrent feelings of self-depreciation, social withdrawal, the alteration of sleeping patterns, of appetite and sexual drive, and so on.

Neuroscientific analysis should shed light not just on the dysfunctions of specific neural pathways, but on the characteristics of the organization of the neural substrate, characteristics which account for a condition of being that represents the first leading cause of years lived with disability (WHO, 2001).[13]

The neuroscientific approach

The perspective that comes closest to this way of understanding depression is that promoted in the neuroscientific field by Helen Mayberg's group, which for years has been working on a model that combines clinical symptoms with a specific functional organization of limbic, subcortical and cortical networks. Multiple sources of evidence suggest that depression cannot be traced back to either the alteration of a specific neurotrasmitter system or one single region of the brain: depression would rather appear to be associated with a number of interconnected functional alterations. Thus, according to Mayberg, a network combination must be sought that can account for both dysfunctions and related compensation processes (Mayberg, 1997, 2003; Mayberg *et al.*, 1999, 2005).

A series of brain-imaging studies have consistently reported: (1) alterations on the cortical level, involving the dorsolateral (BA 9/46), ventrolateral and prefrontal cortex (BA10/47), the orbitofrontal cortex (BA 11) and the parietal cortex (BA 40); (2) changes in limbic-paralimbic regions: the dorsal, rostral and subgenual areas of the cingulate (BA 24b,24a,25), as well as the amygdala, insula and hippocampus; (3) changes in subcortical regions: the caudate, pallidum and anterior thalamus.

The combination of these various dysfunctional focuses in an integrated network of limbic-cortical regions makes it possible to grasp the underlying characteristic of both depressive symptomatology and sadness at the level of the neural substrate, namely the polarization of cognitive resources associated with the painful feelings arising from these conditions. This process is reflected in the *maladaptive* interaction between the limbic and paralimbic component on the one hand, and the cortical component on the other. PET data across different studies point to a decrease in glucose metabolism in dorsal cortical regions – although normal levels of frontal metabolism, as well as frontal hypermetabolism, have also been reported – and a relative increase in ventral limbic and paralimbic areas. The divergent results produced by studies reporting frontal metabolic activity may be understood in the light of this limbic and paralimbic[14] – but also, according to our perspective, subcortical – centrality, which guides subjects' inadequate attempts at cognitive correction. 'For instance, frontal hyperactivity is now viewed as an exaggerated or maladaptive compensatory process resulting in psychomotor agitation and rumination, serving to over-ride a persistent negative mood generated by abnormal chronic activity of limbic-subcortical structures. In contrast, frontal hypometabolism seen with increasing depression severity is the failure to initiate or maintain such a compensatory state, with resulting apathy, psychomotor slowness and impaired executive functioning' (Mayberg, 2003: 197).

The variety of dysfunctional metabolic patterns thus reflects both 'functional lesions' and equally inappropriate ways of coping with these lesions. This opens new perspectives in relation not only to the symptomatological and etiopathogenic variability of depression (reflecting multiple depression phenotypes), but also to the possibility that different metabolic patterns may guide therapeutic intervention. It is important to emphasize, in this respect, that different treatments (CBT, pharmacotherapy, surgery, electroconvulsive therapy) affect similar regions in different ways (Goldapple *et al.*, 2002, 2004; Kennedy *et al.*, 2001; Henry *et al.*, 2001; Mayberg, 2003; Seminowicz *et al.*, 2004).

Another highly interesting element that the studies conducted by Mayberg *et al.* have pointed to is the key role played by the subgenual anterior cingulate cortex (sACC) (BA 25) within the limbic-cortical brain system in the modulation of negative moods. A decrease in sACC activity has been reported in response to different successful treatments of depression, including pharmacological treatment (Mayberg *et al.*, 2000; Drevets, Bogers and Raichle, 2002), electroconvulsive therapy (Nobler *et al.*, 2001) and repetitive transcranial magnetic stimulation (Mottaghy *et al.*, 2002). The sACC is anatomically connected to the cortical regions of the brain, the limbic regions – including the hypothalamus (Barbas *et al.* 2003) and amygdala (Johansen-Berg *et al.*, 2008) – the ventral striatum (Haber *et al.*, 1995, 2006) and the autonomic centres in the brainstem, including the periaqueductal grey (Freedman, Insel and Smith, 2000).

According to our perspective, the leading role played by the anterior cingulated cortex in the modulation of depressive symptoms and its involvement in acute sadness are probably related to the importance of the subgenual cingulate for endogenous pain control (Ploghaus *et al.*, 1999; Bantick *et al.*, 2002; Petrovic *et al.*, 2002; Porro *et al.*, 2003). One study (Bingel *et al.*, 2007), for instance, which investigated habituation to painful stimuli, found that reaction to nociceptive stimuli diminished after repeated exposure in classical pain areas, whereas its activation increased over time in the sACC. These data suggest that habituation to one condition, where continuous nociceptive stimulation cannot be avoided, is associated with an increase in antinociceptive activity – which involves the endogenous opioid system – mediated by the subgenual cingulate. The same area, moreover, is also involved in placebo analgesia (Bingel *et al.*, 2006). It is possible to suggest, therefore, that increased activity in this region during depressive episodes corresponds to an attempt to cope with unavoidable 'psychic pain' by recruiting brain areas similar to those activated in response to physical pain.

By treating depression as the consequence of the dysfunction of an entire system, the approach adopted by Mayberg *et al.* makes it possible to draw on the indications formulated in the clinical field, thus opening the possibility of enquiring after the different personological origins of depression from a neuroscientific perspective.

The personological origins of depression

In this respect, each of the styles of personality we have outlined in the previous chapters may lead to a state of depression in conjunction with life circumstances capable of initiating a downward spiral: a vicious circle of cognition and sadness. For each style of personality, a range of conditions exist that are essential for individual situatedness (and which may change in the course of one's life); it is the loss of these conditions that will trigger a depressive reaction.

In the case of the eating disorder-prone style of personality, for instance, the disorder may arise when the subject finds himself in a confrontational situation – such as job promotion – he is incapable of facing, or following lack of validation at the hands of someone perceived as particularly significant. The feeling of not being able to assume the responsibilities a new position entails in the first case, and one's powerlessness to regain positive acceptance at the hands of the significant other in the second, may trigger a depressive reaction characterized by sadness, as well as feelings of anxiety and emptiness.

In the case of the obsessive-compulsive-prone style of personality, as we have seen, disorders usually emerge in conjunction with situations marked by profound uncertainty. In order to regain their stability, subjects will face these situations through attempts to provide what are often incongruous explanations. Repeated failure in these attempts may lead to the onset of a depressive symptomatology that varies according to the origin of the perceived uncertainty.

If uncertainty concerns the consequences of one's actions, the search for stability will be based on the mental anticipation of dangerous situations, and on an attempt to neutralize the perceived danger by means of rituals or ruminations. Depressive reactions, frequently associated with conditions of anxiety, will be triggered by the failure to regain – through a pervasive increase in compulsions – any kind of certainty.

If uncertainty concerns one's inward states, the search for personal stability will be based on an attempt to realign personal experience to one's own meaning system. Failure in this search will be attributed to intrinsic aspects of one's personality. This process is reminiscent of many of the cases described by Tellenbach (1974).

Finally, if uncertainty concerns one's sense of Self, repeated failure in the attempt to re-situate oneself in relation to reference figures on the basis of which to co-perceive oneself may lead to a depressive condition centred on guilt, emptiness and self-blaming.

In the case of a style prone to hypochondria-hysteria, the increase in emotional intensity beyond a given threshold will be perceived as a threat to one's bodily integrity, a threat that is experienced in different ways in hypochondria and hysteria: hypochondriacs focus personal stability more on bodily states, hysterical subjects on a defining otherness. The depressive states that may emerge as a consequence of the failure of these modes to maintain stability will reflect these different focuses: in the case of hypochondria, they will be characterized by a strong polarization on organic symptoms (limb pain, back pain, gastrointestinal problems, tiredness, etc.); in the case of hysteria – as illustrated by the figure of Wertheimer in Bernhard's story – subjects will instead display a self-pitying attitude.

In the case of the phobia-prone style of personality, phobic disorder may emerge following an unexpected event that is perceived by the subject as an alteration of his own sense of interoceptive stability. In the subjective phenomenology of the patient, this alteration will correspond to a state of acute anxiety and fear, and to a mental anticipation of similar situations in the ineffective attempt to regain control over his emotional sphere. In objective terms, this condition may instead correspond to a strong feeling of frailty and personal weakness, which may even lead to repeated panic attacks. Reiterated failures in the attempt to regain a sense of personal stability may trigger a depressive reaction.

Endnotes

[1] Schneider (1959) and later Tellenbach (1974) described a particular form of illness – that of the 'depressive psychopath' in Schneider and of the 'typus melancholicus' in Tellenbach – whose features appear to be those of a form of depression particularly affecting subjects with an OCP style of personality.

[2] The symptomatological likeness here may be due to common neurobiological factors mediating depression and alcohol dependence. See Markou, Kosten and Koob (1998).

[3] In the German Renaissance, contemplative life was then set in contrast to the *vita speculativa sive studiosa*, and Saturn came to be celebrated as the patron of contemplation.

[4] Parenting practices which may contribute to the development of depression: (1) Most extremely, forms of dysfunctional parenting such as child neglect or maltreatment. (2) A significant attitude of derision or disdain on the parent's part when faced with help requests when the child is in distress (Bretherton, 1985). (3) 'Affectionless control': a parenting style characterized by a lack of warmth and caring and by negative control (criticism, intrusiveness and guilt-induction) (Parker, 1983). (4) Sustained lack of psychological availability on the parent's part, as in the case of depressive episodes that last for some time (Cummings and Cicchetti, 1990).

[5] Genetic association studies of depression have largely yielded inconsistent findings: no evidence has been found linking any particular genotype to a diagnosis of major depressive disorder.

[6] The notion of heredity refers to the stability of each resource present in subsequent generations.

[7] Lazarus, therefore, only takes transitory sadness into account when in the same paragraph he writes: 'I think it is appropriate to call this withdrawal an action tendency' (Lazarus, 1991: 251).

[8] Concerning the socialization of sadness, Stearns (Stearns,1993: 553) writes: 'It appears that how societies think about sadness has something to do with how they think about help'.

[9] In a study analysing the neuropsychological factors that influence homicidal behaviour, Dutton (2002) found that those men who kill their spouses usually do so during periods of perceived or actual abandonment.

[10] The maintenance of self-focus enhances awareness of internal states; in turn, this increased awareness increases the intensity of the negative affect that is being experienced.

[11] No doubt one of the variables that most significantly contribute to the loss of this ability in the course of one's personal development is the intensity of the feeling of rejection experienced.

[12] The amplifying power of cognition and the feeling of possessing a greater degree of autonomy explain why rates of depression rise dramatically during adolescence. The differential rates of depression among girls and boys that are emphasized in various studies (Cole *et al.*, 1999; Hankin and Abramson, 2001) should perhaps also take account of the gender gap in delinquency. Several studies point to a link between child abuse and neglect and elevated rates of criminal offences and social dysfunction.

[13] The World Health Report: http://www.who.int; Cap 2,4.

[14] In chronic pharmacological treatments, limbic and subcortical areas are considered central for drug action (Blier, 2001; Freo *et al.*, 2000).

Message in a Bottle

At the start of our journey we met Robert, whose mode of existence offered us the chance to examine the three assumptions that have informed the perspective on the Self developed in the modern age, assumptions which have become part of the common sense of the West: the interiority of experience, the uniqueness of meaning, the continuity of the Self in heterogeneous circumstances. We have seen how this way of envisaging the problem was based on an ontology that regarded the Self as a thing, applying the same categories to it that are used in the study of objects. An attempt to redefine this problem led us to embrace an ontological perspective that instead stressed the experience of being oneself: ipseity.

With ipseity as our starting point, we addressed the question of personal identity by engaging with developmental psychology and linguistic neuroscience, ultimately reaching a new perspective on the matter: in the footsteps of Ricoeur, we have used the expression 'narrative identity' to describe the process of interpretation of pre-reflexive experience, by means of which the individual recognizes the various emotions and actions characterizing his existence over time as his own. In the narrative process people shape their own uniqueness by the (language-enabled) appropriation of their own experience of being. By telling who he is – thus reconfiguring his own actions and emotions to form a more or less cohesive whole – the individual recognizes and identifies *himself*.

Because identity takes shape as a symbolic reconfiguration of the experience of living, through narratives it can be seen to reflect the various ways in which feeling and action become sedimented over time, becoming fixed in different forms at different moments of one's life. Hence, different narratives of Self reflect different modes of maintaining personal stability, modes which correspond to particular emotional inclinations. It is therefore on the basis of different ways of feeling emotionally situated with respect to the world that we have drawn a distinction between two polarities that frame a range of possible emotional alchemies: one is the Inward tendency, which is associated with a predominantly body-bound emotional polarization; the other is the Outward tendency, which is prevalently characterized by anchoring to external frames of reference. A definition of this ontological foundation has allowed us to outline a psychology of personality and later a psychopathology starting from the pre-reflexive dimension. The

Selfhood, identity and personality styles Giampiero Arciero and Guido Bondolfi

most evident consequence of this change in perspective has been that of re-orienting our understanding of both the genesis of given disorders and of the prospects of clinical and neuroscientific research.

The second part of the book has explored the continuity between normality and neurotic psychopathology by developing this new interpretative perspective through psychology, literature, psychiatry and the neurosciences. These heterogeneous ways of accessing experience, by means of different paths and forms of knowledge, were afforded by the ontological assumption that has always guided us, and according to which human experience corresponds to the way in which life itself unfolds, it being impossible to narrow its totality down to any one discipline. The safeguarding of this ontology, which takes human experience as a whole as its ultimate point of reference, ought to be the pole star guiding free dialogue between disciplines, and informing in particular the new balances and boundaries between psychology, psychopathology, phenomenology and the neurosciences. The dazzling affirmation of the neurosciences cannot lead us to repeat the mistake made by logical positivism, which in the name of mathematical physics attempted to federate all sciences under the leadership of one epistemology. This success must rather induce psychology, psychopathology and phenomenology to reconsider their own foundations and to change in such a way as to become capable of entering the debate on the new themes that the neurosciences have located at the heart of research.

It is this trajectory that our own work is following: for it enables a renewed exchange with the neurosciences starting from a study of the different modes of emotional structuring (Bertolino *et al.*, 2005; Rubino *et al.*, 2007; Mazzola *et al.*, submitted). At the same time, in the light of phenomenological ontology, our work presents the understanding of personal experience and of the unique story of individuals' lives as the central problem in psychology and psychopathology.

It is particularly this second aspect of our work that has not been fully articulated in our book, as we have been guided in the formulation of our arguments by a need to outline a typology and criteriology of personality on the basis of first-person experience, in such a way as to enable a reconfiguration of psychopathology and open a dialogue with the neurosciences. Inevitably, only a fleeting allusion has been made to themes such as the development of sentimental relations, the analysis of unconscious structures and the relation between an individual's story and his memory – elements which play a fundamental role in one's experience of life and in the construction of a narrative of Self. The most precious things at the end of our journey remain precisely these unresolved issues, unanswered questions and foreshadowed topics, and a sighting of new paths.

References

Abela, J.R.Z. and Hankin, B.L. (2008) Cognitive vulnerability to depression in children and adolescents: A developmental psychopathology perspective, in *Handbook of Depression in Children and Adolescents* (eds R.Z. Abela John and L. Hankin Benjamin) Guilford.

Abraham, S.E. and Beumont, E.J.V. (1982) How patients describe bulimia or binge eating. *Psychological Medicine*, **12**, 625–635.

Abramowitz, J.S. (2008) Scrupolosity, in *Clinical Handbook of Obsessive-Compulsive Disorder and Related Problems* (eds J.S. Abramowitz, D. McKay and S. Taylor), The John Hopkins University Press.

Abramowitz, J.S., Whiteside, S.P. and Schwartz, S.A. (2002) A contemporary conceptual model of hypochondriasis. *Mayo Clinic Proceedings*, **77**, 1323–1330.

Abramowitz, J.S., Schwartz, S.A., Moore, K.M. and Luenzmann, K.R. (2003) Obsessive-compulsive symptoms in pregnancy and the puerperium: A review of the literature. *Journal of Anxiety Disorders*, **17** (4), 461–478.

Abramson, Lyn Y., Seligman, Martin E. and Teasdale, John D. (1978) Learned helplessness in humans: critique and reformulation. *Journal of Abnormal Psychology*, **87** (1), 49–74.

Abramson, L.Y., Metalsky, G.I. and Alloy, L.B. (1989) Hopelessness depression: A theory-based subtype of depression. *Psychological Review*, **96**, 358–372.

Akhtar, N., Dunham, F. and Dunham, P. (1991) Directive interactions and early vocabulary development: the role of joint attentional focus. *Journal of Child Language*, **18**, 41–49.

Akiskal, H.S. (1983) Dysthymic disorder: Psychopathology of proposed chronic depressive subtypes. *American Journal of Psychiatry*, **140**, 11–20.

Akiskal, H.S. (2001) Dysthymia and cyclothymia in psychiatric practice a century after Kraepelin. *Journal of Affective Disorders*, **62**, 17–31.

Akiskal, H.S., Bitar, A.H., Puzantian, V.R. *et al.* (1978) The nosological status of neurotic depression: a prospective three-to-four year examination in light of the primary–secondary and unipolar–bipolar dichotomies. *Archives of General Psychiatry*, **35**, 756–766.

Akiskal, H.S., Rosenthal, T.L., Haykal, R.F. *et al.* (1980) Characterological depressions: Clinical and sleep EEG findings separating 'subaffective dysthymias' from 'character-spectrum' disorders. *Archives of General Psychiatry*, **37**, 777–783.

Alloy, L.B., Abramson, L.Y., Smith, J.M. *et al.* (2006) Role of parenting and maltreatment histories in unipolar and bipolar mood disorders: mediation by cognitive vulnerability to depression. *Clinical Child and Family Psychology Review*, **9** (1), 23–64.

Allport, G.W. (1937) *Personality: A Psychological Interpretation*, Holt, Rinehart, & Winston, New York.

American Psychiatric Association (2000) *Diagnostic and Statistical Manual of Mental Disorders*, (4th edn, text revision). Washington, DC.

Selfhood, identity and personality styles Giampiero Arciero and Guido Bondolfi

Amodio, M.D. and Frith, D.C. (2006) Meeting of minds: the medial frontal cortex and social cognition. *Nat. Rev. Neurosci.*, **7**, 268–277.

Anand, P., Aziz, Q., Willert, R. and Van Oudenhove, L. (2007) Peripheral and central mechanisms of visceral sensitization in man. *Neurogastroenterology & Motility*, **19** (Supplement 1), (18), 29–46.

Anderson, J.R. (1984) The development of self recognition: A review. *Developmental Psychobiology*, **17**, 35–49.

Anderson, A.E. and Di Domenico, L. (1992) Diet vs. shape content of popular male and female magazines: A dose response relationship to the incidence of eating disorders. *International Journal of Eating Disorders*, **11**, 283–287.

Andrews, G. and Slade, T. (2002) Agoraphobia without panic disorder is part of the panic disorder syndrome. *Journal of Nervous and Mental Disease*, **190** (9), 624–630.

Arciero, G. (1988) Recent Developments in Evolutionary Accounts of Adaptation, AABT Congress, New York.

Arciero, G. (1989) From epistemology to ontology: A new age of cognition. American Association for the Advancement of Science. San Francisco, CA.

Arciero, G. (2002) *Studi e Dialoghi Sull'identità Personale*, Bollati Boringhieri.

Arciero, G. (2006) *Sulle Tracce Di Sé*, Bollati Boringhieri.

Arciero, G. and Guidano, V.F. (2000) Experience, explanation and the quest for coherence, in *Constructions of Disorder* (eds R.A. Neymeyer and J.D. Raskin), American Psychological Association, Washington, D.C.

Arciero, G., Gaetano, P., Maselli, P. and Gentili, N. (2004) Identity, personality and emotional regulation, in *Cognition and Psychotherapy*, 2 edn (eds A. Freeman, M. Mahoney, P. Devito and D. Martin), Springer, New York.

Arendt, H. (1998) *The Human Condition*, University of Chicago Press.

Arnaud, D. (2004) *Nabuchodonosor*, Roi de Babylone, Fayard Paris.

Arnow, B., Kenardy, J. and Agras, W.S. (1995) The emotional eating scale: The development of a measure to assess coping with negative affect by eating. *International Journal of Eating Disorders*, **18**, 79–90.

Ashton-James, C., van Baaren, R.B., Chartrand, T.L. *et al.* (2007) Mimicry and me: the impact of mimicry on self-construal. *Social Cognition*, **4**, 518–535.

Atance, C.M. and Meltzoff, A.N. (2006) Preschoolers' current desires warp their choices for the future. *Psychological Science*, **17**, 583–587.

Athwal, B.S., Halligan, P.W., Fink, G.R., Marshall, J.C. and Frackowiak, R.S.J. (2001) Imaging hysterical paralysis, in *Contemporary Approaches to the Study of Hysteria* (eds P.W. Halligan, C. Bass and J.C. Marshall), Oxford: Oxford University Press, 216–34.

Attiullah, N., Eisen, J. and Rasmussen, S. (2000) Clinical features of obsessive-compulsive disorder. *Psychiatric Clinics of North America*, **23** (3), 469–491.

Avenanti, A., Bueti, D., Galati, G. and Aglioti, S.M. (2005) Transcranial magnetic stimulation highlights the sensorimotor side of empathy for pain. *Nature Neuroscience*, **8**, 955–960.

Averill, J.R. (1985) The social construction of emotion: with special reference to love, in *The Social Construction of the Person* (eds K. Gergen and K. Davis), Springer-Verlag, New York, pp. 89–109.

Aziz-Zadeh, L., Wilson, S.M., Rizzolatti, G. and Iacoboni, M. (2006) Congruent embodied representations for visually presented actions and linguistic phrases describing actions. *Current Biology*, **16**, 1818–1823.

Bahrke, M.S., Yesalis, C.E., Kopstein, A.N. and Stephens, J.A. (2000) Risk factors associated with anabolic-androgenic steroid use among adolescents. *Sports Medicine*, **29**, 397–405

Bair, M.J., Robinson, R.L., Katon, W. and Kroenke, K. (2003) Depression and pain comorbidity: A literature review. *Archives of Internal Medicine*, **163** (20), 2433–2445.

Bakhtin, M.M. (1984) *Problems of Dostoevsky's Poetics* (ed. and trans. C. Emerson), University of Minnesota Press, Minneapolis.

Balaban, Carey D. (2002) Neural substrates linking balance control and anxiety. *Physiology & Behavior*, **77** (4–5), 469–475.

Balaban, C.D. (2004) Projections from the parabrachial nucleus to the vestibular nuclei: potential substrates for autonomic and limbic influences on vestibular responses. *Brain Research*, **996** (1), 126–137.

Balaban, C.D. and Thayer, J.F. (2001) Neurological bases for balance–anxiety links. *Journal of Anxiety Disorders*, **15**, 53–79.

Baldwin, D.A. (1995) Understanding the link between joint attention and language, in *Joint Attention: Its Origins and Role in Development* (eds C. Moore and P.J. Dunham Lawrence Erlbaum Associates, Inc., Hillsdale, NJ, England, pp. 131–158.

Bantick, S.J., Wise, R.G., Ploghaus, A. *et al.* (2002) Imaging how attention modulates pain in humans using functional MRI. *Brain: A Journal of Neurology*, **125**, 310–319.

Barbas, H., Saha, S., Rempel-Clower, N. and Ghashghaei, T. (2003) Serial pathways from primate prefrontal cortex to autonomic areas may influence emotional expression. *BMC Neuroscience*, **4**, 25.

Barnett, L.R. (1986) Bulimarexia as symptom of sex-role strain in professional women. *Psychotherapy*, **23**, 311–315.

Barnes, J. (1984) *The Complete Works of Aristotle*, vol. **2**, Princeton.

Barrett, M. (1986) Early semantic representation and early word usage, in *The Development of Word Meaning: Progress in Cognitive Development Research* (eds S.A. Kuczaj and M.D. Barrett), Springer Verlag, New York.

Barrett, F.L., Quigley, S.K., Bliss-Moreau, E. and Aronson, R.K. (2004) Interoceptive sensitivity and self-reports of emotional experience. *Journal of Personality and Social Psychology*, **87** (5), 684–697.

Barsky, A.J. (1992) Amplification, somatization, and the somatoform disorders. *Psychosomatics*, **33**, 28–34.

Barsky, A. and Klerman, G. (1983) The amplification of somatic symptoms. *Psychosomatic Medicine*, **50**, 510–519.

Barsky, A.J., Goodson, J.D., Lane, R.S. and Cleary, P.D. (1988) The amplification of somatic symptoms. *Psychosomatic Medicine*, **50**, 510–519.

Barsky, A.J., Cleary, P.D., Sarnie, M.K. and Klerman, G.L. (1993) The course of transient hypochondriasis. *The American Journal of Psychiatry*, **150** (3), 484–488.

Barth, J., Povinelli, D.J. and Cant, J.G.H. (2004) Bodily origins of SELF, in *The Self and Memory* (eds D. Beike, J.L. Lampinen and D.A. Behrend), Psychology Press, New York, pp. 11–43.

Bastiani, A., Rao, R., Weltzin, T. and Kaye, W. (1995) Perfectionism in anorexia nervosa. *International Journal of Eating Disorders*, **17**, 147–152.

Bates, E. (1990) Language about me and you: pronominal reference and the emerging concept of self, in *The Self in Transition* (eds D. Cicchetti and M. Beeghly), University of Chicago Press.

Bates, E., Camaioni, L. and Volterra, V. (1975) The acquisition of performatives prior to speech. *Merrill-Palmer Quaretrly*, **21**, 205–226.

Bateson, C.M. (1979) The epigenesis of conversational interaction: a personal account of research development, in *Before Speech* (ed. M. Bullowa), Cambridge University Press.

Baumann, Z. (2003) *Liquid Love: On the Frailty of Human Bonds*, Polity.

Baumeister, R.E. (1989) *Masochism and the self*, Erlbaum, Hillsdale, NJ.

Baumeister, R.E. (1990) Anxiety and deconstruction: On escaping the self, in *Self-inference Processes: the Ontario Symposium* (eds J.M. Olson and M.P. Zanna), Erlbaum, Hillsdale, NJ.

Baumeister, R.E. and Tice, D.M. (1990) Anxiety and social exclusion. *Journal of Social and Clinical Psychology*, **9**, 165–195.

Baumeister, R.F. and Wotman, S.R. (1992) *Breaking Hearts: The Two Sides of Unrequited Love*, Guilford Press, New York.

Beavin Bavelas, J., Black, A., Lemery, C.R. and Mullett, J. (1986) I show how you feel? *Journal of Personality and Social Psychology*, **50** (2), 322–329.

Beck, A.T. (1967) *Depression: Causes and Treatment*, University of Pennsylvania Press, Pennsylvania.

Beck, U. and Beck-Gernsheim, E. (2002) *Individualization: Institutionalized Individualism and its Social and Political Consequences*, Sage, London.

Beck, A.T., Kovacs, M. and Weissman, A. (1975) Hopelessness and suicidal behavior. *Journal of the American Medical Association*, **234**, 1146–1149.

Beck, A.T., Steer, R., Kovacs, M. and Garrison, B. (1985) Hopelessness and eventual suicide: A 10-year prospective study of patients hospitalized with suicidal ideation. *American Journal of Psychiatry*, **142**, 559–563.

Beck, A.T., Brown, G., Berchick, R.J. *et al.* (1990) Relationship between hopelessness and ultimate suicide: A replication with psychiatric outpatients. *American Journal of Psychiatry*, **147**, 190–195.

Beck, A.T., Steer, R.A., Beck, J.S. and Newman, C.F. (1993) Hopelessness, depression, suicidal ideation, and clinical diagnosis of depression. *Suicide and Life-Threatening Behavior*, **23**, 139–145.

Beckman, M. (2004) Crime, culpability, and the adolescent brain. *Science*, **305**, 596–599.

Belk, R.W. (1988) Possessions and the extended self. *Journal of Consumer Research*, **15** (2), 139–168.

Belk, R.W. (1990) The role of possessions in constructing and maintaining a sense of past. *Advances in Consumer Research*, **17**, 669–676.

Benson, J.B. (1997) The development of planning: It's about time, in *The Developmental Psychology of Planning: Why, How, and When Do We Plan?* (eds S.L. Friedman and E.K. Scholnick), Erlbaum, Hillsdale, NJ, pp. 43–75.

Benveniste, E. (1966) *Problemes De Linguistique Generale 1*, Editions Gallimard.

Benveniste, E. (1974) *Problemes De Linguistique Generale 2*, Editions Gallimard.

Berenthal, B.J. and Fisher, K.W. (1978) Development of self-recognition in the infant. *Developmental Psychology*, **14**, 44–50.

Bertolino, A., Arciero, G., Rubino, V., Latorre, V., De Candia, M., Mazzola, V. *et al.* (2005). Variation of human amygdala response during threatening stimuli as a function of 5'HTTLPR genotype and personality style. *Biol. Psychiatry*, **57**, 1517.

Berman, S.M., Naliboff, B.D., Suyenobu, B. *et al.* (2008) Reduced brainstem inhibition during anticipated pelvic visceral pain correlates with enhanced brain response to the visceral stimulus in women with irritable bowel syndrome. *The Journal of Neuroscience*, **28** (2), 349–359.

Bermudez, J.L. (1998) *The Paradox of Self-Consciousness*, MIT Press, Cambridge, Mass.

Bernardis, P. and Gentilucci, M. (2006) Speech and gesture share the same communication system. *Neuropsychologia*, **44**, 178–190.

Bernhard, T. (1992) *The Loser* (ed. and trans. J. Dawson), Quartet Books, London.

Berthoz, A. (2000) *The Brain's Sense of Movement*, Harvard University Press, Cambridge, USA.

Bertolino, A., Arciero, G., Rubino, V. *et al.* (2005) Variation of human amygdala response during threatening stimuli as a function of 5′HTTLPR genotype and personality style. *Biological Psychiatry*, **57**, 1517.

Bienvenu, O.J., Onyike, C.U., Stein, M.B. *et al.* (2006) Agoraphobia in adults: incidence and longitudinal relationship with panic. *British Journal of Psychiatry*, **188**, 432–438.

Bifulco, A., Brown, W. and Harris, T. (1987) Childhood loss of parent, lack of adequate parental care and adult depression: a replication. *Journal of Affective Disorders*, **12** (2), 115–128.

Bingel, U., Lorenz, J., Schoell, E. *et al.* (2006) Mechanisms of placebo analgesia: rACC recruitment of a subcortical antinociceptive network. *Pain*, **120**, 8–15.

Bingel, U., Schoell, E., Herken, W. *et al.* (2007) Habituation to painful stimulation involves the antinociceptive system. *Pain*, **131** (1–2), 21–30.

Binkofski, F., Buccino, G., Stephan, K.M. *et al.* (1999) A parieto-premotor network for object manipulation: evidence. from neuroimaging. *Experimental Brain Research*, **128**, 210–213.

Birbaumer, N., Grodd, W., Diedrich, O. *et al.* (1998) fMRI reveals amygdala activation to human faces in social phobics. *NeuroReport*, **9**, 1223–1226.

Bishop, S., Duncan, J. and Lawrence, A. (2004) State anxiety modulation of the amygdala response to unattended threat-related stimuli. *The Journal of Neuroscience*, **24**, 10364–10368.

Black, P.H. (2002) Stress and the inflammatory response: a review of neurogenic inflammation. *Brain, Behavior, and Immunity*, **16** (6), 622–653.

Black, D.W. (2007) A review of compulsive buying disorder. *World Psychiatry*, **6**, 14–18.

Blair, R.J.R., Morris, J.S., Frith, C.D. *et al.* (1999) Dissociable neural responses to facial expressions of sadness and anger. *Brain: A Journal of Neurology*, **122** (5), 883–893.

Blier, P. (2001) Crosstalk between the norepinephrine and serotonin systems and its role in the antidepressant response. *Journal of Psychiatry and Neuroscience*, **26** (Suppl), S3–S10.

Bloom, K. (1988) Quality of adult vocalization affects the quality of infant vocalizations. *Journal of Child Language*, **15**, 469–480.

Bondolfi, G. (2004) *Traitement Intégré de la Dépression: De la Résistance à la Prévention de la Rechute*, Steinkopff-Verlag, Darmstadt.

Bondolfi, G., Aubry, J.M., Golaz, J. *et al.* (2006) A stepwise drug treatment algorithm to obtain complete remission in depression: a Geneva study. *Swiss Medical Weekly*, **136** (5–6), 78–85.

Bookheimer, S. (2002) Functional MRI of language: new approaches to understanding the cortical organization of semantic processing. *Annual Review of Neuroscience*, **25**, 151–188.

Bowlby, J. (1940) *Personality and Mental Illness*, Kegan Paul, Trench, Trubner and Co., Ltd, London.

Bowlby, J. (1980) *Attachment and Loss*, vol. **3**, Basic, Loss, New York.

Bradford, J. and Balmaceda, R. (1983) Shoplifting: is there a specific psychiatric syndrome? *Canadian Journal of Psychiatry*, **28**, 248–253.

Brauer, S.J. and Friederici, D.A. (2007) Functional neural networks of semantic and syntactic processes in the developing brain. *Journal of Cognitive Neuroscience*, **19** (10), 1609–1623.

Brehm, S.S. and Brehm, J.W. (1981) *Psychological Reactance: A Theory of Freedom and Control*, Academic Press, New York.

Bretherton, I. (1985) Attachment theory: retrospect and prospect, in *Growing Points of Attachment Theory and Research. Monographs of the Society for Research in Child Development* (eds I. Bretherton and E. Waters), Blackwell, 50, 1-21-2.

Brighton, V., Segal, A., Werther, P. and Steiner, J. (1977) Facial expression and hedonic response to taste stimuli. *Journal of Dental Research*, **56**, B161.

Brown, W. and Harris, T. (1978) *Social Origins of Depression. A Study of Psychiatric Disorder in Women*, Tavistock Publications, London.

Brownell, A.C., Zerwas, S. and Geetha, B.R. (2007) So big: the development of body self-awareness in toddlers. *Child Development*, **78** (5), 1426–1440.

Bruch, H. (1962) Perceptual and conceptual disturbances in anorexia nervosa. *Psychosomatic Medicine*, **24**, 187–194.

Bruner, J. (1983a) The acquisition of pragmatic commitments, in *The Transition from Pre-linguistic to Linguistic Communication* (ed. R. Golinkoff), Erlbaum, Hillsdale, NJ, pp. 27–42.

Bruner, J.S. (1983b) *Child's talk: Learning to use Language*, W.W. Norton, New York.

Bruner, J. 1978. The role of dialogue in language acquisition, in *The Child's Concept of language* (eds A. Sinclair, R.,J. Jarvelle, and W. J. M. Levelt), New York: Springer-Verlag.

Buccino, G., Binkofski, F., Fink, G.R. *et al.* (2001) Action observation activates premotor and parietal areas in a somatotopic manner: an fMRI study. *European Journal of Neuroscience*, **13**, 400–404.

Buccino, G., Lui, F., Canessa, N. *et al.* (2004) Neural circuits involved in the recognition of actions performed by nonconspecifics: An fMRI study. *Journal of Cognitive Neuroscience*, **16**, 114–126.

Buccino, G., Riggio, L., Melli, G. *et al.* (2005) Listening to action-related sentences modulates the activity of the motor system: a combined TMS and behavioral study. Cog. *Brain Research*, **24**, 355–363.

Bulik, C.M., Klump, K.L., Thornton, L. *et al.* (2004) Alcohol Use Disorder Comorbidity in Eating Disorders: A Multicenter Study. *Journal of Clinical Psychiatry*, **65** (7), 1000–1006.

Butterworth, G. (1990) Self-perception in infancy, in *The Self in Transition* (eds D. Cicchetti and M. Beeghly), Chicago University Press.

Byrne, R.W. and Whiten, A. (eds) (1988) *Machiavellian Intelligence: Social Expertise and the Evolution of Intellect in Monkeys, Apes, and Humans*, Oxford University Press, NY.

Calvo-Merino, B., Grèzes, J., Glaser, D.E. *et al.* (2006) Seeing or doing: influence of visual and motor familiarity in action observation. *Current Biology*, **16** (19), 1905–1910.

Camaioni, L. (2001) Early language, in *Infant Development* (eds G. Bremner and A. Fogel), Blackwell.

Carlat, D.J. and Camargo, C.A. (1991) Review of bulimia nervosa in males. *American Journal of Psychiatry*, **148**, 831–843.

Carlat, D.J., Camargo, C.A. and Herzog, D.B. (1997) Eating disorders in males: A report on 135 patients. *American Journal of Psychiatry*, **154**, 1127–1132.

Carlson, S.M., Moses, L.J. and Claxton, L.J. (2004) Individual differences in executive functioning and theory of mind: An investigation of inhibitory control and planning ability. *Journal of Experimental Child Psychology*. **87** (4), 299–319.

Carr, D. (1999) *The Paradox of Subjectivity: The Self in the Transcendental Tradition*, Oxford University Press, New York/Oxford.

Caspi, A., Sugden, K., Moffitt, T.E. *et al.* (2003) Influence of life stress on depression: Moderation by a polymorphism in the 5-HTT gene. *Science*, **301**, 386–389.

Castellanos Margulies, D.F., Kelly, C., Uddin, L. *et al.* (2008) Cingulate-precuneus interactions: a new locus of dysfunction in adult attention-deficit/hyperactivity disorder 2008. *Biological Psychiatry*, **63** (3), 332–337.

Cavanna, A.E. and Trimble, M.R. (2006) The precuneus: a review of its functional anatomy and behavioural correlates. *Brain: A Journal of Neurology*, **129** (3), 564.

Chartrand, T.L. and Bargh, J.A. (1999) The chameleon effect: the perceptionbehavior link and social interaction. *Journal of Personality and Social Psychology*, **76**, 893–910.

Chartrand, T.L., Dalton, A. and Fitzsimons, G.J. (2007) Nonconscious relationship reactance: When significant others prime opposing goals. *Journal of Experimental Social Psychology*, **43** (5), 719–726.

Chekhov, A. (2004) *Three Years*, Hesperus Press.

Cheng, Y., Lin, C.P., Liu, H.L., Hsu, Y.Y., Lim, K.E., Hung, D., and Decety, J. (2007) Expertise modulates pain perception in others. *Curr Biol*; **17** (19), 1708–1713.

Chodoff, P. and Lyons, H. (1958) Hysteria, the hysterical personality and "hysterical" conversion. *The American Journal of Psychiatry*, **114**, 734–740.

Christenson, G.A. and Mansueto, C.S. (1999) Trichotillomania: descriptive characteristics and phenomenology, in *Trichotillomania: New Developments* (eds M.B. Stein G.A. Christenson and E. Hollander), American Psychiatric Pub.

Cioran, M.E. (1990) *Lacrime e Santi*, Adelphi.

Cioran, M.E. (1997) *Cahiers*, Gallimard.

Cioran, M.E. (1998) *Anathemas and Admirations*, Arcade Publishing.

Cioran, M.E. (2001) *Quaderni 1957–1972*, Adelphi.

Clark, D.M. (1986) A cognitive approach to panic. *Behaviour Research and Therapy*, **24** (4), 461–470.

Clark, D.M., Salkovskis, P.M., Ost, L.G. *et al.* (1997) Misinterpretation of body sensations in panic disorder. *Journal of Consulting and Clinical Psychology*, **65** (2), 203–213.

Cloninger, C.R. and Svrakic, D. (1999) Personality disorder, in *Comprehensive Textbook of Psychiatry*, 7th edn (eds B. Sadock and H. Kaplan), Williams & Wilkins.

Cloninger, C.R., Svrakic, D.M. and Przybeck, T.R. (1993) A psychobiological model of temperament and character. *Archives of General Psychiatry*, **50**, 975–990.

Coghill, R.C., McHaffie, J.G. and Yen, Y. (2003) Neural correlates of interindividual differences in the subjective experience of pain. *Proceedings of the National Academy of Sciences of the United States of America*, **100** (14), 8538–8542.

Cole, D.A., Martin, J.M., Peeke, L.G. *et al.* (1999) Children's over- and underestimation of academic competence: A longitudinal study of gender differences, depression and anxiety. *Child Development*, **70**, 459–473.

Collet, C., Vernet-Maury, E., Delhomme, G. and Dittmar, A. (1997) Autonomic nervous system response patterns specificity to basic emotions. *Journal of the Autonomic Nervous System*, **62** (1–2), 45–57.

Cools, R., Calder, A.J., Lawrence, A.D. *et al.* (2005) Individual differences in threat sensitivity predict serotonergic modulation of amygdala response to fearful faces. *Psychopharmacology*, **180**, 670–679.

Cooper, J.L., Morrison, T.L., Bigman, O.L. *et al.* (1988) Bulimia and borderline personality disorder. *International Journal of Eating Disorders*, **7** (1), 43–49.

Costa, P.T. and McCrae, R.R. (1980) Somatic complaints in males as a function of age and neuroticism: a longitudinal analysis. *Journal of Behavioral Medicine*, **3**, 245–255.

Costa, P.T. and McCrae, R.R. (1985) Hypochondriasis, neuroticism, and aging. *American Psychologist*, **40**, 19–28.

Courage, L.M., Edison, C.S. and Howe, L.M. (2004) Variability in the early development of visual self-recognition. *Infant Behavior and Development*, **27** (4), 509–532.

Craig, A.D. (2002) How do you feel? Interoception: the sense of the physiological condition of the body. *Nature Reviews. Neuroscience*, **3**, 655–666.

Craig, A.D. (2003) Interoception: the sense of the physiological condition of the body. *Current Opinion in Neurobiology*, **13**, 500.

Craig, A.D. (2004) Human feelings: why are some more aware than others? *Trends in Cognitive Sciences*, **8**, 239.

Craske, M.G., Mohlman, J., Yi, J. *et al.* (1995) Treatment of claustrophobias and snake/spider phobias: fear of arousal and fear of context. *Behaviour Research and Therapy*, **33** (2), 197–203.

Critchley, H.D. (2004) The human cortex responds to an interoceptive challenge. *Proceedings of the National Academy of Sciences of the United States of America*, **101**, 6333.

Critchley, H.D., Wiens, S., Rotshstein, P. *et al.* (2004) Neural systems supporting interoceptive awareness. *Nature Neuroscience*, **7**, 189–195.

Critchley, H.D., Rothstein, P., Nagai, Y. *et al.* (2005) Activity in the human brain predicting differential heart rate responses to emotional facial expressions. *NeuroImage*, **24**, 751–762.

Crow, S.J., Agras, W.S., Halmi, K. *et al.* (2002) Full syndromal versus subthreshold anorexia nervosa, bulimia nervosa, and binge eating disorder: A multicenter study. *International Journal of Eating Disorders*, **32**, 309–318.

Cummings, E.M. and Cicchetti, D. (1990) Toward a transactional model of relations between attachment and depression, in *Attachment in the Preschool Years: Theory, Research, and Intervention* (eds Mark T. Greenberg, Dante Cicchetti and E. Mark Cummings), University of Chicago Press.

Cunningham, M.R. (1988) What do you do when you're happy or blue? Mood, expectancies, and behavioral interest. *Motivation and Emotion*, **12** (4), 309–331.

Damasio, A.R. (1999) *The Feeling of What Happens: Body, Emotion and the Making of Consciousness*, Heinemann, London.

Damasio, A.R., Grabowski, T.J., Bechara, A. *et al.* (2000) Subcortical and cortical brain activity during the feeling of self-generated emotions. *Nature Neuroscience*, **3**, 1049–1056.

Damon, W. and Hart, D. (1988) *Self Understanding in Childhood and Adolescence*, Cambridge University Press, Cambridge.

Danziger, N., Prkachin, K.M. and Willer, J.C. (2006) Is pain the price of empathy? The perception of others' pain in patients with congenital insensitivity to pain. *Brain: A Journal of Neurology*, **129**, 2494–2507.

Davidson, R.J., Pizzagalli, D., Nitschke, J.B. and Putnam, K. (2002) Depression: perspectives from affective neuroscience. *Annual Review of Psychology*, **53**, 545–574.

Davies, S.J., Jackson, P.R., Lewis, G. *et al.* (2008) Is the association of hypertension and panic disorder explained by clustering of autonomic panic symptoms in hypertensive patients? *Journal of Affective Disorders*, **111** (2–3), 344–350.

Davis, M.H. (1996) *Empathy: A Social Psychological Approach*, Westview Press, Madison, Wisconsin.

De Gucht, V. and Fischler, B. (2002) Somatization: a critical review of conceptual and methodological issues. *Psychosomatics*, **43** (1), 1–9.

de Waelhens, A. (1951) *Une Philosophie de L'ambiguïté: L'existentialisme de Maurice Merleau-Ponty*, Publications universitaires de Louvain.

Deaver, C.M., Miltenberger, R.G., Smyth, J. *et al.* (2003) An evaluation of affect and binge eating. *Behavior Modification*, **27**, 578–599.

Decety, J. and Chaminade, T. (2005) The neurophysiology of imitation and intersubjectivity, in *Perspectives on Imitation: From Neuroscience to Social Science*, vol. **1** (eds S. Hurley and N. Chater), MIT Press, Cambridge, MA.

Decety, J. and Sommerville, A.J. (2003) Shared representations between self and other: a social cognitive neuroscience view. *Trends in Cognitive Sciences*, **7**, 12.

Dehaene-Lambertz, G., Dehaene, S. and Hertz-Pannier, L. (2002) Functional neuroimaging of speech perception in infants. *Science*, **298**, 2013–2015.

Dehaene-Lambertz, G., Hertz-Pannier, L., Dubois, J. *et al.* (2006) Functional organization of perisylvian activation during presentation of sentences in preverbal infants. *PNAS*, **103**, 14240–14245.

Descartes, R. (1650) *The Passions of the Soul*, London.

Devlin, M.J., Goldfein, J.A. and Dobrow, I. (2003) What is this thing called BED?: Current status of binge eating disorder nosology. *International Journal of Eating Disorders*, **34** (suppl.), 2–18.

deWaal, F. (1982) *Chimpanzee Politics: Power and Sex among Apes*, Harper and Row, New York.

Dickhaus, B., Mayer, E.A., Firooz, N. *et al.* (2003) Irritable bowel syndrome patients show enhanced modulation of visceral perception by auditory stress. *The American Journal of Gastroenterology*, **98**, 135–143.

Diderot, D. (1762) Rameau's Nephew. http://records.viu.ca/~Johnstoi/diderot/rameau_E.htm.

Dingemans, A.E., Bruna, M.J. and van Furth, E.F. (2002) Binge eating disorder: a review. *International Journal of Obesity*, **26**, 299–307.

Donnell, C.D. and McNally, R.J. (1990) Anxiety sensitivity and panic attacks in a nonclinical population. *Behaviour Research and Therapy*, **28**, 83–85.

Dostoevsky, F.M. (1953) *Crime and Punishment: A Novel in Six Parts and an Epilogue*, (trans. Jessie Coulson), Oxford University Press, London.

Dostoevsky, F.M. (1998) *Poor Folk and Other Stories*, ('Mr Prokharchin' trans. David McDuff), Penguin Books, London, pp. 215–248.

Dostoevsky, F.M. (2006) *Short Masterpieces of Fyodor Dostoevsky*, Walking Lion Press.

Dougherty, M.L., Abe, A.J. and Izard, E.C. (1996) Differential emotions theory and emotional development in adulthood and later life, in *Handbook of Emotion, Adult Development, and Aging* (eds C. Magai and S.H. McFadden), Academic Press.

Draghi-Lorenz, R., Reddy, V. and Costall, A. (2001) Rethinking the development of "Nonbasic" emotions: a critical review of existing theories. *Developmental Review*, **21**, 263–304.

Drevets, W.C., Videen, T.O., Price, J.L. *et al.* (1992a) A functional anatomical study of unipolar depression. *Journal of Neuroscience*, **12**, 3628–3641.

Drevets, W.C., Bogers, W. and Raichle, M.E. (2002) Functional anatomical correlates of antidepressant drug treatment assessed using PET measures of regional glucose metabolism. *European Neuropsychopharmacology*, **12** (6), 527–544.

Dreyfus, H.L. (1991) *Being-in-the-World: A Commentary on Heidegger's Being and Time, Division I*, MIT Press.

Du Toit, P.L., van Kradenburg, J., Niehaus, D.J.H. and Stein, D.J. (2001) Characteristics and phenomenology of hair-pulling: An exploration of subtypes. *Comprehensive Psychiatry*, **42** (3), 247–256.

Dunn, J. (1988) *The Beginnings of Social Understanding*, Harvard University Press, Cambridge MA.

Dupuy, J. (1985) *L'essor de la Premiere Cybernetique (1943–1953)*, Cahiers du CREA 7.

Dupuy, J. (2000) *The Mechanization of the Mind: On the Origins of Cognitive Science*, Princeton University Press.

Dutton, D.G. (2002) Neurobiology of abandonment homicide. *Aggression and Violent Behavior*, **7** (4), 407–421.

Eddy, K.T., Dorer, D.J., Franko, D.L. *et al.* (2008) Diagnostic crossover in anorexia nervosa and bulimia nervosa. *The American Journal of Psychiatry*, **165** (2), 245–250.

Ehlers, A. and Breuer, P. (1992) Increased cardiac awareness in panic disorder. *Journal of Abnormal Psychology*, **101**, 371–382.

Ehlers, A. and Breuer, P. (1996) How good are patients with panic disorder at perceiving their heartbeats? *Biological Psychology*, **42** (1–2), 165–182.

Eisenberg, N., Fabes, R.A., Miller, P.A. *et al.* (1989) Relation of sympathy and personal distress to prosocial behavior: a multimethod study. *Journal of Personality and Social Psychology*, **57** (1), 55–66.

Eisenberger, N.I. and Lieberman, M.D. (2004) Why rejection hurts: a common neural alarm system for physical and social pain. *Trends in Cognitive Sciences*, **8**, 294–300.

Eisenberger, N., Lieberman, M.D. and Williams, K.D. (2003) Does rejection hurt? An fMRI study of social exclusion. *Science*, **302** (5643), 290–292.

Eisenberger, N.I., Jarcho, J.M., Lieberman, M.D. and Naliboff, B.D. (2006) An experimental study of shared sensitivity to physical pain and social rejection. *PAIN*, **126** (1–3), 132–138.

Ekman, P. (1972) Universal and cultural differences in facial expressions of emotion, in *Nebraska Symposium on Motivation, 1971* (ed. J. Cole), University of Nebraska Press, Licoln, Neb.

Ekman, P. (2003) *Emotions Revealed*, Times Books.

Ekman, P. and Friesen, W.V. (1976) *Pictures of Facial Affect*, Consulting Psychologist Press, Palo Alto, CA.

Eldredge, K., Wilson, G.T. and Whaley, A. (1990) Failure, self-evaluation, and feeling fat in women. *International Journal of Eating Disorders*, **9**, 37–50.

Eley, T.C., Sugden, K., Corsico, A. *et al.* (2004) Gene-environment interaction analysis of serotonin system markers with adolescent depression. *Molecular Psychiatry*, **9**, 908–915.

Eley, T.C., Sugden, K., Gregory, A.M. and Clark, D.M. (2004) Heart-beat perception, panic/ somatic symptoms and anxiety sensitivity in children. *Behaviour Research and Therapy*, **42** (4), 439–448.

Engel, S. (1986) *Learning to Reminisce: a Developmental Study of How Young Children Talk About the Past. (quoted in) K. Nelson. (1996). Language in Cognitive Development*, Cambridge University Press.

Engelberg, M.J., Steiger, H., Gauvin, L. and Wonderlich, S.A. (2007) Binge antecedents in bulimic syndromes: an examination of dissociation and negative affect. *International Journal of Eating Disorders*, **40**, 531–536.

Eppright, T.D., Sanfacon, J.A., Beck, N.C. and Bradley, J.S. (1997) Sport psychiatry in childhood and adolescence: An overview. *Child Psychiatry and Human Development*, **28**, 71–88.

Faber, R.J. (1992) Money changes everything: compulsive buying from a biopsychosocial perspective. *American Behavioral Scientist*, **35** (6), 809–819.

Faber, R.J. and O'Guinn, T.C. (1992) A clinical screener for compulsive buying. *Journal of Consumer Research*, **19**, 459–469.

Faber, R.J. and Vohs, K.D. (2004) To buy or not to buy? in *Handbook of Self-Regulation* (eds R.F. Baumeister and K.D. Vohs), Guilford, NY.

Fadiga, L., Craighero, L., Buccino, G. and Rizzolatti, G. (2002) Speech listening specifically modulates the excitability of tongue muscles: a TMS study. *The European Journal of Neuroscience*, **15**, 399–402.

Fairburn, C.G. and Harrison, P.J. (2003) Eating disorders. *Lancet*, **361**, 407–416.

Fairburn, C.G., Welch, S.L. and Hay, P.J. (1993) The classification of recurrent overeating: the "Binge Eating Disorder" proposal. *International Journal of Eating Disorders*, **13**, 155–159.

Fairburn, C.G., Doll, H.A., Welch, S.L. *et al.* (1998) Risk factors for binge eating disorder. *Archives of General Psychiatry*, **55**, 425–432.

Fairburn, C.G., Cooper, Z., Doll, H.D. and Welch, S.L. (1999) Risk factors for anorexia nervosa: three integrated case-control comparisons. *Archives of General Psychiatry*, **56**, 468–476.

Faravelli, C. and Pallanti, S. (1989) Recent life events and panic disorder. *The American Journal of Psychiatry*, **146**, 622–626.

Fava, G.A. and Wise, T.N. (2007) Issues for DSM-V: psychological factors affecting either identified or feared medical conditions: a solution for somatoform disorders. *The American Journal of Psychiatry*, **164** (7), 1002–1003.

Fava, G.A., Grandi, S., Saviotti, F.M. and Conti, S. (1990) Hypochondriasis with panic attacks. *Psychosomatics*, **31**, 351–353.

Feldner, Matthew T., Zvolensky, Michael J. and Leen-Feldner Ellen, W.A. (2004) A critical review of the empirical literature on coping and panic disorder. *Clinical Psychology Review*, **24**, 123–148.

Ferguson, C.A. (1964) Baby talk in six languages. *American Anthropologist*, **66**, 103–114.

Ferguson, M.L. and Katkin, E.S. (1996) Visceral perception, anhedonia, and emotion. *Biological Psychology*, **42**, 131–145.

Fernald, Simon T. (1984) Expanded intonation contours in mothers' speech to newborns. *Developmental Psychology*, **20**, 104–113.

Fernald, A. (2004) Hearing, listening, and understanding: auditory development in infancy, in *Handbook of Infant Development* (eds G. Bremner and A. Fogel), Blackwell.

Fernandez-Dols, J.M. and Ruiz-Belda, M.A. (1997) Spontaneous facial behavior during intense emotional episodes: Artistic truth and optical truth, in *The Psychology of Facial Expression* (eds J.A. Russell and J.M. Fernández Dols), Cambridge University Press.

Fernández-Dols, J.M. and Ruiz-Belda, M.A. (1995) Are smiles a sign of happiness? Gold medal winners at the Olympic Games. *Journal of Personality and Social Psychology*, **69**, 1113–1119.

Fichter, M.M. and Daser, C. (1987) Symptomatology, psychosexual development and gender identity in 42 anorexic males. *Psychological Medicine*, **17**, 409–418.

Fichter, M.M., Quadflieg, N. and Brandl, B. (1993) Recurrent overeating: an empirical comparison of binge eating disorder, bulimia nervosa and obesity. *International Journal of Eating Disorders*, **14**, 1–16.

Fifer, W.P., Monk, C.E. and Grose-Fifer, J. (2004) Prenatal development and risk, in *Handbook of Infant Development* (eds G. Bremner and A. Fogel), Blackwell.

Fischer, H., Andersson, J.L., Furmark, T. and Fredrikson, M. (1998) Brain correlates of an unexpected panic attack: a human positron emission tomographic study. *Neuroscience Letters*, **251** (2), 137–140.

Fitzgibbon, M.L., Sanchez-Johnsen, L.A.P. and Martinovich, Z. (2003) A test of the continuity perspective across bulimic and binge eating pathology. *International Journal of Eating Disorders*, **34**, 83–97.

Fivush, R. (1991) The social construction of personal narratives. *Merrill-Palmer Quarterly*, **37**, 59–81.

Fivush, R. (2007) Maternal reminiscing style and children's developing understanding of self and emotion. *Clinical Social Work*, **35**, 37–46.

Fivush, R. and Haden, C.A. (2005) Parent–child reminiscing and the construction of a subjective self, in *The Development of Social Cognition and Communication* (eds B.D. Homer and C.S. Tamis-LeMonda), Erlbaum, Mahwah, NJ, pp. 315–335.

Fivush, R. and Nelson, K. (2006) Parent–child reminiscing locates the self in the past. *British Journal of Developmental Psychology*, **24**, 235–251.

Flaubert, G. (1954) *Bouvard et Pécuchet*, Classiques Garnier.

Flaubert, G. (2002) *A Sentimental Education*, Penguin Classics.

Flaubert, G. (2003) *Madame Bovary*, Penguin Classics.

Fogassi, L., Ferrari, P.F., Gesierich, B. *et al.* (2005) Parietal lobe: from action organisation to intention understanding. *Science*, **308**, 662–667.

Fombonne, E., Wostear, G., Cooper, V. *et al.* (2001) The Maudsley long-term follow-up of child and adolescent depression. 2. Suicidality, criminality and social dysfunction in adulthood. *British Journal of Psychiatry*, **179**, 218–223.

Forsyth, J.P., Palav, A. and Du, K. (1999). The absence of relation between anxiety sensitivity and fear conditioning using 20% vs. 13% CO_2 -enriched air as unconditioned stimuli. *Behaviour Research and Therapy*, **37**, 143–153.

Fox, E., Russo, R. and Dutton, K. (2002) Attentional bias for threat: Evidence for delayed disengagement from emotional faces. *Cognition and Emotion*, **16** (3), 355–379.

Fox, M.D., Snyder, A.Z., Vincent, J.L. *et al.* (2005) The human brain is intrinsically organized into dynamic, anticorrelated functional networks. *Proceedings of the National Academy of Sciences of the United States of America*, **102**, 9673–9678.

Fox, M.D., Snyder, A.Z., Vincent, J.L. and Raichle, M.E. (2007) Intrinsic fluctuations within cortical systems account for intertrial variability in human behavior. *Neuron*, **56**, 171–184.

Fraley, R.C. and Davis, K.E. (1997) Attachment formation and transfer in young adults' close friendships and romantic relationships. *Personal Relationships*, **4**, 131–144.

Fraley, R.C., Davis, K.E. and Shaver, P.R. (1998) Dismissing-Avoidance and the defensive organization of emotion, cognition and behavior, in *Attachment Theory and Close Relationships* (eds J.A. Simpson and W.S. Rholes), Guilford Press.

Fredrikson, M., Wik, G., Greitz, T. *et al.* (1993) Regional cerebral blood flow during experimental phobic fear. *Psychophysiology*, **30**, 126–130.

Freed, P.J. and Mann, J.J. (2007) Sadness and loss: Toward a neurobiopsychosocial model. *The American Journal of Psychiatry*, **164** (1), 28–34.

Freedman, L.J., Insel, T.R. and Smith, Y. (2000) Subcortical projections of area 25 (subgenual cortex) of the macaque monkey. *The Journal of Comparative Neurology*, **421**, 172–188.

Freo, U., Ori, C., Dam, M. *et al.* (2000) Effects of acute and chronic treatment with fluoxetine on regional glucose cerebral metabolism in rats: implications for clinical therapies. *Brain Research*, **854** (1–2), 35–41.

Freud, S. (1915) On transience, in *Collected Papers*, vol. **5**, London: Hogarth Press.

Freud, S. (1917) Mourning and melancholia, in *Collected Papers*, vol. **14**, London: Hogarth Press.

Fridlund, A.J. (1994) *Human Facial Expression: An Evolutionary View*, Academic Press, San Diego CA.

Fridlund, A.J. (1997) *The New Ethology of Human Facial Expressions. The Psychology of Facial Expression* (eds J.A. Russell and J.M. Fernández Dols), Cambridge University Press.

Friedman, W.J. (1977) The development of children's knowledge of cyclic aspects of time. *Child Development*, **48**, 1593–1599.

Friedman, W.J. (1990) Children representations of the pattern of daily activities. *Child Development*, **61**, 1399–1412.

Friedman, W.J. (2000) The development of children's knowledge of the times of future events. *Child Development*, **71**, 913–932.

Friedman, W.J. and Brudos, S.L. (1988) On routines and routines: The early development of spatial and temporal representations. *Cognitive Development*, **3**, 167–182.

Frost, R.O. and Gross, R.C. (1993) The hoarding of possessions. *Behaviour Research and Therapy*, **31** (4), 367–381.

Frost, R.O. and Hartl, T.L. (1996) A cognitive-behavioral model of compulsive hoarding. *Behaviour Research and Therapy*, **34** (4), 341–350.

Frost, R.O. and Tolin, D.F. (2008) Compulsive hoarding, in *Clinical Handbook of Obsessive-Compulsive Disorder and Related Problems* (eds J.S. Abramowitz D. McKay and S. Taylor), The John Hopkins University Press.

Frost, R.O., Hartl, T.L., Christian, R. and Williams, N. (1995) The value of possessions in compulsive hoarding: patterns of use and attachment. *Behaviour Research and Therapy*, **33**, 897–902.

Frost, R.O., Steketee, G. and Williams, L. (2000) Hoarding: A community health problem. *Health and Social Care in the Community*, **8**, 229–234.

Furby, L. (1978) Possession in humans: An exploratory study of its meaning and motivation. *Social Behavior and Personality*, **6**, 49–65.

Furmark, T., Tillfors, M., Garpenstrand, H. *et al.* (2004) Serotonin transporter polymorphism related to amygdala excitability and symptom severity in patients with social phobia. *Neuroscience Letters*, **362**, 189–192.

Furnham, A., Badmin, N. and Sneade, I. (2002) Body image dissatisfaction: gender differences in eating attitudes, self-esteem, and reasons for exercise. *The Journal of Psychology*, **136** (6), 581–596.

Galinsky, A.D., Maddux, W.W., Gilin, D. and and White, J.B. (2008) Why it pays to get inside the head of your opponent. *Psychological Science*, **19** (4), 378–384.

Gallagher, S. (2007) Phenomenological and experimental research on embodied experience, in *Body, Language and Mind*, 1 (eds Tom Ziemke, Jordan Zlatev, Roslyn Frank and Rene Dirven), Mouton de Gruyter, Berlin, pp. 241–263.

Gallagher, S. (2007) Introduction: the arts and sciences of the situated body. *Janus Head*, **9.2**, 293–295.

Gallagher, S. and Meltzoff, Andrew (1996) The earliest sense of self and others: Merleau-Ponty and recent developmental studies. *Philosophical Psychology*, **9** (2), 213–236.

Gallese, V. (2001) The "Shared Manifold" Hypothesis: from mirror neurons to empathy. *Journal of Consciousness Studies*, **8** (5–7), 33–50.

Gallese, V. (2003) The manifold nature of interpersonal relations: the quest for a common mechanism. *Philosophical Transactions of the Royal Society of London B*, **358**, 517.

Gallese, V. (2005) "Being Like Me": self-other identity, mirror neurons and empathy, in *Perspectives on Imitation: From Neuroscience to Social Science*, vol. **1** (eds S. Hurley and N. Chater), MIT Press, Cambridge, MA.

Gallese, V. (2007) Before and below theory of mind: embodied simulation and the neural correlates of social cognition. *Philosophical Transactions of the Royal Society of London. Series B, Biological Sciences*, **362**, 659–669.

Gallese, V., Fadiga, L., Fogassi, L. and Rizzolatti, G. (1996) Action recognition in the premotor cortex. *Brain: A Journal of Neurology*, **119**, 593–609.

Gallese, V., Rochat, M., Cossu, G. and Sinigaglia, C. (2009) Motor cognition and its role in the phylogeny and ontogeny of intentional understanding. *Developmental Psychology*, **45**, 103–113.

Gallup, G.G. Jr (1982) Self-awareness and the emergence of mind in primates. *American Journal of Primatology*, **2**, 237–248.

Gallup, G.G. (1994) Self-recognition: Research strategies and experimental design, in *Self-Awareness in Animals and Humans: Developmental Perspectives* (eds S. Parker, R. Mitchell and M. Boccia), Cambridge University Press.

Garner, D.M., Olmsted, M.E. and Polivy, J. (1983) Development and validation of a multidimensional eating disorder inventory for anorexia nervosa and bulimia. *International Journal of Eating Disorders*, **2**, 15–34.

Garner, D.M., Garner, M.V. and Rosen, L.W. (1993) Anorexia nervosa "restricters" who purge: implications for subtyping anorexia nervosa. *International Journal of Eating Disorders*, **13**, 171–185.

Garner, M., Mogg, K. and Bradley, B.P. (2006) Orienting and maintenance of gaze to facial expression in social anxiety. *Journal of Abnormal Psychology*, **115** (4), 760–770.

Gazzaniga, S.M. (1998) *The Mind's Past*, University of California Press.

Gazzola, V., Aziz-Zadeh, L. and Keysers, C. (2006) Empathy and the somatotopic auditory mirror system in Humans. *Current Biology*, **16**, 1824–1829.

Geeraerts, B., van Oudenhove, L., Vos, R. and Tack, J. (2005) Influence of experimentally induced anxiety on rectal sensorimotor function in healthy humans. *Gastroenterology*, **129** (5), 1437–1444.

Gentilucci, M. (2003) Grasp observation influences speech production. *European Journal of Neuroscience*, **17**, 179–184.

Gentilucci, M., Benuzzi, F., Gangitano, M. and Grimaldi, S. (2001) Grasp with hand and mouth: a kinematic study on healthy subjects. *Journal of Neurophysiology*, **86**, 1685–1699.

Gentilucci, M., Santunione, P., Roy, A.C. and Stefanini, S. (2004a) Execution and observation of bringing a fruit to the mouth affect syllable pronunciation. *European Journal of Neuroscience*, **19**, 190–202.

Gentilucci, M., Stefanini, S., Roy, A.C. and Santunione, P. (2004b) Action observation and speech production: study on children and adults. *Neuropsychologia*, **42**, 1554–1567.

Gentilucci, M., Bernardis, P., Crisi, G. and Volta, R.D. (2006) Repetitive transcranial magnetic stimulation of Broca's area affects verbal responses to gesture observation. *Journal of Cognitive Neuroscience*, **18**, 1059–1074.

Gergen, J.K. (1991) *The Saturated Self*, Basic Books, New York.

Gergen, J.K. (1999) *An Invitation to Social Construction*, Sage Publications.

Gergen, J.K. (2001) *Social Construction in Context*, Sage, London.

Gilbert, A.N.A.J., Fridlund, A.J. and Sabini, J. (1987) Hedonic and social determinants of facial displays to odors. *Chemical Senses*, **12**, 355–363.

Ginzburg, C. (2000) *Rapporti Di Forza*, Feltrinelli.

Girard, R. (2006) Eating disorders and mimetic desire. www.uibk.ac.at/theol/cover/contagion/contagion03_Girard.pdf.

Goldapple, K., Segal, Z., Garson, C. *et al.* (2002) Effects of cognitive behavioral therapy on brain glucose metabolism in patients with major depression. *Biological Psychiatry*, **51**, 66.

Goldapple, K., Segal, Z., Garson, C. *et al.* (2004) Modulation of cortical-limbic pathways in major depression: treatment-specific effects of cognitive behavior therapy. *Archives of General Psychiatry*, **61** (1), 34–41.

Goldman, M.J. (1991) Kleptomania: making sense of the nonsensical. *The American Journal of Psychiatry*, **148**, 986–996.

Goldstein, A. and Chambless, D. (1978) A reanalysis of agoraphobia. *Behavior Therapy*, **9**, 47–59.

Goldstein, M.H., King, A.P. and West, M.J. (2003) Social interaction shapes babbling: Testing parallels between birdsong and speech. *PNAS*, **100** (13), 8030–8035.

Goodall, J. (1971) *In the Shadow of Man*, Houghton Mifflin Publishing, Boston.

Goodwin, R.D. and Pine, D.S. (2002) Respiratory disease and panic attacks among adults in the United States. *Chest*, **122**, 645–650.

Gopnik, A. (1984) The acquisition of gone and the development of the object concept. *Journal of Child Language*, **11**, 273–292.

Graybiel, A.M. and Rauch, S.L. (2000) Toward a neurobiology of obsessivecompulsive disorder. *Neuron*, **28**, 343–347.

Graybiel, A.M., Aosaki, T., Flaherty, A.W. and Klmura, M. (1994) The basal ganglia and adaptive motor control. *Science*, **265**, 1826–1831.

Grayson, K. and Shulman, D. (2000) Indexicality and the verification function of irreplaceable possessions: a semiotic analysis. *Journal of Consumer Research*, **27** (June), 17–30.

Greeven, A., Van Balkom, J.L.M., Van Rood, Y.R. *et al.* (2006) The boundary between hypochondriasis and obsessive-compulsive disorder: a cross-sectional study from the Netherlands. *Journal of Clinical Psychiatry*, **67** (11), 1682–1689.

Greicius, M., Krasnow, B., Reiss, A.L. and Vinod Menon, V. (2003) Functional connectivity in the resting brain: A network analysis of the default mode hypothesis. *Proceedings of the National Academy of Sciences of the United States of America*, **100** (1), 253–258.

Griffiths, P.E. (1997) *What Emotions Really Are: The Problem of Psychological Categories*, University of Chicago Press, Chicago.

Griffiths, P. (2004a) Is emotion a natural kind? in *Thinking About Feeling: Contemporary Philosophers on Emotion* (ed R.C. Solomon), Oxford University Press.

Griffiths, P.E. (2004b) Towards a Machiavellian theory of emotional appraisal, in *Emotion, Evolution and Rationality* (eds P. Cruse and D. Evans), Oxford University Press.

Griffiths, P.E. and Gray, R.D. (2001) *Cycles of Contingency: Developmental Systems and Evolution*, MIT Press.

Griffiths, P. and Scarantino, A. (2008) Emotions in the wild: The situated perspective on emotion, in *To Appear in Cambridge Handbook of Situated Cognition* (eds P. Robbins and M. Aydede), Cambridge University Press.

Griffiths, P.E. (2003). Basic Emotions, Complex Emotions, Machiavellian Emotions, in *Philosophy and the Emotions* (ed A. Hatzimoysis), Cambridge, CUP:39–67.

Groesz, L.M., Levine, M.P. and Murnen, S.K. (2002) The effect of experimental presentation of thin media images on body satisfaction: a meta-analytic review. *International Journal of Eating Disorders*, **31**, 1–16.

Gross, J. and Rosen, J.C. (1988) Bulimia in adolescents: Prevalence and psychosocial correlates. *International Journal of Eating Disorders*, **7**, 51–61.

Gu, X. and Han, S. (2007) Attention and reality constraints on the neural processes of empathy for pain. *NeuroImage*, **36**, 256–267.

Guidano, V.F. (1987) *Complexity of the Self*, Guilford, New York.

Guidano, V.F. (1991) *The Self in Process: Toward a Post-Rationalist Cognitive Therapy*, Guilford, New York.

Guidano, V.F. and Liotti, G. (1983) *Cognitive Processes and Emotional Disorders*, Guilford Press, New York.

Gündel, H., O'Connor, M.F., Littrell, L. *et al.* (2003) Functional neuroanatomy of grief: An fMRI study. *The American Journal of Psychiatry*, **160**, 1946–1953.

Gusnard, D.A. and Raichle, M.E. (2001) Searching for a baseline: functional imaging and the resting human brain. *Nature Reviews. Neuroscience*, **2**, 685.

Gusnard, D.A., Akbudak, E., Shulman, G.L. and Raichle, M.E. (2001) Medial prefrontal cortex and self- Gusnard D.A., Akbudak E., Shulman G.L., Raichle M. E. (2001). Medial prefrontal cortex and self-referential mental activity: Relation to a default mode of brain function. *Proceedings of the National Academy of Sciences of the United States of America*, **98**, 4259–4264.

Haber, S.N., Kunishio, K., Mizobuchi, M. and Lynd-Balta, E. (1995) The orbital and medical prefrontal circuit through the primate basal ganglia. *J. Neurosci.*, **15**, 4851–4867.

Haber, S.N., Kim, K.S., Mailly, P. and Calzavara, R. (2006) Reward-related cortical inputs define a large striatal region in primates that interface with associative cortical connections, providing a substrate for incentive-based learning. *J. Neurosci.*, **26**, 8368–8376.

Hacking, I. (1995) *Rewriting the Soul: Multiple Personality and the Sciences of Memory*, Princeton University Press.

Hall, D.A., Fussell, C. and Summerfield, A.Q. (2005) Reading fluent speech from talking faces: typical brain networks and individual differences. *Journal of Cognitive Neuroscience*, **17** (6), 939–953.

Halliday, M.A.K. (1975) *Learning How to Mean*, Elsevier, New York.

Halliday, M.A.K. (1985) *Spoken and Written Language*, Deakin University, Victoria.

Halligan, P.W., Athwal, B.S., Oakley, D.A. *et al.* (2000) Imaging hypnotic paralysis: implications for conversion hysteria. *Lancet*, **355**, 986–987.

Halmi, K.A., Sunday, S.R., Strober, M. *et al.* (2000) Perfectionism in anorexia nervosa: variation by clinical subtype, obsessionality, and pathological eating behavior. *The American Journal of Psychiatry*, **157**, 1799–1805.

Hamlin, K.J., Wynn, K. and Bloom, P. (2007) Social evaluation by preverbal infants. *Nature*, **450**, 557–559.

Hammad, M.A., Barsky, A.J. and Regestein, Q.R. (2001) Correlation between somatic sensation inventory scores and hyperarousal scale scores. *Psychosomatics*, **42**, 29–34.

Hankin, B.L. and Abramson, L.Y. (2001) Development of gender differences in depression: An elaborated cognitive vulnerability-transactional stress theory. *Psychological Bulletin*, **127** (6), 773–796.

Hariri, A.R., Mattay, V.S., Tessitore, A. *et al.* (2002) Serotonin transporter genetic variation and the response of the human amygdala. *Science*, **297**, 400–403.

Harkness, K.L. and Lumley, M.N. (2008) Child abuse and neglect and the development of depression in children and adolescents, in *Handbook of Depression in Children and Adolescents* (eds R.Z. Abela John and L. Hankin Benjamin), Guilford.

Harré, R. (1986) An outline of the social constructionist viewpoint, in *The Social Construction of Emotions* (ed. R. Harré), Basil Blackwell, New York.

Harrè, J. (1986) *The Social Construction of Emotions*, Basil Backwell, Oxford.

Harris, T., Brown, W. and Bifulco, A. (1986) Loss of parent in childhood and adult psychiatric disorder: the role of lack of adequate parental care. *Psychological Medicine*, **16** (3), 641–659.

Harrison, B.J., Pujol, J., Lopez-Solà, M. *et al.* (2008) Consistency and functional specialization in the default mode brain network. *Proceedings of the National Academy of Sciences of the United States of America*, **105**, 9781–9786.

Hart, S. and Carrington, H. (2002) Jealousy in 6-month-old infants. *Infancy*, **3** (3), 395–402.

Hart, S., Field, T., Del Valle, C. and Letourneau, M. (1998) Infants protest their mothers attending to an infant-size doll. *Social Development*, **7**, 54–61.

Hasler, G., Gergen, P.J., Kleinbaum, D.G. *et al.* (2005) Asthma and panic in young adults. A 20-year prospective community study. *American Journal of Respiratory and Critical Care Medicine*, **171**, 1224–1230.

Hauk, O., Johnsrude, I. and Pulverm¸ller, F. (2004) Somatotopic representation of action words in human motor and premotor cortex. *Neuron*, **41** (2), 301–307.

Hay, P.J. and Fairburn, C.G. (1998) The validity of the DSM-IV scheme for classifying bulimic eating disorders. *International Journal of Eating Disorders*, **23**, 7–15.

Hay, P.J., Fairburn, C.G. and Doll, H.A. (1996) The classification of bulimic eating disorders: a community-based cluster analysis study. *Psychological Medicine*, **26**, 801–812.

Hayek, F.A. (1978) *New Studies in Philosophy, Politics, Economics and History of Ideas*, University of Chicago Press.

Heatherton, T.F. and Baumeister, R.F. (1991) Binge eating as escape from self-awareness. *Psychological Bulletin*, **110**, 86–108.

Heatherton, T.E., Polivy, J. and Herman, C.E. (1989) Restraint and internal responsiveness: Effects of placebo manipulations of hunger state on eating. *Journal of Abnormal Psychology*, **98**, 89–92.

Heatherton, T.E., Herman, C. and Polivy, E.J. (1991) Effects of physical threat and ego threat on eating behavior. *Journal of Personality and Social Psychology*, **60**, 138–143.

Heidegger, M. (1962) *Being and Time*, Blackwell Publishing.

Heidegger, M. (1984) *The Metaphysical Foundations of Logic*, Indiana University Press.

Heidegger, M. (1986) *Logica. Il problema della verita'*, Mursia (Gesamtausgabe Abt. 2 Vorlesungen Bd. 21. Logik, die Frage nach der Wahrheit Marburger Vorlesung Wintersemester 1925/26).

Heidegger, M. (1987) *Seminari di Zollikon*, Guida.

Heidegger, M. (1988) *The Basic Problems of Phenomenology*, First Midland Book.

Heidegger, M. (2001a) *The Fundamental Concepts of Metaphysics*, Indiana University Press.

Heidegger, M. (2001b) *Phenomenological Interpretations of Aristotle: Initiation Into Phenomenological Research*, Indiana University Press.

Heidegger, M. (2001c) *Zollikon Seminars. Protocols – Conversations – Letters*, Northwestern University Press.

Heims, S.J. (1991) *Constructing a Social Science for Postwar America: The Cybernetics Group, 1946–1953*, MIT Press.

Henry, M.E., Schmidt, M.E., Matochik, J.A. *et al.* (2001) The effects of ECT on brain glucose: A pilot FDG PET study. *The Journal of ECT*, **17** (1), 76–82.

Herzog, D.B., Norman, D.K., Gordon, C. and Pepose, M. (1984) Sexual conflict and eating disorders in 27 males. *The American Journal of Psychiatry*, **141**, 989–990.

Hewitt, P.L. and Flett, G.L. (1991) Perfectionism in the self and social contexts: conceptualization, assessment, and association with psychopathology. *Journal of Personality and Social Psychology*, **60**, 456–470.

Hewitt, P.L., Flett, C.L. and Ediger, E. (1995) Perfectionism traits and perfectionistic self-presentation in eating disorder attitudes, characteristics, and symptoms. *International Journal of Eating Disorders*, **18**, 317–326.

Hinde, R.A. (1985a) Expression and negotiation, in *The Development of Expressive Behavior* (ed. G. Zivin), Academic Press, New York, pp. 103–116.

Hinde, R.A. (1985b) Was "the expression of emotions" a misleading phrase? *Animal Behaviour*, **33**, 985–992.

Hobson, A.R. and Aziz, Q. (2003) Central nervous system processing of visceral pain in health and disease. *News in Physiological Science*, **18**, 109–114.

Hodson, G. and Costello, K. (2007) Interpersonal disgust, ideological orientations, and dehumanisation as predictors of intergroup attitudes. *Psychological Science*, **18** (8), 691–698.

Hofmann, S.G. and Barlow, D.H. (2002) Social phobia (social anxiety disorder), in *Anxiety and Itsdisorders: The Nature and Treatment of Anxiety and Panic*, 2nd Edn (ed. D.H. Barlow), Guilford Press, New York.

Hofmann, S.G., Lehman, C.L. and Barlow, D.H. (1997) How specific are specific phobias? *Journal of Behavior Therapy and Experimental Psychiatry*, **28** (3), 233–240.

Hofmann, S.G., Heinrichs, N. and Moscovitch, D.A. (2004) The nature and expression of social phobia: toward a new classification. *Clinical Psychology Review*, **24** (7), 769–797.

Holland, A. and Andre, T. (1994) Athletic participation and the social status of adolescent males and females. *Youth and Society*, **25**, 388–407.

Homae, F., Watanabe, H., Nakano, T. *et al.* (2006) The right hemisphere of sleeping infant perceives sentential prosody. *Neurosci Research*, **54**, 276–280.

Hudson, J.A. (1990) The emergence of autobiographic memory in mother–child conversation, in *Knowing and Remembering in Young Children* (eds R. Fivush and J.A. Hudson), Cambridge University Press, New York, pp. 166–196.

Hudson, J.A. (2002) "Do you know what we're going to do this summer?" Mothers' talk to young children about future events. *Journal of Cognition and Development*, **3**, 49–71.

Hudson, J.A. (2006) The development of future time concepts through mother–child conversation. *Merrill-Palmer Quarterly*, **52** (1), 70–95.

Hudson, J.A., Shapiro, L.R. and Sosa, B.B. (1995) Planning in the real world: Preschool children's scripts and plans for familiar events. *Child Development*, **66** (4), 984–998.

Huprich, S.K. (1998) Depressive personality disorder: theoretical issues, clinical findings, and future research questions. *Clinical Psychology Review*, **18**, 477–500.

Hurley, S. (2006) Active perception and perceiving action: The shared circuits hypothesis, in *Perceptual Experience* (eds T. Gendler and J. Hawthorne), Oxford University Press.

Husserl, E. (1962) *Ideas*, Collier Books.

Hyatt, C.W. and Hopkins, W.D. (1994) Self-awareness in bonobos and chimpanzees: a comparative perspective, in *Self-Awareness in Animals and Humans* (eds S.T. Parker, R.W. Mitchell and M.L. Boccia), Cambridge University Press.

Hyman, P.E. and Cocjin, J. (2005) Colon motility during a panic attack. *Psychosomatic Medicine*, **67** (4), 616–617.

Hynes, A.C., Baird, A.A. and Grafton, T.S. (2005) Differential role of the orbital frontal lobe in emotional versus cognitive perspective-taking. *Neuropsychologia*, **44** (3), 374–383.

Iacoboni, M., Woods, R.P., Brass, M. *et al.* (1999) Cortical mechanisms of human imitation. *Science*, **286** (5449), 2526–2528.

Iacoboni, M., Molnar- Szakacs, I., Gallese, V. *et al.* (2005) Grasping the intentions of others with one's owns mirror neuron system. *PLOS Biology*, **3**, 79.

Ibsen, H. (1919) *The Collected Works of Henrik Ibsen*, vol. **2** (ed. and trans. Archer William), William Heinemann, London.

Irving, L.M., Wall, M., Neumark-Sztainer, D. and Story, M. (2002) Steroid use among adolescents: Findings from project EAT. *Journal of Adolescent Health*, **30**, 243–252.

Izard, C.E. (1991) *The Psychology of Emotions*, Plenum Press.

Izard, C.E., Libero, D.Z., Putnam, P. and Haynes, O.M. (1993) Stability of emotion experiences and their relation to traits of personality. *Journal of Personality and Social Psychology*, **64**, 847–860.

Jackson, P.L., Meltzoff, A.N. and Decety, J. (2005) How do we perceive the pain of others? A window into the neural processes involved in empathy. *NeuroImage*, **24**, 771–779.

Jackson, P.L., Brunet, E., Meltzoff, A.N. and Decety, J. (2006) Empathy examined through the neural mechanisms involved in imagining how I feel versus how you feel pain. *Neuropsychologia*, **44**, 752–761.

Jackson, P.L., Rainville, P. and Decety, J. (2006) To what extent do we share the pain of others? Insight from the neural bases of pain empathy. *Pain*, **125** (1–2), 5–9.

Jacob, R.G. and Furman, J.M. (2001) Psychiatric consequences of vestibular dysfunction. *Current Opinion in Neurology*, **14** (1), 41–46.

Jacob, P. and Jeannerod, M. (2005) The motor theory of social cognition: a critique. *Trends in Cognitive Sciences*, **9** (1), 21–25.

Jacob, R.G., Furman, J.M., Joseph, M. *et al.* (1997) Surface dependence: a balance control strategy in panic disorder with agoraphobia. *Psychosomatic Medicine*, **59**, 323–330.

Jacobs, D.F. (1989) A general theory of addictions: Rationale for and evidence supporting a new approach for understanding and treating addictive behaviors, in *Compulsive Gambling: Theory, Research, and Practice* (eds H.J. Shaffer, S.A. Stein, B. Gambino and T.N. Cummings), Lexington Books/D.C., Lexington (MA), pp. 35–64.

Jacobsen, J.P. (2008) *Niels Lyhne*, Dodo Press.

James, W. (1884) What is an emotion? *Mind*, **9**, 188–205.

James, W. (1890) *The Principles of Psychology*, Holt, NY.

James, W. (1894) The physical basis of emotion. *Psychological Review*, **1**, 516–529.

James, W. (1950) *The Principles of Psychology*, vol. **2**, Dover, New York.

Janet, P. (1898) *Névroses et Idées Fixes*, Alcan, Paris.

Janet, P. (1904) Les obsessions et al Psychastenie (2 vol.), reprinted by L'Harmattan, Paris.

Janet, P. (1907) *The Major Symptoms of Hysteria*, The Macmillian Company, NY.

Jansen, A., Smeets, T., Martijn, C. and Nederkoorn, C. (2006) I see what you see: the lack of a self-serving body-image bias in eating disorders. *British Journal of Clinical Psychology*, **45** (1), 123–135.

Janssen, S.A. (2002) Negative affect and sensitization to pain. *Scandinavian Journal of Psychology*, **43**, 131–137.

Jaspers, K. (1964) *Psicopatologia Generale*, Il Pensiero Scientifico.

Jeannerod, M. (2006) *Motor Cognition*, Oxford University Press.

Johansen-Berg, H., Gutman, D.A., Behrens, T.E.J. *et al.* (2008) Anatomical connectivity of the subgenual cingulate region targeted with deep brain stimulation for treatment-resistant depression. *Cerebral Cortex*, **18** (6), 1374–1383.

Johnson, D.B. (1983) Self-recognition in infants. *Infant Behavior and Development*, **6**, 211–222.

Johnson, C., Lewis, C. and Hagman, J. (1984) The syndrome of bulimia. Review and synthesis. *Psychiatric Clinics of North America*, **7** (2), 247–273.

Jones, S.S., Collins, K. and Hong, H. (1991) An audience effect on smile production in 10-month-old infants. *Psychological Science*, **2**, 45–49.

Joyce, J. (1993) *Dubliners: An Annotated Edition* (eds John Wyse Jackson and Bernard McGinley), Sinclair-Stevenson, London, pp. 95–104.

Kafka, F. (1966) *Letter to His Father* (bilingual edition), Schocken, New York.

Kafka, F. (1995) *The Complete Stories* (ed. N. Nahum), Schocken, New York.

Kalin, N.H., Shelton, S.E. and Davidson, R.J. (2007) Role of the primate orbitofrontal cortex in mediating anxious temperament. *Biological Psychiatry*, **62** (10), 1134–1139.

Kant, I. (1967) *Kritik der reinen Vernuft*, (trad. it. di P. Chiodi), UTET, Torino.

Kant, I. (1977) *I progressi della metafisica*, vol. **VIII**, (trad. it. P. Manganaro), Bibliopolis Napoli.

Kant, I. (1980) *Fondazione Della Metafisica Dei Costumi*, vol. **IV**, (trad. it. P. Chiodi) Laterza Bari. Werke.

Kanwisher, N., McDermott, J. and Chun, M.M. (1997) The fusiform face area: a module in human extrastriate cortex specialized for face perception. *The Journal of Neuroscience*, **17**, 430–4311.

Katkin, E.S., Wiens, S. and Öhman, A. (2001) Nonconscious fear conditioning, visceral perception, and the development of gut feelings. *Psychological Science*, **12**, 366–370.

Katzman, D.K. *et al.* (1997) A longitudinal magnetic resonance imaging study of brain changes in adolescents with anorexia nervosa. *Archives of Pediatrics & Adolescent Medicine*, **151**, 793–797.

Kaufman, J., Yang, B.Z., Douglas-Palumberi, H. *et al.* (2004) Social supports and serotonin transporter gene moderate depression in maltreated children. *Proceedings of the National Academy of Sciences of the United States of America*, **101**, 17316–17321.

Kaufman, J., Yang, B.Z., Douglas-Palumberi, H. *et al.* (2006) Brain-derived neurotrophic factor–5-HTTLPR gene interactions and environmental modifiers of depression in children. *Biological Psychiatry*, **59**, 673–680.

Keenan, J.P., Wheeler, M.A. *et al.* (2000) Self-recognition and the right prefrontal cortex. *Trends in Cognitive Sciences*, **4** (9), 338–344.

Keenan, J.P., Nelson, A. *et al.* (2001) Self-recognition and the right hemisphere. *Nature*, **409** (6818), 305.

Keenan, J.P., Wheeler, M. *et al.* (2003) Self-face processing in a callosotomy patient. *The European Journal of Neuroscience*, **18** (8), 2391–2395.

Kellner, R., Slocumb, J., Wiggins, R.G. *et al.* (1985) Hostility, somatic symptoms, and hypochondriacal fears and beliefs. Article. *Journal of Nervous & Mental Disease*, **173** (9), 554–560.

Kendler, K.S. (2005) "A gene for...": The nature of gene action in psychiatric disorders. *The American Journal of Psychiatry*, **162**, 1243–1252.

Kendler, K.S., Kuhn, J.W., Vittum, J. *et al.* (2005) The interaction of stressful life events and a serotonin transporter polymorphism in the prediction of episodes of major depression: A replication. *Archives of General Psychiatry*, **62**, 529–535.

Kennedy, S.H., Evans, K., Kruger, S. *et al.* (2001) Changes in regional glucose metabolism with PET following paroxetine treatment for major depression. *The American Journal of Psychiatry*, **158**, 899–905.

Kern, S. (1983) *The Culture of Time and Space 1880–1918*, Harvard University Press, Cambridge, Massachusetts.

Kikuchi, M., Komuro, R., Oka, H. *et al.* (2005) Relationship between anxiety and thyroid function in patients with panic disorder. *Progress in Neuro-Psychopharmacology & Biological, Psychiatry*, **29**, 77–81.

Kindlundh, A.M.S., Hagekull, B., Isacson, D.G.L. and Nyberg, F. (2001) Adolescent use of anabolic-androgenic steroids and relations to self-reports of social, personality and health aspects. *European Journal Public of Health*, **11**, 322–328.

Klein, D.N. (1990) Depressive personality: reliability, validity, and relation to dysthymia. *Journal of Abnormal Psychology*, **99**, 412–421.

Klein, D.N. and Miller, G.A. (1993) Depressive personality in nonclinical subjects. *The American Journal of Psychiatry*, **150**, 1718–1724.

Kleine, S.S. and Baker, S.M. (2004) An integrative review of material possession attachment. *Academy of Marketing Science Review*, **1**, Retrieved from http://www.amsreview.org/articles/kleine01-2004.pdf.

Kleist, H. (1997) *Selected Writings* (ed. and trans. David Constantine) J.M. Dent, London.

Klibansky, R., Panofsky, E. and Saxl, F.I. (1964) *Saturn and Melancholy: Studies in the History of Natural Philosophy, Religion and Art*, Basic Books.

Knapp, M., McCrone, P., Fombonne, E. *et al.* (2002) The Maudsley long-term follow-up of child and adolescent depression: 3. Impact of comorbid conduct disorder on service use and costs in adulthood. *British Journal of Psychiatry*, **180**, 19–23.

Koselleck, R. (2004) *Futures Past: On the Semantics of Historical Time (Studies in Contemporary German Social Thought)*, Columbia University Press.

Koyama, T., McHaffie, J.G., Laurienti, P.J. and Coghill, R.C. (2005) The subjective experience of pain: Where expectations become reality. *Proceedings of the National Academy of Sciences of the United States of America*, **102** (36), 12950–12955.

Kraepelin, E. (1893) *Psychiatrie. Ein Kurzes Lehrbuch fur Studierende and Aerzte, IV Auflage*, Abel, Leipzig.

Kraepelin, E. (1921) *Manic Depressive Insanity and Paranoia*, Livingstone, Edinburgh, UK.

Kraut, R.E. and Johnston, R.E. (1979) Social and emotional messages of smiling: an ethological approach. *Journal of Personality and Social Psychology*, **37**, 1539–1553.

Kretschmer, E. (1926) *Hysteria; Nerv. & Meet. Dis. Mono. Ser. #44*, Nerv. & Men. Dis. Pub. Co, New York.

Kretschmer, E. (1936) *Physique and Character*, Harcourt Brace, New York.

Kringelbach, M.L. and Rolls, E.T. (2004) The functional neuroanatonomy of the human orbitofrontal cortex: evidence from neuroimaging and neuropsychology. *Progress in Neurobiology*, **72**, 341–372.

Kroenke, K., Sharpe, M. and Sykes, R. (2007) Revising the classification of somatoform disorders: key questions and preliminary recommendations. *Psychosomatics*, **48** (4), 277–285.

Kubzansky, L.D., Kawachi, I., Weiss, S.T. and Sparrow, D. (1997) Anxiety and coronary heart disease: a synthesis of epidemiological, psychological and experimental evidence. *Annals of Behavioral Medicine*, **20** (2), 47–58.

Kuchinad, A., Schweinhardt, P., Seminowicz, D.A. *et al.* (2007) Accelerated brain gray matter loss in fibromyalgia patients: premature aging of the brain? *The Journal of Neuroscience*, **27** (15), 4004–4007.

Kuhl, P.K. (2000) A new view of language acquisition. *Proceedings of the National Academy of Science*, **97** (22), 11850–11857.

Kuhl, P.K. and Meltzoff, A.N. (1982) The bimodal perception of speech in infancy. *Science*, **218**, 1138–1141.

Kuhl, P.K. and Meltzoff, A.N. (1996) Infant vocalizations in response to speech: Vocal imitation and developmental change. *The Journal of the Acoustical Society of America*, **100**, 2425–2438.

Kuhl, P.K., Williams, K.A., Lacerda, F. *et al.* (1992) Linguistic experience alters phonetic perception in infants by 6 months of age. *Science*, **255**, 606–608.

Kuhl, K.P. *et al.* (1997) Cross-language analysis of phonetic units in language addressed to infants. *Science*, **277**, 684–686.

Ladee, C.A. (1966) *Hypochondriacal Syndromes*, American Elsevier Publishing Co., Inc, New York.

Lambe, E.K. *et al.* (1997) Cerebral gray matter volume deficits after weight recovery from anorexia nervosa. *Archives of General Psychiatry*, **54**, 537–542.

Lamm, C., Batson, C.D. and Decety, J. (2007) The neural substrate of human empathy: effects of perspective-taking and cognitive appraisal. *Journal of Cognitive Neuroscience*, **19** (1), 42–58.

Larson, C.L., Schaefer, H.S., Siegle, G.J. *et al.* (2006) Fear is fast in phobic individuals: amygdala activation in response to to Fear-Relevant Stimuli. *Biological Psychiatry*, **60**, 410–417.

Latner, J.D. and Clyne, C. (2008) The diagnostic validity of the criteria for binge eating disorder. *The International Journal of Eating Disorders*, **41** (1), 1–14.

Lazarus, R.S. (1991) *Emotion and Adaptation*, Oxford University Press.

Leckman, J.F., Grice, D.E., Boardman, J. *et al.* (1997) Symptoms of obsessive compulsive disorder. *The American Journal of Psychiatry*, **154**, 911–917.

LeDoux, J. (1998) Fear and the brain: where have we been, and where are we going? *Biological Psychiatry*, **44**, 1229–1238.

Leit, A., Pope, H.G. Jr and Gray, J.J. (2001) Cultural expectations of muscularity in men: The evolution of Playgirl centerfolds. *The International Journal of Eating Disorders*, **29** (1), 90–93.

Leslie, K.R., Johnson-Frey, S.H. and Grafton, S.T. (2004) Functional imaging of face and hand imitation: towards a motor theory of empathy. *NeuroImage*, **21**, 601–607.

Levinas, E. (1961) *Totalite' et Infini. Essai sur l'exteriorite'*, Nijhoff. Le Haye.

Levine, J.D., Gordon, N.C., Smith, R. and Fields, H.L. (1982) Post-operative pain: effect of extent of injury and attention. *Brain Research*, **234** (2), 500–504.

Levy, R.I. (1973) *Tahitians*, University of Chicago Press, Chicago.

Levy, E. and Nelson, K. (1994) Words in discourse: A dialectical approach to the acquisition of meaning and use. *Journal of Child Language*, **21**, 367–389.

Lewis, M. (1987) Social development in infancy and early childhood, in *Handbook of Infant Development*, 2nd edn (ed. J. Osofsky), Wiley, New York, pp. 419–493.

Lewis, M. (1992a) Self-conscious emotions and the development of self, in *Affect: Psychoanalytic Perspectives* (eds T. Shapiro and R.N. Emde), International Universities Press, Madison, pp. 45–73.

Lewis, M. (1992b) *Shame: The Exposed Self*, The Free Press, New York.

Lewis, M. (1993a) The emergence of human emotions, in *Handbook of Emotions* (eds M. Lewis and J.M. Haviland), Guildford, New York, pp. 223–235.

Lewis, M. (1993b) Self-conscious emotions: Embarrassment, pride, shame and guilt, in *Handbook of Emotions* (eds M. Lewis and J. Haviland), Guilford, New York, pp. 563–573.

Lewis, M. (1995) Self-conscious emotions. *American Psychologist*, **63**, 68–78.

Lewis, M.D. (2005) Bridging emotion theory and neurobiology through dynamic systems modeling. *Behavioral and Brain Sciences*, **28**, 169–194.

Lewis, M. and Brooks-Gunn, J. (1979) *Social Cognition and the Acquisition of Self*, Plenum Publishing Corporation.

Lewis, M. and Brooks-Gunn, J. (1979) *Social Cognition and the Acquisition of Self*, Plenum, New York.

Lewis, M. and Ramsay, D. (2004) Development of self-recognition, personal pronoun use, and pretend play during the 2nd year. *Child Development*, **75** (6), 1821–1831.

Liberman, A.M. and Whalen, D.H. (2000) On the relation of speech to language. *Trends in Cognitive Sciences*, **4**, 187–196.

Lifton, R.J. (1993) *The Protean Self*, Basic Books, New York.

Lifton, R.J. (1993) *The Protean Self: Human Resilience in an Age of Fragmentation*, Basic Books, New York.

Liotti, M., Mayberg, H.S., McGinnis, S. *et al.* (2002) Unmasking disease-specific cerebral blood flow abnormalities: Mood challenge in patients with Remitted unipolar depression. *The American Journal of Psychiatry*, **159** (11), 1830–1840.

Lipowski, Z.J. (1988) Somatization: The concept and its clinical application. *The American Journal of Psychiatry*, **145**, 1358–1368.

Livet, P. (2006) La fascination de l'auto-organization. Debat, in *L'auto-Organisation* (eds P. Dumouchel and J-.P. Dupuy), Seuil.

Lochner, C. and DaStein, D.J. (2003) Heterogeneity of obsessive-compulsive disorder: a literature review. *Harvard Review of Psychiatry*, **11**, 113–132.

Locke, J.L. (1993) *The Child's Path to Spoken Language*, Harvard University Press, Cambridge, MA.

Locke, G.R., Weaver, A.L., Melton, L.J. and Talley, N.J. (2004) Psychosocial factors are linked to functional gastrointestinal disorders: A population based nested case-control study. *The American Journal of Gastroenterology*, **99** (2), 350–357.

Lorberbaum, J.P. *et al.* (1999) Feasibility of using fMRI to study mothers responding to infant cries. *Depress. Anxiety*, **10**, 99–104.

Lorberbaum, J.P. *et al.* (2002) A potential role for thalamocingulate circuitry in human maternal behavior. *Biological Psychology*, **51**, 431–445.

Lutz, A.C. (1988) *Unnatural Emotions*, The University of Chicago Press.

MacDonald, G. and Leary, M.R. (2005) Why does social exclusion hurt? the relationship between social and physical pain. *Psychological Bulletin*, **131** (2), 202–223.

MacIntyre, A. (1981) *After Virtue*. University of Notre Dame Press. Notre Dame, Indiana.

MacNeilage, F.P. and Davis, L.B. (2000) On the origin of internal structure of word forms. *Science*, **288** (5465), 527–531.

Maddux, W.W., Mullen, E. and Galinsky, A.D. (2008) Chameleons bake bigger pies and take bigger pieces: Strategic behavioral mimicry facilitates negotiation. *Journal of Experimental Social Psychology*, **44** (2), 461–468.

Magai, C. and McFadden, S.H. (1995) *The Role of the Emotion in Social and Personality Research: History, Theory and Research*, Plenum Press, New York.

Mailis-Gagnon, A., Giannoylis, I., Downar, J. *et al.* (2003) Altered central somatosensory processing in chronic pain patients with "hysterical" anesthesia. *Neurology*, **60** (9), 1501–1507.

Maj, M. (2008) Depression, bereavement, and 'understandable' intense sadness: should the DSM-IV approach be revised? *The American Journal of Psychiatry*, **165**, 1373–1375.

Malatesta, C.Z. (1990) The role of emotion in the development and the organization of personality, in *Nebraska Symposium on Motivation*, vol. **36** (ed. R. Thompson), Socioemotional development, University of Nebraska Press, Lincoln, pp. 1–56.

Malatesta, C.Z. and Wilson, A. (1988) Emotion, cognition, interaction in personality development: a discrete emotions, functionalist analysis. *British Journal of Social Psychology*, **27**, 91–112.

Malatesta, C.Z., Fiore, M.J. and Messina, J. (1987) Affect personality and facial expressive charateristics of older individuals. *Psychology and Aging*, **1**, 64–69.

Marcuse, H. (1964) *One Dimensional Man: The Ideology of Industrial Society*, Routledge.

Marin, C. and Carron, R. (2002) The origin of the concept of somatization. *Psychosomatics*, **43** (3), 249–250.

Markou, A., Kosten, T.R. and Koob, G.F. (1998) Neurobiological similarities in depression and drug dependence: a self-medication hypothesis. *Neuropsychopharmacology*, **18**, 135–174.

Markus, H.R. and Kitayama, S. (1991) Culture and the self: Implications for cognition, emotion, and motivation. *Psychological Review*, **98**, 224–253.

Marshall, J.C., Halligan, P.W., Fink, G.R. *et al.* (1997) The functional anatomy of a hysterical paralysis. *Cognition*, **64** (1), B1–B8.

Masataka, N. (1993) Effects of contingent and noncontingent maternal simulation on the vocal behaviour of three- to four-month-old Japanese infants. *Journal of Child Language*, **20**, 303–312.

Masataka, N. (1995) The relation between index-finger extension and the acoustic quality of cooing in three-month-old infants. *Journal of Child Language*, **22** (2), 247–257.

Mataix-Cols, D., Rauch, S.L., Baer, L. *et al.* (2002) Symptom stability in adult obsessive-compulsive disorder: data from a naturalistic two-year follow-up study. *The American Journal of Psychiatry*, **159** (2), 263–268.

Mataix-Cols, D., Wooderson, S., Lawrence, N. *et al.* (2004) Distinct neural correlates of washing, checking, and hoarding symptom dimensions in obsessive-compulsive disorder. *Archives of General Psychiatry*, **61**, 564–576.

Mataix-Cols, D., Rosario-Campos, M.C. and Leckman, J.F. (2005) A multidimensional model of obsessive-compulsive disorder. *The American Journal of Psychiatry*, **162** (2), 228–238.

Mathews, A., Yiend, J. and Lawrence, A.D. (2004) Individual differences in the modulation of fear-related brain activation by attentional control. *Journal of Cognitive Neuroscience*, **16**, 1683–1694.

Maturana, H.R. (1988) Ontology of observing. The biological foundations of self consciousness and the physical domain of existence. Conference Workbook: Texts in Cybernetics, American Society For Cibernetics Conference, Felton, CA. 18–23 October, 1988.

Maturana, R.H. (1994) Reality: the search for objectivity, or the quest for a compelling argument, Unpublished manuscript.

Mayberg, H.S. (1997) Limbic-cortical dysregulation: a proposed model of depression. *Journal of Neuropsychiatry and Clinical Neurosciences*, **9**, 471–481.

Mayberg, H.S. (2003) Modulating dysfunctional limbic-cortical circuits in depression: towards development of brain-based algorithms for diagnosis and optimised treatment. *British Medical Bulletin*, **65**, 193–207.

Mayberg, H.S., Liotti, M., Brannan, S.K. *et al.* (1999) Reciprocal limbic-cortical function and negative mood: converging PET findings in depression and normal sadness. *The American Journal of Psychiatry*, **156**, 675–682.

Mayberg, H.S., Brannan, S.K., Mahurin, R.K. *et al.* (2000) Regional metabolic effects of fluoxetine in major depression: serial changes and relationship to clinical response. *Biological Psychiatry*, **48**, 830–843.

Mayberg, H.S., Lozano, A.M., Voon, V. *et al.* (2005) Deep brain stimulation for treatment-resistant depression. *Neuron*, **45** (5), 651–660.

Mayou, R., Kirmayer, L.J., Simon, G. *et al.* (2005) Somatoform disorders: time for a new approach in DSM-V. *The American Journal of Psychiatry*, **162** (5), 847–855.

Mazzola, V., Latorre, V., Tomasevic, L. *et al.* (2009) Two self-referential modes of processing modulate the affective component of pain (submitted).

McCabe, R.E. and Boivin, M. (2008) Eating disorders, in *Clinical Handbook of Obsessive-Compulsive Disorder and Related Problems* (eds J.S. Abramowitz, D. McKay and S. Taylor), The John Hopkins University Press.

McCarthy, G., Puce, A., Gore, J.C. and Allison, T. (1997) Face-specific processing in the human fusiform gyrus. *Journal of Cognitive Neuroscience*, **9**, 605–610.

McCulloch, S.W. (1965) *Embodiments of Mind*, MIT.

McDermut, W., Zimmerman, M. and Chelminski, I. (2003) The construct validity of depressive personality disorder. *Journal of Abnormal Psychology*, **112**, 49–60.

McKay, D., Abramowitz, J.S., Calamari, J.E. *et al.* (2004) A critical evaluation of obsessive–compulsive disorder subtypes: Symptoms versus mechanisms. *Clinical Psychology Review*, **24**, 283–313.

McMurray, B. (2007) Defusing the childhood vocabulary explosion. *Science*, **317**, 631.

McNally, R.J. (2002) Anxiety sensitivity and panic disorder. *Biological Psychiatry*, **52**, 938–946.

Meister, G., Wilson, S.M., Deblieck, C. *et al.* (2007) The essential role of premotor cortex in speech perception. *Current Biol.*, **17**, 1692–1696.

Meltzoff, A.N. (1990) Foundations for developing a concept of self: The role of imitation in relating self to other and the value of social mirroring, social modeling, and self practice in infancy, in *The Self in Transition: Infancy to Childhood* (eds D. Cicchetti and M. Beeghly), University of Chicago Press, Chicago.

Meltzoff, N.A. (2007) Like Me: a foundation for social cognition. *Developmental Science*, **10** (1), 126–134.

Meltzoff, A.N. and Moore, M.K. (1977). Imitation of facial and manual gestures by human neonates, *Science*, **198**, 75–78.

Meltzoff, A.N. and Moore, M.K. (1983). Newborn infants imitate adult facial gestures, *Child Development*, **54**, 702–709.

Merckelbach, De Jong, Muris and Van den Hout, (1996), The etiology of specific phobias: A review.*Psychology Review*, **1–6**, 337–361.

Merleau-Ponty, M. (1945) *Phenomenologie de la Perception*, Gallimard, Paris.

Merleau-Ponty, M. (1962) *Phenomenology of Perception*, Routledge & Kegan Paul.

Merleau-Ponty, M. (1969) *La Prose Du Monde*, Gallimard.

Merskey, H. (1995) *The Analysis of Hysteria: Understanding Conversion and Dissociation*, Gaskell, London.

Messner, R. (2006) *La Mia Vita al Limite*, Corbaccio.

Mestrovic, G.S. (1997) *Postemotional Society*, Sage, London.

Miller, P.A. and Eisenberg, N. (1988) The relation of empathy to aggressive and externalizing/antisocial behavior. *Psychological Bulletin*, **103** (3), 324–344.

Miltenberger, R.G., Redlin, J., Crosby, R. *et al.* (2003) Direct and retrospective assessment of factors contributing to compulsive buying. *Journal of Behavior Therapy and Experimental Psychiatry*, **34**, 1–9.

Mink, O.L. (1970) History and fiction as modes of comprehension. *New Literary History*, **1**, 541–558.

Mink, O.L. (1972) Interpretation and narrative understanding. *The Journal of Philosophy*, **69** (9), 735–737.

Mitchell, J.E., Hatsukami, D., Eckert, E.D. and Pyle, R.L. (1985) Characteristics of 275 patients with bulimia. *The American Journal of Psychiatry*, **142** (4), 482–485.

Mizes, J.S. (1988) Personality characteristics of bulimic and noneating-disordered female controls: A. cognitive behavioral perspective. *International Journal of Eating Disorders*, **7** (4), 541–550.

Mobbs, D., Petrovic, P., Marchant, J.L. *et al.* (2007) When fear is near: threat imminence elicits prefrontal-periaqueductal gray shifts in humans. *Science*, **317** (5841), 1079.

Molnar-Szakacs, I., Iacoboni, M., Koski, L. *et al.* (2002) Action observation in the pars opercularis: evidence from 58 subjects studied with fMRI. Annual Meeting of the Cognitive Neuroscience Society, 2002.

Moore, C., Mealiea, J., Garon, N. and Povinelli, D.J. (2007) The development of body self-awareness. *Infancy*, **11** (2), 157–174.

Mori, D., Chaiken, S. and Pliner, P. (1987) "Eating lightly" and the self-presentation of femininity. *Journal of Personality and Social Psychology*, **53**, 693–702.

Moriguchi, Y., Decety, J., Ohnishi, T. et al. (2006) *Empathy and Judging Other's Pain: An fMRI Study of Alexithymia*, Cerebral Cortex.

Mottaghy, F.M., Keller, C.E., Gangitano, M. *et al.* (2002) Correlation of cerebral blood flow and treatment effects of repetitive transcranial magnetic stimulation in depressed patients. *Psychiatry Research*, **115**, 1–14.

Mounier, E. (1946) *Traité du Caractère*, Ed. du Seuil.

Mountz, J.M., Modell, J.G., Wilson, M.W. *et al.* (1989) Positron emission tomographic evaluation of cerebral blood flow during state anxiety in simple phobia. *Archives of General Psychiatry*, **46**, 501–504.

Muhlau, M. *et al.* (2007) Gray matter decrease of the anterior cingulate cortex in anorexia nervosa. *The American Journal of Psychiatry*, **164**, 1850–1857.

Muir, D. and Hains, S. (1999) Young infants' perception of adult intentionality: Adult contingency and eye direction, in *Early Social Cognition: Understanding Others in the First Months of Life* (ed. P. Rochat), Lawrence Erlbaum, Mahwah, NJ, pp. 155–187.

Mumford, D.B., Bavington, K.S., Hussain, B.Y. *et al.* (1991) the Bradford somatic inventory. a multi-ethnic inventory of somatic symptoms reported by anxious and depressed patients in Britain and the indo-pakistan subcontinent. *British Journal of Psychiatry*, **158**, 379–386.

Murphy, M.R. *et al.* (1981) Species-typical behavior of hamsters deprived from birth of the neocortex. *Science*, **213**, 459–461.

Murray, E.A., O'Doherty, J.P. and Schoenbaum, G. (2007) What we know and do not know about the functions of the orbitofrontal cortex after 20 years of cross-species studies. *The Journal of Neuroscience*, **27**, 8166–8169.

Najib, A., Lorberbaum, J.P., Kose, S. *et al.* (2004) Regional brain activity in women grieving a romantic relationship. *The American Journal of Psychiatry*, **161** (12), 2245–2256.

Neisser, U. (1994) Self perception and self knowledge. *Psyche & Logos*, **15**, 392–407.

Nelson, K. (1985) *Making Sense: The Acquisition of Shared Meaning*, Academic Press.

Nelson, K. (1993) The psychological and social origins of autobiographical memory. *Psychological Science*, **4**, 1–8.

Nelson, K. (1996) *Language in Cognitive Development: The Emergence of the Mediated Mind*, Cambridge University Press, Cambridge.

Nelson, K. (2001) Language and the self: from the "Experiencing I" to the "Continuing Me", in *The Self in Time* (eds C. Moore and K. Lemmon), Erlbaum, Hillsdale, NJ, pp. 15–34.

Nelson, K. (2006) *Narratives from the Crib*, Harvard University Press.

Nelson, K. and Fivush, R. (2004) The emergence of autobiographical memory: a social cultural developmental theory. *Psychological Review*, **111**, 486–511.

Neumeister, A., Nugent, A.C., Waldeck, T. *et al.* (2004) Neural and behavioral responses to tryptophan depletion in unmedicated patients with remitted major depressive disorder and controls. *Archives of General Psychiatry*, **61** (8), 765–773.

Niedenthal, M.P. (2007) Embodying emotion. *Science*, **316**, 1002–1005.

Niedenthal, P.M., Barsalou, L.W. and Winkielman, P. (2005) Embodiment in attitudes, social perception, and emotion. *Personality and Social Psychology Review*, **9**, 184–211.

Nielsen, M., Suddendorf, T. and Slaughter, V. (2006) Mirror self-recognition beyond the face. *Child Development*, **77** (1), 176–185.

Nishitani, N., Schurmann, M., Amunts, K. and Hari, R. (2005) Broca's region: From action to language. *Physiology*, **20**, 60–69.

Nobler, M.S., Oquendo, M.A., Kegeles, L.S. *et al.* (2001) Decreased regional brain metabolism after ECT. *The American Journal of Psychiatry*, **158**, 305–308.

Noë, A. (2004) *Action in Perception*, MIT.

Northoff, G., Heinzel, A., de Greck, M. *et al.* (2006) Self- referential processing in our brain: A meta-analysis of imaging studies on the self. *NeuroImage*, **31**, 440–457.

Norwood, R. (1985) *Women Who Love Too Much*, Jeremy P, Los Angeles, CA.

O'Doherty, J., Kringelbach, M.L., Rolls, E.T. *et al.* (2001) Abstract reward and punishment representations in the human orbitofrontal cortex. *Nature Neuroscience*, **4**, 95–102.

O'Guinn, T.C. and Faber, R.J. (1989) Compulsive buying: a phenomenological exploration. *Journal of Consumer Research*, **16** (2), 147–157.

Öhman, A. and Mineka, S. (2001) Fears, phobias, and preparedness: toward an evolved module of fear and fear learning. *Psychological Review*, **108**, 483–522.

Olivardia, R., Pope, H.G. and Hudson, J.I. (2000) Muscle dysmorphia in male weightlifters: A case-control study. *American Journal of Psychiatry*, **157**, 1291–1296.

Olivardia, R., Pope, H.G. Jr, Borowiecki, J.J. III and Cohane, G.H. (2004) Biceps and body image: the relationship between muscularity and self-esteem, depression, and eating disorder symptoms. *Psychology of Men & Masculinity*, **5** (2), 112–120.

Otto, M.W., Pollack, M.H., Sachs, G.S. and Rosenbaum, J.F. (1992) Hypochondriacal concerns, anxiety, sensitivity, and panic disorder. *Journal of Anxiety Disorders*, **8**, 97–99.

Panksepp, J. (1998) *Affective Neuroscience*, Oxford University Press.

Panksepp, J. (2005) Why does separation distress hurt? comment on Macdonald and Leary. *Psychological Bulletin*, **131** (2), 224–230.

Pannekamp, A., Weber, C. and Friederici, D.A. (2006) Prosodic processing at the sentence level in infants. *Neuroreport*, **17** (6), 675–678.

Papousek, M. and Papousek, H. (1989) Forms and functions of vocal matching in interactions between mothers and their precanonical infants. *First Language*, **9** (6), 137–157.

Paquette, V., Levesque, J., Mensour, B. *et al.* (2003) Change the mind and you change the brain: effects of cognitive–behavioral therapy on the neural correlates of spider phobia. *NeuroImage*, **18**, 401–409.

Parker, G. (1983) Parental 'affectionless control' as an antecedent to adult depression. *Archives of General Psychiatry*, **34**, 138–147.

Parker, G., Hadzi-Pavlovic, D., Greenwald, S. and Weissman, M. (1995) Low parental care as a risk factor to lifetime depression in a community sample. *Journal of Affective Disorders*, **33**, 173–180.

Parkinson, B., Fischer, H.A. and Manstead, S.R.A. (2005) *Emotion in Social Relations*, Psychology Press.

Parkinson, B. (1995). *Ideas and realities of emotion*. London: Routledge.

Paul, T., Schroeter, K., Dahme, B. and Nutzinger, D.O. (2002) Self-injurious behavior in women with eating disorders. *The American Journal of Psychiatry*, **159**, 408–411.

Pennebaker, J.W., Gonder-Frederick, L., Cox, D.J. and Hoover, C.W. (1985) The perception of general vs. specific visceral activity and the regulation of health-related behavior. *Advances in Behavioral Medicine*, **1**, 165–198.

Perlman, D. and Peplau, L.A. (1981) Towards a social psychology of loneliness, in *Personal Relationships in Disorder* (eds S. Duck and R. Gilmour), Academic Press.

Perna, G., Bertani, A., Politi, E. *et al.* (1997) Asthma and panic attacks. *Biological Psychiatry*, **42** (7), 625–630.

Pessoa, F. (1989) *Faust*, Einaudi.

Pessoa, L. (2008) On the relationship between emotion and cognition. *Nature Reviews. Neuroscience*, **9**, 148–158.

Petrovic, P., Kalso, E., Petersson, K.M. and Ingvar, M. (2002) Placebo and opioid analgesia – imaging a shared neuronal network. *Science*, **295**, 1737–1740.

Phan, K.L., Fitzgerald, D.A., Nathan, P.J. and Tancer, M.E. (2006) Association between amygdala hyperactivity to harsh faces and severity of social anxiety in generalized social phobia. *Biological Psychiatry*, **59**, 424–429.

Phillips, K.A., Hirschfeld, R.M.A., Shea, M.T. and Gunderson, J.G. (1993) Depressive personality disorder: Perspectives for DSM-IV. *Journal of Personality Disorders*, **7**, 30–42.

Phillips, K.A., Gunderson, J.G., Triebwasser, J. *et al.* (1998) Reliability and validity of depressive personality disorder. *The American Journal of Psychiatry*, **155**, 1044–1048.

Phillips, M.L., Marks, I.M., Senior, C. *et al.* (2000) A differential neural response in obsessive-compulsive disorder patients with washing compared with checking symptoms to disgust. *Psychological Medicine*, **30**, 1037–1050.

Picardi, A. (2003) First step in the assessment of cognitive-emotional organisations within the framework of Guidano's model of the self. *Psychoter Psychosom*, **72**, 363–365.

Pies, R. (2007) The historical roots of the "bipolar spectrum": Did Aristotle anticipate Kraepelin's broad concept of manic-depression? *Journal of Affective Disorders*, **100** (1–3), 7–11.

Pieters, G.L., de Bruijn, E.R., Maas, Y. *et al.* (2007) Action monitoring and perfectionism in anorexia. *Brain and Cognition*, **63**, 42–50.

Pirandello, L. (1994) *Novelle per un anno* (3 vol.), Giunti.

Platek, S.M., Myers, T.E. and Gallup, G.G. Jr (2004) Cross-modal self-recognition: The role of visual, auditory, and olfactory primes. *Consciousness and Cognition*, **13**, 197–210.

Platek, M.S., Loughead, W.J., Gur, C.R. *et al.* (2006) Neural substrates for functionally discriminating self-face from personally familiar faces. *Human Brain Mapping*, **27** (2), 91–98.

Ploghaus, A., Tracey, I., Gati, J.S. *et al.* (1999) Dissociating pain from its anticipation in the human brain. *Science*, **284**, 1979–1981.

Polanyi, M. (1958) *Personal Knowledge: Towards a Post-Critical Philosophy*, Routledge & Kegan Paul, London.

Polanyi, M. (1966) *The Tacit Dimension*, Anchor Books, New York.

Polanyi, M. (1969) *Knowing and Being*, The University of Chicago Press.

Polivy, J. and Herman, C.P. (1985) Dieting and binging: A causal analysis. *American Psychologist*, **40** (2), 193–201.

Pollard, A.C., Pollard, H.J. and Corn, K.J. (1989) Panic onset and major events in the lives of agoraphobics: a test of contiguity. *Journal of Abnormal Psychology*, **3**, 318–321.

Pollatos, O., Kirsch, W. and Schandry, R. (2005) On the relationship between interoceptive awareness, emotional experience, and brain processes. *Brain Research. Cognitive Brain Research*, **25** (3), 948–962.

Pollatos, O., Kurz, A., Albrecht, J. *et al.* (2008) Reduced perception of bodily signals in anorexia nervosa. *Eating Behaviours*, **9** (4), 381–388.

Pope, H.G. Jr and Katz, D.L. (1994) Psychiatric and medical effects of anabolic- androgenic steroid use: a controlled study of 160 athletes. *Archives of General Psychiatry*, **51**, 375–382.

Pope, H.G. Jr, Katz, D.L. and Hudson, J.I. (1993) Anorexia nervosa and "reverse anorexia" among 108 male bodybuilders. *Comprehensive Psychiatry*, **34**, 406–409.

Pope, H.G. Jr, Olivardia, R., Gruber, A. and Borowiecki, J. (1999) Evolving ideals of male body image as seen through action toys. *The International Journal of Eating Disorders*, **26** (1), 65–72.

Pope, H.G., Phillips, K.A. and Olivardia, R. (2000) *The Adonis Complex: The Secret Crisis of Male Body Obsession*, Free Press, New York.

Pope, H.G. Jr, Lalonde, J.K., Pindyck, L.J. *et al.* (2006) Binge eating disorder: a stable syndrome. *The American Journal of Psychiatry*, **163** (12), 2181–2183.

Porges, S.W. (1993) *Body Perception Questionnaire. Laboratory of Developmental Assessment*, University of Maryland.

Porro, C.A., Cettolo, V., Francescato, M.P. and Baraldi, P. (2003) Functional Activity Mapping of the Mesial Hemispheric Wall During Anticipation of Pain. *NeuroImage*, **19**, 1738–1747.

Post, R.M. (1992) Transduction of psychosocial stress into the neurobiology of recurrent affective disorder. *The American Journal of Psychiatry*, **149** (88), 999–1010.

Povinelli, D.J. (2000) *Folk Physics for Apes: The Chimpanzee's Theory of How the World Works*, Oxford University Press, Oxford.

Povinelli, D.J. and Cant, J.G.H. (1995) Arboreal clambering and the evolution of self-conception. *Quarterly Review of Biology*, **70**, 393–421.

Povinelli, D.J. and Prince, C.G. (1998) When self met other, in *Self-Awareness: Its Nature and Development* (eds M. Ferrari and R.J. Sternberg), Guilford Press, New York, pp. 37–107

Povinelli, D.J. and Simon, B.B. (1998) Young children's understanding of briefly versus extremely delayed images of the self: Emergence of the autobiographical stance. *Developmental Psychology*, **34**, 188–194.

Povinelli, D.J., Landau, K.R. and Perilloux, H.K. (1996) Self-recognition in young children using delayed versus live feedback: Evidence of a developmental asynchrony. *Child Development*, **67**, 1540–1554.

Povinelli, D.J., Landry, A.M., Theall, L.A. *et al.* (1999) Development of young children's understanding that the recent past is causally bound to the present. *Developmental Psychology*, **35**, 1426–1439.

Power, M.J. and Dalgleish, T. (2007) *Cognition and Emotion*, Psychology Press.

Premack, D. and Woodruff, G. (1978) Does the chimpanzee have a theory of mind? *The Behavioral and Brain Sciences*, **1** (4), 515.

Preston, S.D. and de Waal, F.B.M. (2002) Empathy: Its ultimate and proximate bases. *The Behavioral and brain sciences*; **25** (1), 1–20

Prinz, J. (2003) Emotion, psychosemantics, and embodied appraisals, in *Philosophy and the Emotions* (ed. A. Hatzimoysis), Cambridge University Press.

Prinz, J. (2004a) Embodied emotions, in *Thinking About Feeling: Contemporary Philosophers on Emotions* (ed. R.C. Solomon), Oxford University Press, Oxford, pp. 89–105.

Prinz, J. (2004b) *Gut Reactions: A Perceptual Theory of Emotion*, Oxford University Press, Oxford.

Prkachin, K., Mass, H. and Mercer, S. (2004) Effects of exposure on perception of pain expression. *PAIN*, **111** (1–2), 8–12.

Probst, M., Vandereycken, W., Vanderlinden, J. and Van Coppenolle, H. (1998) The significance of body size estimation in eating disorder: its relationship with clinical and psychological variables. *The International Journal of Eating Disorders*, **24** (2), 167–174.

Proust, M. (1927) A propos du "style" de Flaubert, in *Chroniques*, Gallimard, Paris.

Pulvermuller, F. (2001) Braian reflections of words and their meaning. *Trends in Cognitive Sciences*, **5**, 517–524.

Pulvermuller, F. (2002) *The Neuroscience of Language*, Cambridge University Press, Cambridge, UK.

Pulvermuller, F. (2005) Brain mechanism linking language and action. *Nature Neurosc, Reviews*, **6**, 576–582.

Pulvermüller, F., Huss, M., Kherif, F. *et al.* (2006) Motor cortex maps articulatory features of speech sounds. *Proceedings of the National Academy of Sciences of the United States of America*, **103** (20), 7865–7870.

Pyszczynski, T. and Greenberg, J. (1987) Self-regulatory perseveration and the depressive self-focusing style: A self-awareness theory of reactive depression. *Psychological Bulletin*, **102** (1), 122–138.

Pyszczynski, T., Hamilton, J.C., Herring, F.H. and Greemberg, J. (1989) Depression, self focused attention, and the negative memory bias. *Journal of Personality and Social Psychology*, **57** (2), 351–357.

Quevedo, A.S. and Coghill, R.C. (2007) Attentional modulation of spatial integration of pain: evidence for dynamic spatial tuning. *Journal of Neuroscience*, **27** (43), 11635–11640.

Rachilde (2004) *Monsieur Venus: A Materialist Novel* (MLA Texts and Translations), The Modern Language Association of America, New York.

Raffoul, F. (2004) A chaque fois mien. Editions Galilee. Paris

Raichle, M.E., MacLeod, A.M., Snyder, A.Z. *et al.* (2001) A default mode of brain function. *Proceedings of the National Academy of Sciences of the United States of America*, **98**, 676–682.

Rainville, P. (2002) Brain mechanisms of pain affect and pain modulation. *Current Opinion in Neurobiology*, **12**, 195–204.

Rainville, P. (2008) Hypnosis and the analgesic effect of suggestions. *Pain*, **134**, 1.

Rainville, P., Duncan, G.H., Price, D.D. *et al.* (1997) Pain affect encoded in human anterior cingulate but not somatosensory cortex. *Science*, **277**, 968–971.

Rainville, P., Bechara, A., Naqvi, N. and Damasio, A.R. (2006) Basic emotions are associated with distinct patterns of cardiorespiratory activity. *International Journal of Psychophysiology*, **61**, 5–18.

Rasmussen, S.A. and Eisen, J.L. (1989) Clinical features and phenomenology of obsessive-compulsive disorder. *Psychiatric Annals*, **19**, 67–72.

Rasmussen, S. and Eisen, J.L. (1991) Phenomenology of OCD: clinical subtypes, heterogeneity and coexistence, in *The Psychobiology of Obsessive–Compulsive Disorder* (eds J. Zohar, T. Insel and S.A. Rasmussen), Springer, New York.

Rasmussen, S. and Eisen, J. (1992) The epidemiology and differential diagnosis of obsessive compulsive disorder. *The Journal of Clinical Psychiatry*, **53**, 4–10.

Rauch, S.L., Savage, C.R., Alpert, N.M. *et al.* (1995) A positron emission tomographic study of simple phobic symptom provocation. *Archives of General Psychiatry*, **52**, 20–28.

Rauch, S.L., Whalen, P.J., Shin, L.M. *et al.* (2000) Exaggerated amygdala response to masked facial stimuli in posttraumatic stress disorder: a functional MRI study. *Biological Psychiatry*, **47**, 769–776.

Reddy, V. (2003) On being the object of attention: implications for self–other consciousness. *Trends in Cognitive Science*, **9**, 397–402.

Reddy, V. (2005) Feeling shy and showing-off; self-conscious emotions must regulate self-awareness, in *Emotional Development* (eds J. Nadel and D. Muir), Oxford University Press.

Reese, E. (2002) Social factors in the development of autobiographical memory: The state of the art. *Social Development*, **11**, 124–142.

Reiman, E.M. (1997) The application of positron emission tomography to the study of normal and pathologic emotions. *Journal of Clinical Psychiatry*, **58** (Suppl 16), 4–12.

Reisman, D. (1961) *The Lonely Crowd*, Yale University Press, New Haven and London.

Reiss, S. (1991) Expectancy theory of fear, anxiety, and panic. *Clinical Psychology Review*, **11**, 141–153.

Reiss, S. and McNally, R.J. (1985) Expectancy model of fear, in *Theoretical Issues in Behavior Therapy* (eds S. Reiss and R.R. Bootzin), Academic Press, New York, pp. 107–121.

Reiss, S., Peterson, R.A., Gursky, D.M. and McNally, R.J. (1986) Anxiety sensitivity, anxiety frequency, and the prediction of fearfulness. *Behaviour Research and Therapy*, **24**, 1–8.

Ribot, T. (1904) Les Maladies de la Volonte. Paris, Alcan.

Ricciardelli, L.A. and McCabe, M.P. (2001) Self-esteem and negative affect as moderators of sociocultural influences on body dissatisfaction, strategies to decrease weight, and strategies to increase muscles among adolescent boys and girls. *Sex Roles*, **44**, 189–207.

Ricciardelli, L.A. and McCabe, M.P. (2004) A biopsychosocial model of disordered eating and the pursuit of muscularity in adolescent boys. *Psychological Bulletin*, **130** (2), 179–205.

Richards, J., Cooper, A. and Winkelman, J. (2003) Interoceptive accuracy in nonclinical panic. *Cognitive Therapy and Research*, **27** (4), 447–461.

Ricoeur, P. (1969) *Le conflit des interpretations*, (trad it. Balzaotti, Botturi, Colombo), Edition du Seuil, Paris.

Ricoeur, P. (1976) *Interpretation Theory*, Texas Christian University Press.

Ricoeur, P. (1980) *Narrative time. On Narrative* (ed. W.J.T. Mitchell), The University of Chicago Press.

Ricoeur, P. (1984) *Time and Narrative*, vol. 1, Univ. of Chicago Press.

Ricoeur, P. (1990) *Soi-Meme Comme un Autre*, Edition du Seuil, Paris.

Ricoeur, P. (1995) *Oneself as Another*, University of Chicago Press.

Riegler, A. (2003) The Key to Radical Constructivism. http://www.univie.ac.at/Constructivism/key.html.

Rilke, R.M. (1939) *Duino Elegies*, Norton, New York.

Rilke, R.M. (2003) *Die Erzälungen*, Insel, Frankfurt.

Rizzolatti, G. (2005) The mirror neuron system and imitation, in *Perspectives on Imitation: from Neuroscience to Social* (eds S. Harley and N. Chater), MIT Press.

Rizzolatti, G. and Craighero, L. (2004) The mirror neuron system. *Annual Review of Neuroscience*, **27**, 169–192.

Rizzolatti, G. and Gallese, V. (1997) From action to meaning, in *Les Neurosciences et la Philosohie de L'action* (ed. Jean-Luc Petit) VRIN.

Rizzolatti, G. and Sinigaglia, C. (2006) *So Quel che Fai. Il Cervello Che Agisce e i Neuroni Specchio*, Raffaello Cortina. Editore, Milano.

Rizzolatti, G. *et al.* (1996) Premotor cortex and the recognition of motor actions, Cognitive. *Brain Research*, **3**, 131–141.

Rizzolatti, G., Fadiga, L., Gallese, V. and Fogassi, L. (1996) Premotor cortex and the recognition of motor actions. *Cognitive Brain Research*, **3**, 131–141.

Rogoff, B. *et al.* (1996) Developmental transitions in children's partecipation in sociocultural activities, in *The Five to Seven Year Shift* (eds A.J. Sameroff and M.H. Haith), University of Chicago Press, Chicago.

Ron, M.A. (1996) Somatisation and conversion disorders, in *Neuropsychiatry* (eds B.S. Fogel, R.B. Schiffer in S.M. Rao), Williams and Williams, Baltimore, MD.

Rosen, B.C. (2001) *Masks and Mirrors: Generation X and the Chameleon Personality*, Westport, London.

Rosen, B.C. and Aneshensel, C.S. (1976) The chameleon syndrome: a social dimension of the female sex role. *Journal of Marriage and the Family*, **38**, 605–617.

Roy, A., Adinoff, B., Roehrich, L. *et al.* (1988) Pathological gambling. A psychobiological study. *Archives of General Psychiatry*, **45** (4), 369–373.

Roy-Byrne, P., Geraci, M. and Uhde, T. (1986) Life events and the onset of panic disorder. *The American Journal of Psychiatry*, **143** (11), 1424–1427.

Rubin, D.C. (ed.) (1986) *Autobiographical Memory*, Cambridge University Press, New York.

Rubin, D.C. (ed.) (1996) *Remembering Our Past*, Cambridge University Press.

Rubino, V., Blasi, G., Latorre, V., Fazio, L. *et al.* (2007) Activity in medial prefrontal cortex during cognitive evaluation of threatening stimuli as a function of personality style. *Brain Research Bulletin*, **74**, 250.

Ruby, P. and Decety, J. (2004) How would you feel versus how do you think she would feel? A neuroimaging study of perspective taking with social emotions. *Journal of Cognitive Neuroscience*, **16**, 988–999.

Ruby, P., Decety, J. Effect of subjective perspective taking during simulation of action: a PET investigation of agency. *Nature Neuroscience*, 2001, **4** (5), 546–550.

Ruby, P., Decety, J. What do you believe versus what do you think they believe: A neuroimaging study of conceptual perspective taking. *European Journal of Neuroscience*, 2003, **17** (11), 2475–2480.

Rufer, M., Grothusen, A., Maß, R. *et al.* (2005) Temporal stability of symptom dimensions in adult patients with obsessive–compulsive disorder. *Journal of Affective Disorders*, **88**, 99–102.

Ruiz-Belda, M.A., Fernández-Dols, J.-M., Carrera, P. and Barchard, K. (2003) Spontaneous facial expressions of happy bowlers and soccer fans. *Cognition & Emotion*, **17**, 315–326.

Russell, J.A. and Fernández-Dols, J.M. (1997) What does a facial expression mean? in *The Psychology of Facial Expression* (eds J.A. Russell and J.M. Fernández Dols), Cambridge University Press.

Russell, J., Bachorowski, J. and Fernandez-Dols, J.-M. (2003) Facial and vocal expressions of emotion. *Annual review of psychology*. **54**, 329–349.

Ryder, A.G. and Bagby, R.M. (1999) Diagnostic viability of depressive personality disorder: theoretical and conceptual issues. *Journal of Personality Disorders*, **13**, 99–117.

Ryder, A.G., Bagby, R.M. and Schuller, D.R. (2002) Differentiating depressive personality disorder and dysthyrnia: a categorical problem with a dimensional solution. *Harvard Review of Psychiatry*, **10**, 337–352.

Ryder, A.G., Bagby, R.M., Marshall, M. and Costa, P.T. Jr (2005) The Depressive personality: psychopathology, assessment and treatment, in *Depression and Personality: Conceptual and Clinical Challenges* (eds M. Rosenbluth, S.H. Kennedy and R.M. Bagby), American Psychiatric Press, Washington, DC.

Salkovskis, P.M. (1985) Obsessional-compulsive problems: a cognitive-behavioural analysis. *Behaviour Research and Therapy*, **23**, 71–583.

Salkovskis, P.M. (1989) Cognitive-behavioural factors and the persistence of intrusive thoughts in obsessional problems. *Behaviour Research and Therapy*, **27** (6), 677–682.

Salkovskis, P.M., Clark, D.M. and Gelder, M.G. (1996) Cognition-behaviour links in the persistence of panic. *Behaviour Research and Therapy*, **34** (5–6), 453–458.

Santonastaso, P., Ferrara, S. and Favaro, A. (1999) Differences between binge eating disorder and nonpurging bulimia nervosa. *International Journal of Eating Disorders*, **25**, 215–218.

Saper, C. (2002) The central autonomic nervous system: conscious visceral perception and autonomic pattern generation. *Annual Review of Neuroscience*, **25**, 433–469.

Sarkar, S., Aziz, Q., Woolf, C.J. *et al.* (2000) Contribution of central sensitization to the development of non-cardiac chest pain. *Lancet*, **356**, 1154–1159.

Sartre, J.-P. (1948) The emotions, in *Outline of a Theory*, Philosophical Library, NY.

Saxena, S., Brody, A.L., Schwartz, J.M. and Baxter, L.R. (1998) Neuroimaging and frontal–subcortical circuitry in obsessive-compulsive disorder. *British Journal of Psychiatry*, (Supplement), 26–37.

Saxena, S., Bota, R.G. and Brody, A.L. (2001) Brain–behavior relationships in obsessive-compulsive disorder. *Seminars in Clinical Neuropsychiatry*, **6**, 82–101.

Saxena, S., Brody, A.L., Maidment, K.M. *et al.* (2004) Cerebral glucose metabolism in obsessive-compulsive hoarding. *The American Journal of Psychiatry*, **161**, 1038–1048.

Scaife, M. and Bruner, S.J. (1975) The capacity for joint visual attention in the infant. *Nature*, **253**, 265–266.

Scarantino, A. (2005) Explicating Emotions, http://etd.library.pitt.edu.

Schachter, S. and Singer, J.E. (1962) Cognitive, social and physiological determinants of emotional state. *Psychological Review*, **69**, 379–399.

Schacter, L.D., Addis, R.D. and Buckner, L.R. (2007) Remembering the past to imagine the future: the prospective brain. *Nature Reviews Neuroscience*, **8**, 657–660.

Schaible, H.G., Ebersberger, A. and Von Banchet, G.S. (2002) Mechanismsof pain in arthritis. *Annals of the New York Academy of Sciences*, **966**, 343–354.

Schapp, W. (1976) Geschichten verstrickt, in *Zum Sein von Mensch und Ding*, B. Heymann, Wiesbaden.

Scher, C.D., Ingram, R.E. and Segal, Z.V. (2005) Cognitive reactivity and vulnerability: empirical evaluation of construct activation and cognitive diatheses in unipolar depression. *Clinical Psychology Review*, **25**, 487–510.

Scherhorn, G., Reisch, L.A. and Raab, G. (1990) Addictive buying in West Germany: An empirical study. *Journal of Consumer Policy*, **13**, 355–388.

Schlesier-Stropp, B. (1984) Bulimia: A review of the literature. *Psychological Bulletin*, **95**, 247–257.

Schmidt, N.B., Lerew, D.R. and Joiner, T.E. Jr (2000) Prospective evaluation of the etiology of anxiety sensitivity: Test of a scar model. *Behaviour Research and Therapy*, **38** (11), 1083–1095.

Schmidt, N.B., Lerew, D.R. and Jackson, R.J. (1997). The role of anxiety sensitivity in the pathogenesis of panic: Prospective evaluation of spontaneous panic attacks during acute stress. *Journal of abnormal psychology*. 1997, **106** (3), 355–364.

Schmidt, N.B., Lerew, D.R., and Jackson, R.J. (1999). Prospective evaluation of anxiety sensitivity in the pathogenesis of panic: replication and extension. *Journal of abnormal psychology*. **108** (3), 532–537.

Schmidt, N.B. and Trakowski, J.H. (1999). Attentional focus and fearful responding in patients with panic disorder during a 35% CO_2 challenge. *Behavior therapy*, **30** (4), 623–640.

Schneider, K. (1959) *Clinical Psychopathology*, Grune & Stratton, London.

Schneider, J.A. and Agras, W.S. (1987) Bulimia in males: a matched comparison with females. *International Journal of Eating Disorders*, **6**, 235–242.

Schneider, K. and Unzner, L. (1992) Preschoolers' attention and emotion in an achievement and an effect game: A longitudinal study. *Cognition & Emotion*, **6**, 37–63.

Sedikides, C. (1992) Mood as a determinant of attentional focus. *Cognition & Emotion*, **6** (22), 129–148.

Selvini Palazzoli, M. (1963–1981) *L'anoressia Mentale*, Feltrinelli, Milano.

Semerano, G. (1994) *Le origini della cultura europea*, vol. **2/1**, Dizionari etimolgici. Basi semantiche delle lingue indeuropee. Dizionari della lingua greca. Dizionari della lingua latina, Olschki.

Semin, G.R. and Manstead, A.S.R. (1982) The social implications of embarassment displays and restitution behaviour. *European Journal of Social Psychology*, **12**, 367–377.

Seminowicz, D.A., Mayberg, H.S., McIntosh, A.R. *et al.* (2004) Limbic-frontal circuitry in major depression: a path modeling metanalysis. *NeuroImage*, **22**, 409–418.

Sharma, D.D., Kumar, R. and Sharma, R.C. (2006) Starvation in obsessive-compulsive disorder due to scrupulosity. *Indian Journal of Psychiatry*, **48**, 265–266.

Sharpe, M. and Mayou, R. (2004) Somatoform disorders: A help or hindrance to good patient care? *British Journal of Psychiatry*, **1** (84), 465–467.

Shin, L.M., Wright, C.I., Cannistraro, P.A. *et al.* (2005) A functional magnetic resonance imaging study of amygdala and medial prefrontal cortex responses to overtly presented fearful faces in posttraumatic stress disorder. *Archives of General Psychiatry*, **62**, 273–281.

Shotter, J. (1998) Agency and identity: A relational approach, in *The Social Child* (eds A. Campbell and S. Muncer), Psychology Press, Hove, UK, pp. 271–291.

Simon, C.E., VonKorff, M., Piccinelli, M. *et al.* (1999) An international study of the relation between somatic symptoms and depression. *The New England Journal of Medicine*, **341** (18), 1329–1335.

Singer, G.H. and Singer, L.J. (2001) *Handbook of Children and the Media*, Sage, London.

Singer, T. and Frith, C. (2005) The painful side of empathy. *Nature Neuroscience*, **8**, 845–846.

Singer, T., Seymour, B., O'Doherty, J. *et al.* (2004) Empathy for pain involves the affective but not the sensory components of pain. *Science*, **303**, 1157–1161.

Singer, T., Seymour, B., O'Doherty, J.P. *et al.* (2006) Empathic neural responses are modulated by the perceived fairness of others. *Nature*, **439**, 466–469.

Skipper, J.I., Nusbaum, H.C. and Small, S.L. (2005) Listening to talking faces: motor cortical activation during speech perception. *NeuroImage*, **25** (1), 76–89.

Skoog, G. and Skoog, I. (1999) A 40-year follow-up of patients with obsessive-compulsive disorder. *Disorder Arch Gen Psychiatry*, **56**, 121–127.

Smith, C., Adamson, L. and Bakeman, R. (1988) Interactional predictors of early language. *First Language*, **8**, 143–156.

Solomon, R. (1976) *The Passions*, Doubleday, New York.

Solomon, R.C. (2003a) *Not Passion's Slave: Emotions and Choice*, Oxford University Press, Oxford; New York.

Solomon, R.C. (2003b) Emotions, thoughts and feelings: what is a 'cognitive theory' of the emotions and does it neglect affectivity?, in *Philosophy and the Emotions* (ed. A. Hatzimoysis), Cambridge University Press.

Solomon, R.C. (ed.) (2004) *Thinking about Feelings: Contemporary Philosophers on Emotion*, Oxford University Press, Oxford and New York.

Sollier, P. (1891) Anorexie hystérique (sitiergie hystérique): forms pathogéniques-traitment moral. *Revue de Médecine*, **11**, 625–650.

Sonnby-Borgström, M. (2002) Automatic mimicry reactions as related to differences in emotional empathy. *Scandinavian Journal of Psychology*, **43**, 433–443.

Soussignan, R. and Schaal, B. (1996) Forms and social signal value of smiles associated with pleasant and unpleasant sensory experience. *Ethology*, **102**, 1020–1041.

Spence, S.A. (1999) Hysterical paralyses as disorders of action. *Cognitive Neuropsychiatry*, **4**, 203–226.

Spence, S.A., Crimlisk, H.L., Cope, H. *et al.* (2000) Discrete neurophysiological correlates in prefrontal cortex during hysterical and feigned disorder of movement. *Lancet*, **355**, 1243–1244.

Spitzer, R.L., Delvin, M., Walsh, B.T. *et al.* (1992) Binge eating disorder: A multisite field trial of the diagnostic criteria. *International Journal of Eating Disorders*, **11**, 191–203.

Spitzer, R.L., Stunkard, A.J., Yanovski, S. *et al.* (1993) Binge eating disorder should be included in DSM-IV: a reply to Fairburn *et al.* the classification of recurrent overeating: the binge eating disorder proposal. *International Journal of Eating Disorders*, **13**, 161–169.

Spitzer, R.L., Henderson, K.A. and Zivian, M.T. (1999) Gender differences in population versus media body sizes: A comparison over four decades. *Sex Roles*, **40**, 545–565.

Staab, J.P. (2006) Chronic dizziness: the interface between psychiatry and neuro-otology. *Current Opinion in Neurology*, **19** (1), 41–48.

Staab, J.P. and Ruckenstein, M.J. (2007) Expanding the differential diagnosis of chronic dizziness. *Archives of Otolaryngology–Head & Neck Surgery*, **133** (2), 170–176.

Stapel, D. and Koomen, W. (2001) I, we, and the effects of others on me: How self-construal level moderates social comparison effects. *Journal of Personality and Social Psychology*, **80**, 766–781.

Staud, R., Cannon, R.C., Mauderli, A.P. *et al.* (2003) Temporal summation of pain from mechanical stimulation of muscle tissue in normal controls and subjects with fibromyalgia syndrome. *PAIN*, **102**, 87–95.

Stearns, C.Z. (1993) Sadness, in *Handbook of Emotion* (eds M. Lewis and J.M. Haviland), Guilford Press.

Stein, M.B., Shea, C.A. and Uhde, T.W. (1989) Social phobic symptoms in patients with panic disorder: practical and theoretical implications. *The American Journal of Psychiatry*, **146** (2), 235–238.

Stein, N.L., Trabasso, T. and Liwag, M. (1993) The representation and organization of emotional experience: unfolding the emotion episode, in *Handbook of Emotions* (eds M. Lewis and J.M. Haviland), Guildford Press, New York, pp. 279–300.

Stein, M.B., Goldin, P.R., Sareen, J. *et al.* (2002) Increased amygdala activation to angry and contemptuous faces in generalized social phobia. *Archives of General Psychiatry*, **59**, 1027–1034.

Stein, R.I., Kenardy, J., Wiseman, C.V. *et al.* (2007) What's driving the binge in binge eating disorder? A prospective examination of precursors and consequences. *International Journal of Eating Disorders*, **40**, 195–203.

Stengers, I. (1985) *Généalogies De L'auto-Organisation*, Cahiers du CREA, 8.

Steptoe, A. and Noll, A. (1997) The perception of bodily sensations, with special reference to hypochondriasis. *Behaviour Research and Therapy*, **35** (10), 901–910.

Stewart, S.H., Buffett-Jerrott, S.E. and Kokaram, R. (2001) Heartbeat awareness and heart rate reactivity in anxiety sensitivity: A further investigation. *Journal of Anxiety Disorders*, **15** (6), 535–553.

Stilger, V.G. and Yesalis, C.E. (1999) Anabolic-androgenic steroid use among high school football players. *Journal of Community Health*, **24**, 131–145.

Straube, T., Glauer, M., Dilger, S. *et al.* (2006) Effects of cognitive–behavioral therapy on brain activation in specific phobia. *NeuroImage*, **29**, 125–135.

Straube, T., Mentzel, H.-J. and Miltner, W.H.R. (2007) Waiting for spiders: Brain activation during anticipatory anxiety in spider phobics. *NeuroImage*, **37**, 1427–1436.

Strawson, G. (1999) The self, in *Models of the Self* (eds S. Gallagher and J. Shear), Imprint Academic.

Strawson, G. (2007) Episodic ethics, in *Narrative and Understanding Persons* (ed. D.D. Hutto), Cambridge University Press.

Striegel-Moore, R.H. and Franko, D.L. (2003) Epidemiology of binge eating disorder. *International Journal of Eating Disorders*, **34** (Suppl), S19–S29.

Striegel-Moore, R.H., McAvay, G. and Rodin, J. (1986) Psychological and behavioral correlates of feeling fat in women. *International Journal of Eating Disorders*, **5**, 935–947.

Striegel-Moore, R.H., Wilson, G.T., Wilfley, D.E. *et al.* (1998) Binge eating in an obese community sample. *International Journal of Eating Disorders*, **23**, 27–37.

Sturges, L.V., Goetsch, V.L., Ridley, J., and Whittal, M. (1998) Anxiety sensitivity and response to hyperventilation challenge: Physiologic arousal, interoceptive acuity, and subjective distress. *Journal of anxiety disorders*, **12** (2), 103–115.

Sturges, L.V. and Goetsch, V.L., 1996. Psychophysiological reactivity and heartbeat awareness in anxiety sensitivity. *Journal of Anxiety Disorders* 10, **44**, 283–294.

Sugiura, M. *et al.* (2005) Cortical mechanisms of visual self-recognition. *NeuroImage*, **24**, 143–149.

Summerfeldt, L.J. and Endler, N.S. (1998) Examining the evidence for anxiety-related cognitive biases in obsessive-compulsive disorder. *Journal of Anxiety Disorders*, **12**, 579–598.

Szmukler, G., McCance, C., McCrone, L. and Hunter, D. (1986) Anorexia nervosa: a psychiatric case register study from Aberdeen. *Psychological Medicine*, **16**, 49–58.

Taylor, S. (1995) Anxiety sensitivity: Theoretical perspectives and recent findings. *Behaviour Research and Therapy*, **33**, 243–258.

Tellenbach, H. (1974) *Melancholy*, 2nd edn, Springer, Berlin.

Tettamanti, M., Buccino, G., Saccuman, M.C. *et al.* (2005) Listening to action-related sentences activates fronto-parietal motor circuits. *Journal of Cognitive Neuroscience*, **17**, 273–281.

Thelen, E. (1979) Rhythmical behavior in infancy: an ethological perspective. *Animal Behavior*, **27**, 699–715.

Thelen, E. (2002) Self-organization in developmental processes: Can systems approaches work, in *Brain Development and Cognition. A Reader* (eds M.H. Johnson, Y. Munakata and R.O. Gilmore), Blackwell.

Thelen, E. and Smith, L.B. (1994) *A Dynamics Systems Approach to the Development of Perception and Action*, MIT Press.

Thomas, K.M., Drevets, W.C., Dahl, R.E. *et al.* (2001) Amygdala response to fearful faces in anxious and depressed children. *Archives of General Psychiatry*, **58**, 1057–1063.

Thompson, E. and Varela, F.J. (2001) Radical embodiment: neural dynamics and consciousness. *Trends in Cognitive Sciences*, **5**, 418–425.

Tiihonen, J., Kuikka, J., Viinamaki, H. *et al.* (1995) Altered cerebral blood flow during hysterical paresthesia. *Biological Psychiatry*, **37**, 134–135.

Tomasello, M. (2003) *Constructing a Language: A Usage-based Theory of Language Acquisition*, Harvard University Press.

Tomasello, M. and Farrar, M.J. (1986) Joint Attention and Early Language. *Child Development*, **57** (6), 1454–1463.

Tomasello, M. and Todd, J. (1983) Joint attention and early lexical acquisition style. *First Language*, **4**, 197–212.

Tomasello, M., Farrar, M.J. and Dines, J. (1984) Children's speech revisions for a familiar and an unfamiliar adult journal of speech. *Language and Hearing Research*, **27**, 359–363.

Tomkins, S.S. and McCarter, R. (1964) What and where are the primary affects? Some evidence for a theory. *Perceptual and Motor Skills*, **18**, 119.

Treede, R.D., Meyer, R.A., Raja, S.N. and Campbell, J.N. (1992) Peripheral and central mechanisms of cutaneous hyperalgesia. *Progress in Neurobiology*, **38**, 397–421.

Trevarthen, C. (1977) Descriptive analyses of infant communication behavior, in *Studies in Mother-Infant Interaction. The Loch Lomond Symposium* (ed. H.R. Schaffer), Academic Press, London.

Trevarthen, C. (1979) Communication and cooperation in early infancy, in *Before Speech* (ed. M. Bullowa), Cambridge University Press, Cambridge.

Trevarthen, C. (1992) An infant's motives for speaking and thinking in the culture, in *The Dialogical Alternative* (ed. A.H. Wold), Scandinavian Univ. Press, Oslo, pp. 99–137.

Trevarthen, C. (2004) *Learning About Ourselves from Children Why a growing Human Brain Needs Interesting Companions*, Perception-in-Action Publications.

Trevarthen, C. and Aitken, K.J. (2001) Infant intersubjectivity: research, theory, and clinical applications. *Journal of Child Psychology and Psychiatry*, **42** (1), 3–48.

Trevarthen, C. and Hubley, P. (1978) Secondary intersubjectivity: confidence, confiding and acts of meaning in the first year, in *Action, Gesture and Symbol: The Emergence of Language* (ed. A. Lock), Academic Press.

Trevarthen, C. and Logotheti, K. (1989) Child and culture: genesis of cooperative knowing, in *Cognition and Social Words* (eds A. Cellatiy, D. Rogers in J.A. Sloboda), Oxford University Press, Oxford.

Trevarthen, C., Kokkinaki, T. and Fiamenghi, G.A. (1999) What infants' imitations communicate: with mothers, with fathers, and with peers, in *Imitation in Infancy* (eds J. Nadel and G. Butterworth), Cambridge University Press, Cambridge UK.

Trivedi, M.H. (2004) The Link Between Depression and Physical Symptoms. *The Primary Care Companion to the Journal of Clinical Psychiatry*, **6** (Suppl 1), 12–16.

Turk, D.J., Heatherton, T.F., Kelley, W.M. *et al.* (2002) Mike or me? Self-recognition in a split-brain patient. *Nature Neuroscience*, **5** (9), 841–842.

Turk, D.J., Heatherton, T.F., Macrae, C.N. *et al.* (2003) Out of contact, out of mind: the distributed nature of the self. *Annals of the New York Academy of Sciences*, **1001**, 65–78.

Tylee, André P. and Ghandi, Paul (2005) The importance of somatic symptoms in depression in primary care. *Primary Care Companion to the Journal of Clinical, Psychiatry*, **7** (4), 167–176.

Uddin, L.Q. *et al.* (2005) Self-face recognition activates a frontoparietal'mirror' network in the right hemisphere: an event-related fMRI study. *NeuroImage*, **25**, 926–935.

Uddin, Q.L., Kaplan, T.J., Molnar-Szakacs, I. *et al.* (2005) Self-face recognition activates a frontoparietal "mirror" network in the right hemisphere: an event-related fMRI study. *Neuroimage*, **25** (3), 926–935.

Uddin, Q.L., Iacoboni, M., Lange, C. and Keenan, J. (2007) The self and social cognition: the role of cortical midline structures and mirror neurons. *Trends in Cognitive Sciences*, **11**, 153–157.

Uher, R., Murphy, T., Brammer, M.J. *et al.* (2004) Medial Prefrontal Cortex Activity Associated With Symptom Provocation in Eating Disorders. *The American Journal of Psychiatry*, **161**, 1238–1246.

Valet, M., Sprenger, T., Boecker, H. *et al.* (2004) Distraction modulates connectivity of the cingulo-frontal cortex and the midbrain during pain–an fMRI analysis. *PAIN*, **109**, 399–408.

Van Baaren, R.B., Maddux, W.W., Chartrand, T.L. *et al.* (2003) It takes two to mimic: Behavioral consequences of self-construals. *Journal of Personality and Social Psychology*, **84**, 1095–1102.

Van Den Broeck, H., Vanderheyden, K. and Cools, E. (2006) The field of cognitive styles: from a theoretical review to the construction of the cognitive style inventory. Vlerick Leuven Gent Working Paper Series, 2003/26.

Van der Does, A.J.W., Willem, A.J., Van Dyck, R. and Spinhoven, P. (1997) Accurate heartbeat perception in panic disorder: Fact and artefact. *Journal of Affective Disorders*, **43**, 121–130.

Van der Does, A.J.W., Antony, M.M., Ehlers, A. and Barsky, A.J. (2000) Heartbeat perception in panic disorder: a reanalysis. *Behaviour Research & Therapy*, **38**, 47–62.

Van Hanswijck de, Jonge P., Waller, G., Fiennes, A. *et al.* (2003) Reported sexual abuse and cognitive content in the morbidly obese. *Eating Behaviours*, **2003**, **4**, 315–322.

Van Oudenhove, L., Demyttenaere, K., Tack, J. and Aziz, Q. (2004) Central nervous system involvement in functional gastrointestinal disorders. *Best Practice & Research. Clinical Gastroenterology*, **18** (4), 663–680.

Van Oudenhove, L., Vandenberghe, J., Geeraerts, B. *et al.* (2005) Influence of anxiety on gastric sensorimotor function in humans. *Gastroenterology*, **129** (5), 1437–1444.

Vandereycken, W. and van Deth, R. (1990) From Fasting Saints to Anorexic Girls: The History of Self-Starvation.

Varela, F.J. (1979) *Principles of Biological Autonomy*, Elsevier/North-Holland, New York.

Varela, F.J. (1983) L'auto-organisation: De l'apparence au mécanisme, in *L'Auto-Organisation: De la Physique au Politique* (eds P. Dumouchel and J.P. Dupuy), Editions du Seuil, Paris, pp. 147–165.

Varela, F.J. (1999) The specious present: the neurophenomenology of time consciousness, in *Naturalizing Phenomenology* (eds J. Petitot, F.J. Varela, B. Pachoud and J.M. Roy), Stanford University Press, Stanford, CA, pp. 266–314.

Varela, F.J. and Shear, J. (1999) The view from within: first-person methodologies in the study of consciousness. special issue. *Journal of Consciousness Studies*, **6** (2–3), 299–306.

Varela, F.J., Thompson, E. and Rosch, E. (1991) *The Embodied Mind: Cognitive Science and Human Experience*, MIT Press, Cambridge, MA.

Vervaet, M., van Heeringen, C. and Audenaert, K. (2004) Binge eating disorder and non-purging bulimia: More similar than different? *European Eating Disorders Review*, **2004** (12), 27–33.

Vitousek, K. and Manke, F. (1994) Personality variables and disorders in anorexia nervosa and bulimia nervosa. *Journal of Abnormal Psychology*, **103**, 137–147.

Vogt, B.A. (2005) Pain and emotion interactions in subregions of the cingulate gyrus. *Nature Reviews. Neuroscience*, **6** (7), 533–544.

Volpi, F. (1996) La question du logos dans l'articulation de la facticité chez le jeune Heidegger, lecteur d'Aristote, in *Heidegger 1919–1929. De l'herméneutique de la Facticité à la Métaphysique du Dasein* (ed. Jean-François Courtine), Vrin, Paris.

Von Wright, G.H. (1971) *Explanation and Understanding*, Routledge & Kegan Paul, London.

Vuilleumier, P., Chicherio, C., Assal, F. *et al.* (2001) Functional neuroanatomical correlates of hysterical sensorimotor loss. *Brain: A Journal of Neurology*, **124** (6), 1077–1090.

Waelhens de, A. (1951) *Une Philosophie de L'ambiguite'*, Pub. Universiste' de Louvain.

Wagner, A., Aizenstein, H., Venkatraman, V.K., Fudge, J. *et al.* (2007) Altered reward processing in women recovered from anorexia nervosa. *The American Journal of Psychiatry*, **164**, 1842–1849.

Walsh, B.T. and Devlin, M.J. (1998) Eating disorders: progress and problems. *Science*, **280**, 1387–1390.

Warren, E.J., Sauter, A.D., Eisner, F. *et al.* (2006) Positive emotions preferentially engage an auditory–motor "Mirror" system. *The Journal of Neuroscience*, **26** (50), 13067–13075.

Watkins, K. *et al.* (2003) Seeing and hearing speech excites the motor system involved in speech production. *Neuropsychologia*, **41**, 989–994.

Watkins, K. *et al.* (2004) Modulation of motor excitability during speech perception:the role of Broca's area. *Journal of Cognitive Neuroscience*, **16** (6), 978–987.

Watson, L. (1992) *The Secret Life of Inanimate Objects*, Destiny Books, Rochester, Vermont.

Weber, M. (1997) *The Methodology of the Social Sciences*, (Edward A. Shils and Henry A. Finch, trans. & foreword by Shils), Free Press, New York, pp. 1903–1917.

Wegner, K.E., Smyth, J.M., Crosby, R.D. *et al.* (2002) An evaluation of the relationship between mood and binge eating in the natural environment using ecological momentary assessment. *The International Journal of Eating Disorders*, **32** (3), 352–361.

Weil, E. (1974) *Logique de la Philosophie*, Vrin, Paris.

Weissman, M.M., Wolk, S., Goldstein, R.B. *et al.* (1999) Depressed adolescents grown up. *The Journal of the American Medical Association*, **281**, 1707–1713.

Welch-Ross, M. (2001) Personalizing the temporally extended self:Evaluative self-awareness and the development of autobiographical memory, in *The Self in time:Developmental Perspectives* (eds C. Moore and K. Lemmon), Lawrence Erlbaum, Hillsdale, NJ.

Whalen, P.J., Rauch, S.L., Etcoff, N.L. *et al.* (1998) Masked presentations of emotional facial expressions modulate amygdala activity without explicit knowledge. *The Journal of Neuroscience*, **18**, 411–418.

White, H.S. (1996) The child's entry into the "age of reason", in *The Five to Seven Year Shift* (eds A.J. Sameroff and M.H. Haith), University of Chicago Press, Chicago.

Whitehead, W.E. and Drescher, V.M. (1980) Perception of gastric contractions and self-control of gastric motility. *Psychophysiology*, **17**, 552–558.

Whiteside, U., Chen, E., Neighbors, C. *et al.* (2007) Difficulties regulating emotions: Do binge eaters have fewer strategies to modulate and tolerate negative affect? *Eating Behaviours*, **8**, 162–169.

WHO (2001). The World Health Report (2001) Mental health: new understanding, new hope.

Wichstrom, L. and Pedersen, W. (2001) Use of anabolic-androgenic steroids in adolescence: Winning, looking good or being bad? *Journal of Studies on Alcohol*, **62**, 5–13.

Wiederman, M.W. and Pryor, T. (1996) Substance use among women with eating disorders. *The International Journal of Eating Disorders*, **20** (2), 163–168.

Wiens, S. and Palmer, N.S. (2001) Quadratic trend analysis and heartbeat detection. *Biological Psychology*, **58**, 159–175.

Wiens, S., Mezzacappa, S.E. and Katkin, S.E. (2000) Heartbeat detection and the experience of emotions. *Cognition & Emotion*, **14**, 417–427.

Wilson, S.M. and Iacoboni, M. (2006) Neural responses to non-native phonemes varying in producibility: evidence for the sensorimotor nature. *NeuroImage*, **33**, 316–325.

Wilson, S.M., Saygin, A.P., Sereno, M.I. and Iacoboni, M. (2004) Listening to speech activates motor areas involved in speech production. *Nature Neuroscience*, **7**, 701–702.

Wimmer, H. and Perner, J. (1983) Beliefs about beliefs: Representation and constraining function of wrong beliefs in young children's understanding of deception. *Cognition*, **13**, 41–68.

Winnicott, D.W. (1965) *The Maturational Process and the Facilitating Environment*, International Universities Press, New York.

Wise, T.N. and Birket-Smith, M. (2002) The somatoform disorders for DSM-V: the need for changes in process and content. *Psychosomatics*, **43**, 437–440.

Witkin, H.A. (1978) Cognitive styles in personal and cultural adaptation, in *The 1977 Heinz Werner Lectures*, Clark university Press, Worcester, Mass.

Witkin, H.A. and Goodenough, D.R. (1977) Field dependence and interpersonal behavior. *Psychological Bulletin*, **84**, 661.

Wittchen, H.U., Nelson, C.B. and Lachner, G. (1998) Prevalence of mental disorders and psychosocial impairments in adolescents and young adults. *Psychological Medicine*, **28** (1), 109–126.

Wonderlich, S.A., Crosby, R.D., Joiner, T. *et al.* (2005) Personality subtyping and bulimia nervosa: Psychopathological and genetic correlates. *Psychological Medicine*, **35**, 649–657.

Wonderlich, S., Crosby, R., Engel, S. *et al.* (2007) Personality-based clusters in bulimia nervosa: differences in clinical variables and ecological momentary assessment. *Journal of Personality Disorders*, **21** (3), 340–357.

Woodside, D.B., Garfinkel, P.E., Lin, E. *et al.* (2001) Comparisons of men with full or partial eating disorders, Men without eating disorders, and women with eating disorders in the community. *The American Journal of Psychiatry*, **158** (4), 570–574.

Woolf, C.J. (1983) Evidence for a central component of post-injury pain hypersensitivity. *Nature*, **306**, 686–688.

Woolf, C.J. (1991) Generation of acute pain: central mechanisms. *British Medical Bulletin*, **47**, 523–533.

Woolf, C.J. (1995) An overview of the mechanisms of hyperalgesia. *Pulmonary Pharmacology*, **8**, 161–167.

Woolf, C.J. and Salter, M.W. (2000) Neuronal plasticity: increasing the gain in pain. *Science*, **288**, 1765–1769.

Woolf, V. (2000) *The Mark on the Wall (Collected Works of Virginia Woolf)*, Classic Books.

Yates, E. (1986) The influence of psycho-social factors on non-sensical shoplifting. *International Journal of Offender Therapy and Comparative Criminology*, **30**, 203–211.

Yates, J.A., Jones, E.K., Marie, V.G. and Hogben, H.J. (1985) detection of the heartbeat and events in the cardiac cycle. *Psychophysiology*, **22**, 561–567.

Yerevanian, B.I. and Akiskal, H.S. (1979) Neurotic, characterological, and dysthymic depressions. *Psychiatric Clinics of North America*, **2**, 595–617.

Young, M.A., Fogg, L.F., Scheftner, W. *et al.* (1996) Stable trait components of hopelessness: Baseline and sensitivity to depression. *Journal of Abnormal Psychology*, **105** (2), 155–165.

Zahavi, D. (2003) Phenomenology of self, in *The Self* (eds T. Kircher and A. David), Cambridge University Press.

Zaner, R.M. (1971) *The Problem of Embodiment*, Martinus Nijhoff, The Hague.

Zoellner, A. and Craske, M. (1999) Interoceptive accuracy and panic. *Behaviour Research and Therapy*, **37** (12), 1141–1158.

Zvolensky, M.J. and Forsyth, J.P. (2002) Anxiety sensitivity dimensions in the prediction of body vigilance and emotional avoidance. *Cognitive Therapy and Research*, **26** (4), 449–460.

Zvolensky, M.J., Eifert, G.H. and Lejuez, C.W. (2001). Emotional control during recurrent 20% carbon dioxide-enriched air induction: Relation to individual difference variables. *Emotion*, **2**, 148–165.

Index